# NURSING PROCESS

Application
of
Conceptual
Models

# NURSING PROCESS

## Application of Conceptual Models

EDITED BY

**PAULA J. CHRISTENSEN, RN, PhD**

Professor and Chair
Department of Nursing
Rockford College, Rockford, Illinois

**JANET W. KENNEY, RN, PhD**

Associate Professor
Arizona State University College of Nursing
Tempe, Arizona

THIRD EDITION

*Illustrated*

**THE C. V. MOSBY COMPANY**

ST. LOUIS • BALTIMORE • PHILADELPHIA • TORONTO   1990

*Editor:* Nancy L. Coon
*Developmental Editor:* Susan R. Epstein
*Project Manager:* Patricia Tannian
*Editing and Production:* Editing, Design & Production, Inc.
*Design:* Liz Fett

**THIRD EDITION**

The C.V. Mosby Company
11830 Westline Industrial Drive, St. Louis, Missouri 63146

**Library of Congress Cataloging in Publication Data**
Nursing process: application of conceptual models / edited by Paula
 J. Christensen, Janet W. Kenney.—3rd ed.
     p.     cm.
   Includes bibliographical references.
   ISBN 0-8016-3271-4
   1. Nursing.  2. Nursing—Philosophy.  I. Christensen, Paula J.
 II. Kenney, Janet W.
   [DNLM:  1. Nursing Process.    WY 100 N9759]
 RT42.N87   1990
 610.73—dc20
 DNLM/DLC                                                    90-5417
 for Library of Congress                                      CIP

C/VH/VH  9  8  7  6  5  4  3  2  1

# Contributors

**JUDITH A. BARTON, RN, PhD**
Assistant Professor
University of Colorado
School of Nursing
Denver, Colorado

**JOANNE R. CROSS, RN, MSN, NCC**
Assistant Professor
Wright State University
School of Nursing
Dayton, Ohio

**LINDA J. DRIES, RN, MS, CDE**
Clinical Nurse Specialist
Swedish American Hospital
Rockford, Illinois

**ELIZABETH S. FAYRAM, RN, MSN**
Assistant Professor of Nursing
Edgewood College
Department of Nursing
Madison, Wisconsin

**CYNTHIA MAKIELSKI MARTZ, RNC, MSN**
Staff Nurse in Labor and Delivery
Humana Hospital
Overland Park, Kansas

**CATHY D. MEADE, RN, PhD**
Assistant Professor
University of Wisconsin–Milwaukee
School of Nursing
Milwaukee, Wisconsin

**PHYLLIS BAKER RISNER, RN, PhD**
Assistant Professor
Wright State University
School of Nursing
Dayton, Ohio

**KAREN A. SAUCIER, RN, PhD**
Dean and Professor
Delta State University
School of Nursing
Cleveland, Mississippi

*To all professional nurses and nursing students*
*who aspire to integrate theories in the nursing process*
*within contemporary nursing practice*

# Preface

Nursing theories continue to be developed and refined as nurse leaders write about their perspectives of nursing practice in today's health care environment. Each vision of nursing ultimately focuses on the consumers of health care, the clients. Thus, all of the theories address how nurses strive to enhance clients' well-being and how nursing responds to society's ever-expanding health care needs. Nursing theories complement the use of the nursing process, the profession's accepted systematic guide to nursing care. The integration of nursing theories with the nursing process provides a consistent yet flexible methodology. The nursing process ensures consistency while the nursing theories, with their unique applications, allow nurses a choice of approaches in which to frame their clinical practice.

This book was written primarily to help nursing students, practitioners, and educators understand theoretical approaches and apply them to the nursing process. The way nurses use the nursing process and nursing theories depends on their level of proficiency in practice. Novice practitioners follow a more structured approach. As expertise develops, nurses rely more on their own experience and internalize the nursing process and theories as part of their empirical and personal knowledge. Delineation of the levels of nurses' proficiency was the result of a research project by Patricia Benner. Her work is introduced in the first chapter of this edition and is integrated throughout the chapters on the nursing process components.

Nursing judgment is based on both empirical, or scientific, knowledge and personal knowledge, which includes self-awareness and intuition. Many in the nursing profession are challenging the adherence of nurse researchers, practitioners, and theorists to a scientific paradigm that recognizes only limited sources of knowledge. The newer view of nursing practice honors the personal element, which develops as creativity and trust in one's own judgment grow. Nurses possess a wealth of empirical as well as personal knowledge, and both are essential to clinical expertise. This recognition is threaded throughout the text in discussions of the use of the nursing process. The nursing process is a vehicle by which the totality of nurses' knowledge is applied to enhance the quality of care.

## FEATURES OF THIS EDITION

This third edition of *Nursing Process: Application of Conceptual Models* incorporates major recent developments in the nursing profession. By recognizing the levels of nursing proficiency, for example, we can understand the relative importance of the nursing process and nursing theories at different stages in the development of a nurse's expertise. Acknowledging the essential contribution of personal as well as empirical knowledge to clinical expertise expands our visions of nursing practice.

In addition to theoretical and philosophical changes, the third edition offers some practical features. Section I first discusses the importance of a theoretical approach as the basis for professional nursing practice. The evolution of the nursing process and theory development in nursing are described. An overview of theories, models, and frameworks currently used in nursing and other disciplines is presented. These theoretical approaches serve both as an introduction to different models and frameworks and as a reference for understanding their application in subsequent chapters.

Section II describes the nursing process in detail. The basic components—assessment, analysis and diagnosis, planning, implementation, and evaluation—are illustrated with different frameworks and models. Guidelines for applying each component and examples of using them with the individual, family, and community client are also given. The nursing and biomedical domains are defined and discussed primarily in the chapters on nursing diagnosis. The juxtaposition of nursing and medicine is an interesting and challenging one, because it highlights the difference between nursing diagnoses and medical diagnoses and treatment. The community as a client is seen as both a geographic population and an aggregate group with similar interests or needs. In keeping with trends in community health nursing, the community assessment chapter focuses on aggregate groups. Finally, several useful nursing intervention strategies have been updated and a few new ones added. A variety of strategies are presented to enhance nursing care with individuals, families, and communities.

Section III consists of five case studies: two individual clients, two family clients, and one community client. The format for each case study is identical to that described in the components chapters and follows the guidelines for developing and writing a comprehensive nursing process.

We recommend that the reader begin with Chapter 1 and proceed in sequence through Chapter 12. It is important that the reader understand the rationale for a theoretical approach and the interrelationships of the components. The 10 chapters in Section II provide the foundation for understanding the case studies in Section III. Appendix A is a glossary of important terms, and Appendix B is a complete list of the guidelines from the components chapters.

• • •

We have been excited about the evolution of this edition as we wove the threads of new thinking within nursing into the fabric of the nursing process. Our goal has been to show how the nursing process can be used to guide nursing practice while recognizing nurses as individuals with different talents and abilities. Nurses' uniqueness, levels of proficiency, and ways of knowing contribute to the richness of our profession and to the potential quality of care for our clients.

PAULA J. CHRISTENSEN
JANET W. KENNEY

# Contents

**NURSING PROCESS**
Application
of
Conceptual
Models

SECTION

I

# Theory-Based Nursing Practice

CHAPTER

1

# Relevance of Theoretical Approaches in Nursing Practice

JANET W. KENNEY

## NURSING AS A DISCIPLINE

Nursing is recognized as an emerging scientific discipline with a unique perspective of persons, their health, the environment, and the nurse. Nursing's perspective has developed over the past four decades and is based on an evolving philosophy and history, former practice, theory, research, and emerging ideas of nursing scholars. As each discipline develops, it directs the way that its domain, or field of knowledge, will develop. In the development of nursing knowledge, Meleis (1985) identified four major areas that are addressed:

- Major concepts and problems of nursing
- Assessment, diagnosis, and intervention processes
- Tools to assess, diagnose, and intervene
- Research designs and methods congruent with nursing

Nursing has made tremendous progress in each of these areas. The major concepts identified by the discipline are *client, health, environment,* and *nursing.* Determining the nurse's role in facilitating the client's health in the environment is the complex problem on which nursing focuses. The nursing process, along with new assessment tools and diagnoses, has evolved and continues to be refined. New research designs and methods also continue to be explored.

During the 1960s, the nursing discipline sought to define itself as a true profession, with a scientific base for its practice and emerging theories. Empirical knowledge became the dominant pattern, and traditional nursing followed the male medical model, which embodied the empirical scientific approach. The empirical method focuses on observ-

able, objective, logical hard data, and an analytical, verbal, and linear line of reasoning. Other ways of knowing, especially personal knowledge, which includes subjectivity, sensing, feeling, intuition, emotion, and experience, were devalued or discredited. Science, or "true" knowledge, was based on the superiority of empirical validation; all other forms of knowledge were considered mere speculation.

In 1978, Carper described four "patterns of knowing" within nursing; these are also used in most other disciplines. Each pattern requires a specific process of discovery and has its own method for determining credibility of knowledge in each field. The four patterns of knowing are described by Carper:

*Empirical knowledge* is based on objective evidence obtained by the senses; it requires validation and verification by others.

*Ethical knowledge* examines philosophical premises of justice and seeks credibility through logical justification.

*Esthetics* judges creativity, form, structure, and beauty through criticism of the meaning of the creative process and product.

*Personal knowledge* integrates and analyzes current interpersonal situations with past experience and knowledge.

Since the 1980s, there has been a growing awareness that too much reliance on empirical knowledge has led to a distorted view of the world. Each discipline's body of knowledge would be incomplete if it were based only on empirical, observable evidence. Whereas some disciplines rely more heavily on one pattern of knowing, other disciplines, especially nursing, integrate all four patterns of knowing for a more complete picture of reality. Empirical, ethical, esthetic, and personal knowledge all are valid ways of knowing and are useful for certain purposes.

Within the developing nursing discipline, various facts have been organized into a scientific body of knowledge. Several models have emerged that relate concepts, order knowledge, and describe, explain, and predict the field of nursing knowledge and practice. These nursing models serve to guide inquiry and understanding of the nursing domain. The development of different models or views of nursing leads to the formulation of different theories, which enhance the discipline.

Theories are based on specific models and their beliefs and provide specific tools that can guide practice and research. Theory, research, and practice are integrally related. Whereas the primary use of theory is to guide research, theory interacts with and guides practice; research validates and modifies theory and changes practice.

## NURSING PRACTICE

The practice of nursing is based on the synthesis and application of knowledge from the biophysical, behavioral, and humanistic sciences. This knowledge base rapidly changes and expands as research and new theories provide additional information. Knowledge and values about life, people, and events influence each person's perception, understanding, and behavior in the world. Viewing life events and people as separate "bits and pieces" limits one's understanding of the world. Therefore, disciplines construct theories, frameworks, and models to show relationships among events and people, to organize information, and to apply in practice. Nursing models represent several different views of nursing: perspectives about who is the client, what is health, what is the nurse's role or actions, and what is the environment in which nursing occurs.

A *science* is an organized body of knowledge, composed of specialized concepts and terminology, interrelated beliefs, facts, principles, laws, theories, and methodologies which are used in education, research, and practice. Nursing is a science and an art that applies cognitive, psychomotor, and interpersonal skills to assist clients to achieve their optimum health potential. The science of nursing incorporates the study of relationships among nurses, their clients, and environments within the context of health. The art of nursing is the interpersonal relationship and interaction process between the person and the nurse within a social environ-

ment during delivery of nursing care. The science and art of nursing are integrated within the nursing process.

The nursing profession believes that nurses are client advocates. Clients are encouraged to actively participate in providing information about themselves and their views of health and illness, and in decision-making. The nurse assumes responsibility and accountability to the client, team members, other health care providers, the agency, and the state. The nurse is a team member in the health care system and assumes a variety of roles and responsibilities. Some of these roles are practitioner, educator, researcher, collaborator, advocate, role model, evaluator, and leader/manager.

Before the 1960s, nursing practice was based on apprenticeship learning, performance of technical skills, and application of isolated facts and principles, such as aseptic technique and principles of mobility. Since the 1980s, nursing practice has been guided by the application of theories and models in the nursing process. Many nurses are familiar with some models, such as Maslow's (1970) hierarchy of needs and Erikson's (1963) developmental stages. Other nurses are familiar with nursing models, such as Orem's (1980) self-care model and Roy's (1984) adaptation model.

Some nurses consistently use nursing models in their practice. There are many unique nursing and developmental models that are applicable in nursing practice. These models provide a frame of reference that can be applied to each component of the nursing process. Nurses use these models to

- Collect, organize, and classify data
- Understand, analyze, and interpret client's health situations
- Guide nursing diagnoses
- Plan, implement, and evaluate nursing care
- Explain nursing actions and interactions with clients
- Describe, explain, and possibly predict client's responses
- Demonstrate responsibility and accountability
- Achieve desired outcomes for clients

## LEVELS OF NURSING PROFICIENCY

In 1984, Benner examined different ways in which practicing nurses think, and identified five levels of nursing proficiency: novice, advanced beginner, competent, proficient, and expert.

The first level, novice or student, operates from a set of rules in a context-free situation. Guidelines are used to determine the course of actions: Experience is needed to make judgments. Benner's study showed that the level of nursing practice is directly related to the practitioner's level of knowledge, experience, and expertise. With increasing experience, proficient and expert nurses perceive the client situation as a gestalt. They do not rely on rules; they have an intuitive grasp of the situation based on personal knowledge and experience. These nurses are able to take appropriate actions without analyzing each factor in the client situation separately. The thinking process is internalized because expert practitioners use a holistic approach and see the possibilities for their clients.

The nursing process provides a systematic guide or method to assist beginners. It helps the student and novice develop a style of thinking that leads to appropriate clinical judgments. Nurse educators originally developed the nursing process as a teaching tool to guide students in learning the practice of nursing. Nurse leaders believed that the scientific approach of the nursing process would raise nursing to a recognized profession in the 1960s. However, Benner's research (1984) also implied that too much reliance on the nursing process may reduce the proficient and expert nurse's intuitive and creative approach to nursing practice.

The nursing process and the various models can be considered the "training wheels" of practice. They guide and direct the student and beginning practitioner who depend on more structured methods. Nursing models provide a viewpoint for the components of the nursing process and assist the beginner to define nursing and direct the goals of nursing care. Expert nurses have internalized the nursing process and various models; therefore, they combine their experience with theoretical knowledge to analyze and identify the rationale underlying their apparently intuitive decisions. Models help the expert nurse to consider the interrelationship of data and to explain the basis for their judgments.

This chapter begins with a historical overview of trends in nursing. A description of the structural and functional components of theory follows. Terms such as *assumptions, concepts, propositions, conceptual model, theoretical framework,* and *theory* are explained. General perspectives of nursing models are discussed, along with the purpose of and criticisms concerning each. The chapter concludes with an overview of how to choose and apply a model within the nursing process.

The perspective taken in this book is that existing nursing conceptualizations are models with varying degrees of specification and that these models can be used in each component of the nursing process. Therefore, the term *model* includes theories, frameworks, and models, unless otherwise specified. Also, because the models present different perspectives, they are considered complementary, rather than competitive. Throughout this book, the term *client* refers to the individual, family, or community, unless specifically identified.

## HISTORICAL PERSPECTIVES
### Nursing and the Nursing Process

Prior to the 1960s, nursing practice was generally based on apprenticeship learning and the application of isolated principles. Nurses depended on the physician's diagnosis and orders, which usually consisted of vital signs and simple treatments. Hygienic and comfort measures were initiated by nurses. The medical model, which views separation of the body and mind, and focuses on cure and treatment of pathological problems, was adopted by nurses. Also, nurses, like physicians, believed they knew what was best for the patient. Only ill patients—those under a physician's care—were considered the passive recipients of nursing care.

In the 1960s, the scientific era stimulated development of the nursing profession, with the aim of creating a science of nursing. The interpersonal, intellectual, and scientific aspects of nursing were emphasized by the profession. Early nurse theorists viewed nursing as an interaction process and focused on the process and methods of assessment. Orlando (1961) addressed the interpersonal aspects of the nurse-client relationship. She also emphasized the need to deliberate and to validate patient needs, rather than the use of an intuitive approach. Knowles (1967) applied the scientific approach to her definition of nursing, which included discovery, delving, doing, and discrimination. With continued focus on the scientific approach, nursing leaders explained how to apply this approach in the nursing process. In 1966, Kelly described available data for nursing assessment as the client's physical signs and symptoms, the medical history and diagnosis, the social history and cultural background, and the physical or psychological factors in the environment. Johnson (1967) stressed the importance of systematically collecting data and rigorously analyzing it. Nursing diagnosis was defined at that time as determining the etiology of a symptom and its alleviation.

In 1967, Yura and Walsh wrote the first comprehensive book describing four components of the nursing process. These authors emphasized the intellectual, interpersonal, and technical skills of nursing practice. Since the nursing process has been developed and refined, it has become the primary method and focus of nursing practice; however, the number and definition of components lack complete consensus among nurses. In 1973, the American Nurses' Association adopted and legitimized the components of the nursing process in their *Standards of Nursing Practice.* The manual of the Joint Commission on Accreditation of Hospitals requires documentation of the nursing process. Since 1975, most states have revised their nurse practice acts to reflect this broader scope of nursing practice. State board examinations currently test knowledge of assessment, analyzing, planning, implementing, and evaluating—the five major components of the nursing process.

By the 1970s, the profession viewed nursing as a scientific discipline evolving toward a theoretically based practice that focused on the client. Many nursing theorists, such as Abdellah, Hall, Henderson, Johnson, King, Levine, Neuman, Orlando, Orem, Rogers, and Roy, had published their beliefs and ideas about nursing, and some had developed conceptual models. These theorists' views of nursing often were more idealistic than practical and realistic.

### Current Trends in Nursing

Over the last 10 years, there has been a trend in the nursing profession to adopt some new views in nursing practice and theory development. These broader beliefs, which represent new world views, are client advocacy, holism, intuition, and the phenomenological approach.

*Advocacy* means adequately *informing* the client and family about all relevant health or illness areas so that they can make knowledgeable decisions and *supporting* their decisions. Most clients do not want to be passive recipients of care; they prefer to receive sufficient accurate information so that they can make decisions that affect their lives. The Patient's Bill of Rights is an example of the shift in the decision-making power of clients, along with the explanation and signing of "informed consent" for all treatments and operations.

However, it cannot be assumed that all clients want to take responsibility for decisions about their health care. Some clients prefer not to make decisions, leaving their choices to health care professionals. *Supporting* means preserving the client's right to choose and respecting the client's decision without giving approval or disapproval.

Advocacy is not without risks. Nurses who inform clients may be seen as interfering with the established medical treatment by physicians, team members, and sometimes the client's family. Informed clients may choose treatment options con-

trary to health team members' views. This may create conflict between the client and the health team members. Effective nurse advocates are well aware of these risks both to the client and the nurse, and they try to balance the client's personal rights with those of other health care professionals and the institution.

*Holism* refers to a philosophy in which humans are viewed in their entirety, as a unit that cannot be separated into parts without destroying its integrity. A person's extended family, lifestyle, community, socioeconomic status, and religion, as well as all factors that have meaning for that person, are considered interrelated. Holism is not merely a comprehensive collection of the parts, for the total is greater than the sum of parts.

The nursing assessment uses a reductionistic approach to examine separate parts of a person for problem identification, and the overall picture may be missed. With increasing experience, nurses understand that these separate parts all are interrelated and that the interrelationship provides a holistic picture of the client's situation. Expert nurses readily see both the separate parts and the gestalt, or combined interrelationship of the parts, thereby using a holistic approach to view the clients in the context of their living experience.

*Intuition* is an awareness of meanings, relationships, and possibilities by way of insight, without conscious knowledge. It can be a sudden perception of a pattern in a seemingly unrelated series of events or a creative discovery. Intuition is a form of personal knowledge that may reflect a synthesis of past experiences. It is also described as a process of reaching accurate conclusions with inadequate information or perceiving "wholes" rather than "bits and pieces," characteristic of linear reasoning. Expert nurses are open to perceiving a client's subtle behaviors and meanings and have an intuitive grasp, based on their experience, in understanding the client's situation and recognizing patterns. However, these experts do not overlook important facts, nor do they rely solely on their intuition to make decisions or take actions. After years of practice, nurses begin to develop and trust their intuition, and thus make accurate decisions.

The *phenomenological approach* means that the nurse integrates the client's perception of reality and meaning as a personal, complex, subjective experience to develop insight into the client's living experience of well-being and illness. This approach emphasizes understanding clients in terms of their lived experience and focuses on the meaning of the

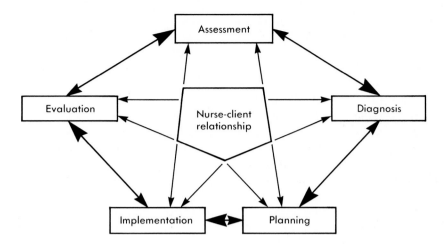

**Fig. 1-1.** Nursing process: feedback system. (Developed by P.J. Christensen.)

experience from the client's frame of reference. The nurse encourages clients to reveal their inner awareness and the contextual meaning of their daily life, including past-present-future meanings and interpretations. The phenomenological approach analyzes the client situation in the living context without isolating any interacting variables. The nurse seeks to comprehend the essence and soul of clients and to understand their view of the total complex situation. Simplistically, the nurse is asking the client, "What does this health concern mean to you in relation to your life experiences (past and present) and what is the perceived impact on your future?" The proficient or expert nurse, according to Benner (1984), recognizes the effect of the interacting meanings on the client and develops a plan that takes these meanings into account.

## THE NURSING PROCESS

The nursing process is a deliberate activity whereby the practice of nursing is performed in a systematic manner. Throughout the nursing process, the nurse uses a comprehensive knowledge base to assess the client's health status, to make judicious judgments and diagnoses, and to plan, implement, and evaluate appropriate nursing actions. As the core of nursing practice, the nursing process provides the structure for nursing care.

### Description of Nursing Process Components

The nursing process has five components, which are interactive and sequential, as shown in Fig. 1-1. Each component has several phases. A nursing

model is selected to guide each component. Additional models are often used to supplement the nursing model. The five components of the nursing process are described here and explained and illustrated more fully in Section II.

*Assessment* is a continuous process of collecting data about the client's human responses, health status, strengths, and concerns. After initial information about the client's situation is obtained, a nursing model is chosen to guide the comprehensive data collection. The data should be multifocal, reflecting historical and current data and representing a variety of sources. Interview, direct observation, and measurement are used to gather data. Data are systematically recorded and serve as the database for all other components in the nursing process. Data collection is ongoing throughout the nursing process. Because new data may alter other components, they should be reported and communicated appropriately.

*Diagnosis* involves two phases: analysis/synthesis and diagnostic statements. After the database is collected, the analysis begins by sorting the data into categories represented in the chosen model to identify behavioral patterns. The client's behavioral patterns, including cues, signs, and symptoms, are compared with the model, health standards, and scientific or developmental norms to identify health concerns, strengths, and resources. The underlying etiology of the client's health concerns is identified and forms the basis for the nursing diagnosis. Each diagnosis is validated with the client or health care professionals to verify the accuracy of the data interpretation.

The nursing diagnostic statements are written in clear, concise language. Each diagnosis should be client-centered, specific, and accurate, and should include an etiological or descriptive statement. Nursing diagnoses reflect only those health concerns that can be treated by nurses. They provide direction for nursing interventions. The list of medical and nursing diagnoses represents the client's current health status and should be updated as the client's condition changes.

The nursing diagnosis differentiates the practice of nursing from medicine. Medical care focuses on the disease pathology and a curative approach, whereas nursing focuses on human responses. Nursing emphasizes the whole unique person, who is interacting with the environment and whose health state—not just the illness or disease—requires nursing intervention. Although the nursing and medical diagnoses are independent of one another, they are interrelated and should not be isolated from each other.

*Planning* occurs when the client and nurse identify activities to prevent, reduce, or correct the nursing diagnoses. The phases in planning are prioritize nursing diagnoses, establish client goals and objectives/outcomes, identify strategies, determine nursing orders and scientific rationale, and write the nursing care plan. The setting of the nurse-client interaction, whether it is the emergency room, clinic, hospital unit, home, or another site, directly influences planning. Initially, the diagnoses are *prioritized* according to their seriousness or life-threatening nature; then goals and objectives are mutually established by the nurse and client. Both goals and objectives describe the client's expected behavioral outcomes. However, goals are usually broad, long-term statements, whereas objectives are discrete, short-term steps leading to achievement of a specific goal. The chosen nursing model guides the direction of goals, objectives, and strategies.

Each *goal* is based on a specific nursing diagnosis and reflects realistic resolution of the diagnosis. Goals must be achievable within the client's capabilities and limitations. Goals and objectives describe the expected client outcomes, and include broad or specific criteria to measure the client's behavior during or after implementation of the plans.

Several *objectives* are usually written as steps to achieve each goal. Objectives are client focused and reflect mutual planning with the client. They include specific criteria to measure the client's behavior and are written in the sequence in which they will be performed. Objectives must be realistic because they serve as the criteria against which nursing actions will be evaluated.

After objectives are identified, the nurse determines which nursing *strategies* will most effectively achieve the objectives and goals. Strategies are designed to prevent, reduce, or correct a nursing diagnosis. The choice of a strategy is based on anticipated effectiveness in achieving the client's outcomes, the benefits and risks for the client, and the available resources, including people, equipment, time, finances, and facilities.

*Nursing orders* state who will do what within a given time period. They describe the client and nursing actions to achieve each objective. Nursing orders are stated in concise, specific terms, and in the appropriate sequence. They may include maintenance, promotion, and restorative aspects of care, along with coordination and collaboration with other health team members. The client's individuality and autonomy are incorporated in the nursing orders. The nursing orders support the medical regimen of care and are kept current and revised, and describe alternate plans as necessary.

*Scientific rationale* describes the scientific basis for planning. The reason for each nursing order is clearly identified. The rationale may include principles, theory, research findings, and current literature.

*Implementation* is performing the nursing orders designated in the plan by the client, nurse, or others. It may include collaboration with other health care providers in performing responsibilities. The client's physical and psychological safety is considered and protected. Each action is performed with skill and efficiency, and includes ongoing assessment. The nursing actions and the client's reactions or behaviors are recorded to verify that the plan was implemented and to evaluate the effectiveness of the plan.

*Evaluation* is comparing the client's health status with the objectives and goals and determining the client's progress or lack of progress toward goal achievement. Criteria for measuring the client's level of achievement are stated in each objective. Evaluation is a continuous process that occurs during ongoing assessment and implementation of nursing care. While implementing the orders, the nurse makes formative evaluative judgments that describe the client's response or reaction to each nursing action and the respective objective. The formative evaluation provides continuous data that may be used to change or modify the nursing diagnosis, plans, and implementation. Periodically, a

**Table 1-1** Components, Definitions, and Activities in the Nursing Process

| Components | Definitions | Activities |
|---|---|---|
| Assessment | An ongoing process of data collection to determine the client's strengths and health concerns | Collect data<br>  Interview<br>  History<br>  Examination<br>  Review records |
| Diagnosis | The analysis/synthesis of data to identify patterns, and compare with norms and models | Analyze and synthesize data<br>  Identify gaps<br>  Categorize<br>  Recognize patterns<br>  Compare with norms and models |
| | A clear, concise statement of client's health status and concerns appropriate for nursing intervention | Develop diagnostic statements<br>  Actual concerns<br>  Potential concerns<br>  Etiology |
| Planning | Determination of how to assist client in resolving concerns related to restoration, maintenance, or promotion of health | Establish priorities<br>Set goals/objectives<br>Select strategies<br>Write nursing orders<br>Describe rationale |
| Implementation | The carrying out the plan of care by the client and nurse | Perform interventions<br>Collaborate<br>Make ongoing assessment<br>Update/revise plan<br>Document responses |
| Evaluation | A systematic, continuous process of comparing the client's response with written goals/objectives. | Compare responses with objectives/goals<br>Determine progress<br>Revise plan of care |

summative evaluation is performed that compares the client's overall progress or lack of progress toward meeting the goal.

A summation of the nursing process is shown in Table 1-1. Each component of the nursing process is explained in detail with examples in the chapters in Section II. Specific guidelines for each component and their phases are provided in Appendix A. A model of the nursing process, illustrating the feedback system between each component, is shown in Fig. 1-1.

The nursing process model in Fig. 1-1 depicts the typical flow of information by the dark lines and heavy arrows clockwise from assessment to diagnosis, plan, implementation, evaluation, and back to assessment. The small arrows in the opposite direction show that information from the succeeding components affects previous components by providing feedback. The lighter lines intersecting with the nurse-client relationship show that this relationship affects each component of the nursing process and that each component is interdependent on all other components.

## Purposes of the Nursing Process

The nursing process serves many purposes. The main purpose is to provide a systematic methodology for nursing practice: it unifies, standardizes, and directs nursing practice. The nurse's roles and functions are defined, and communication, collaboration, and synchronization of health team members are enhanced by the nursing process. Emphasis is placed either on health promotion, maintenance, and restoration or on enhancing a peaceful death, depending on the client's situation. Other purposes of the nursing process are to

- Facilitate documentation of data, diagnoses, plans, client responses, and evaluation
- Evaluate the efficiency and effectiveness of care
- Give direction, guidance, and meaning to nursing care
- Provide for continuity of care and to reduce omissions
- Individualize client participation in care
- Promote creativity and flexibility in nursing practice

Accountability and responsibility to clients and the nursing profession can be demonstrated by the nursing process. As health care costs increase, both consumers and administrators of health care agencies are concerned about cost effectiveness and accountability. Service providers, including nurses, are watched by those paying for their services, namely, consumers and third party payors, to determine the worth of their services. Nurses are expected to be accountable for their actions and to evaluate the effectiveness of their care. The nursing process enhances accountability to the client, service providers, and the agency/institution, and may be used to demonstrate cost effectiveness in these times of scarce resources.

### Characteristics of the Nursing Process

Seven major characteristics of the nursing process enhance its usefulness in practice:
1. It is goal-directed toward client-centered health care.
2. It is systematic and provides an organized approach to nursing.
3. It is dynamic by focusing on the changing responses of the client during the ongoing process.
4. It is applicable to individuals, families, and community groups at any level of health.
5. It is adaptable to any practice setting or specialization, and the components may be used sequentially or concurrently.
6. It is interpersonal and based on the nurse-client relationship.
7. It is useful with any type of model, especially nursing.

## HISTORY OF THEORY DEVELOPMENT IN NURSING

Until the 1960s, nursing was principally derived from social, biological, and medical theories. With the exception of Florence Nightingale's work, nursing theory had its beginnings with the publication of Peplau's (1952) book, which described the interpersonal process between the nurse and the patient. The nature of the nurse's role came under scrutiny during this decade as nurse leaders debated the nature of nursing practice and theory development. Thereafter, several nurse leaders, namely Abdellah, Orlando, Wiedenbach, Hall, Henderson, Levine, and Rogers, developed and published their views of nursing, as shown in Table 1-2. Their descriptions of nursing and nursing models evolved from their personal, professional, and educational experiences and reflected their perception of "ideal" nursing practice. Several

themes emerged as to the nature of nursing: it was described as an interpersonal process, as meeting the client's needs, or as providing nursing care.

During the 1970s, a consensus developed among nursing leaders that the common elements of nursing include the nature of nursing (role/actions), the individual recipient of care (client), the context of nurse-client interactions (environment), and health (Fawcett, 1978). Nurses debated whether there should be one conceptual model for nursing or several models to describe the relationships among the nurse, client, environment, and health.

Several methods have been used to develop nursing models. Initially, as nurses acquired advanced education and became familiar with theories in other disciplines, they recognized that these theories would be useful in explaining nursing actions. Thus, theories were borrowed from other disciplines. An example of this approach is the use of systems theory as the basis for Johnson's behavioral system model for nursing (1980). With recognition of the importance that theory plays in developing a scientific discipline, and awareness that theories in other disciplines were insufficient to describe nursing, nurses began to develop their own theories. Dickoff, James, and Weidenbach (1968) stimulated this trend by describing how theory is developed for a practice discipline. Although their approach has been debated, it sparked a growing commitment by nurses to develop their own models and theories. Some nurse theorists expanded or extended theories in other disciplines, such as Roy's (1984) work based on Helson's theory of adaptation. Other nurse theorists analyzed nursing practice situations to determine the theoretical underpinnings. King's (1981) work is representative of this approach, whereas Martha Rogers' (1970) work evolved from a philosophical and physics background.

Borrowing theories from other disciplines was criticized by some nurses as lacking originality and novelty. Also, some holistic nurses argued that current nursing models inadequately address the whole client and that a broader, phenomenological model was needed in nursing. Another criticism of nursing models is that they are relatively underdeveloped as theories in the strictest sense of the term. This may be related to the lack of clarity about what constitutes theory and theory testing in general, and the paucity of theory testing in nursing. Therefore, although some nursing models can describe and explain the nature of nursing, their ability to control and predict client outcomes is yet to be achieved. This is the aim of some nurse theorists, but presently nursing models reflect a synthe-

**Table 1-2** History of Nursing Theory Development

| Events | Year | Nurse Theorists |
|---|---|---|
| | 1860 | Florence Nightingale<br>Described nursing and environment |
| | 1952 | Hildegard E. Peplau<br>Nursing as an interpersonal process: patients with felt needs |
| Scientific era: nurses questioned purpose of nursing | 1960 | Faye Abdellah (also 1965; 1973)<br>Patient-centered approaches |
| | 1961 | Ida Jean Orlando<br>Nurse-patient relationship; deliberative nursing approach |
| Process of theory development discussed among professional nurses | 1964 | Ernestine Wiedenbach (also 1970; 1977)<br>Nursing: philosophy, purpose, practice, and art |
| | 1966 | Lydia E. Hall<br>Core (patient), care (body), cure (disease) |
| | 1966 | Virginia Henderson (also 1972; 1978)<br>Nursing assists patients with 14 essential functions toward independence |
| Symposium: theory development in nursing | 1967 | Myra Estrin Levine (also 1973)<br>Four conservation principles of nursing |
| Symposium: nature of science and nursing<br>Dickoff, James, and Weidenbach wrote "Theory in a Practice Discipline," in *Nursing Research* | 1968 | |
| Symposium: nature of science in nursing.<br>First nursing theory conference | 1969 | |
| Second nursing theory conference | 1970 | Martha E. Rogers (also 1980)<br>Science of unitary man: energy fields, openness; pattern, and organization |
| Consensus on nursing concepts: Nurse/nursing, health, client/patient/individual, society/environment | 1971 | Dorothea E. Orem (also 1980; 1985)<br>Nursing facilitates patients' self-care |
| Discussion on what is theory: the elements, criteria, types and levels, and the relation to research | 1971 | Imogene King (also 1975; 1981)<br>Theory of goal attainment through nurse-client transactions |
| NLN required conceptual frameworks in nursing education | 1973 | |
| Borrowed theories from other disciplines<br>Expanded theories from other disciplines. | 1974 | Sister Callista Roy (also 1976; 1980; 1984)<br>Roy's adaptation model: nurse adjusts patient's stimuli (focal, contextual, or residual). |
| Recognized problems in practice and developed theories to test and use in practice. | 1976 | Josephine Paterson and L. Zderad<br>Humanistic nursing |
| Second nurse educator conference on nursing theory | 1978 | Madeleine Leininger (also 1980; 1981)<br>Transcultural nursing<br>Caring nursing |
| Articles on theory development in *ANS, Nursing Research,* and *Image* | 1978 | Jean Watson (also 1985) |
| | 1979 | Philosophy and science of caring; humanistic nursing |
| Books written for nurses on how to critique theory, how to develop theory, and describing application of nursing theories | 1980 | Dorothy E. Johnson<br>Behavioral system model for nursing |
| Graduate schools of nursing develop courses in how to analyze and apply nursing theories | | Betty Neuman<br>Health-care systems model: a total person approach |
| Research studies in nursing identified nursing theories as framework for study | 1981 | Rosemarie Rizzo Parse (also 1987)<br>Man-living-health: a theory of nursing |
| Numerous books published on analysis, application, evaluation, and/or development of nursing theories | 1982–present | |

**Table 1-3**   Theory Development System: Process, Activities, and Product

| Process | Activities | Product |
|---|---|---|
| Exploration | Identifies values, beliefs, and assumptions: <br> What do nurses do (actions, skills) and for whom (individuals, families, community)? <br> When (under what conditions)? <br> Where (in what settings)? <br> How (roles—practitioner, research)? | Philosophy of nursing |
| Concept analysis | Define and describe major concepts: <br> Nursing—action, interactions, process <br> Clients—individual, family, community <br> Health—maintenance, prevention, restoration <br> Environment—hospital, community, clinic | Concept identification |
| Construct relationships | Descriptive theory <br> Describes some relationships between concepts, but the relationship is not clearly defined among *all* the concepts | Conceptual model |
| Test relationships | Explanatory theory <br> Explains the interrelationship among the major concepts; however, the logical and empirical adequacy of the relationships requires further explication | Theoretical framework |
| Validate relationships in practice | Predictive and prescriptive theory <br> Provides a set of interrelated concepts and relational statements that are logical and amenable to empirical testing, and explain or predict phenomena | Theory |

sis of the first two approaches. Table 1-2 presents a chronology of events related to nursing theory development and nurse theorists' work.

## DESCRIPTION OF THEORY
### Structural Components

The terms *theory, theoretical framework,* and *conceptual model* are frequently used indiscriminately and interchangeably in nursing and other disciplines. These terms have been defined differently by various writers, which has led to much confusion. Different definitions of theory arise from a lack of consensus on what constitutes theory and what criteria must be met for something to be considered a theory. Although there is general agreement on the structural criteria required for a theory, there is less consensus on functional criteria, which are based on values and beliefs.

Nursing theory development has been described as a system by Chinn (1987). Theory development is considered both a process, with numerous activities, and a product, as shown in Table 1-3. The *process* of theory development includes four interacting, sequential phases: analyze concepts, construct relationships, test relationships, and validate relationships in practice. Each phase influences both preceding and succeeding phases. There are five *products* of theory development: a philosophy

of nursing, concept identification, conceptual model, theoretical framework, and theories.

Initially, theorists begin by defining their values, beliefs, and assumptions, which are expressed as their philosophy of nursing. Next, the major concepts in the philosophy are identified and defined. When the relationship among some concepts is explained by propositions or relational statements, the theorist's work is considered a conceptual model. As a network of concepts that are interrelated by relational statements is developed, the model may be called a theoretical framework, although further refinement is required for logical and empirical adequacy. Finally, when a theorist's work consists of a set of concepts logically interrelated and amenable to testing, it is considered a theory. However, the theory must be tested and validated in a variety of practice settings for support and acceptance. The terms commonly used to describe the system of theory development are explained in the following paragraphs and the process, activities, and products are shown in Table 1-3.

### Philosophy

Theory development begins with an examination and analysis of what a theorist believes about the nature of nursing: what is nursing, what does the nurse do, how, and to whom? A philosophy is the theorist's viewpoint: what the theorist assumes, believes and values, or holds to be true in relation to nursing.

*Assumptions* are beliefs, which may have been tested or accepted as givens in other theories, but are taken for granted by a theorist. They are the basis for the theorist's view and serve as a point of reference. Theorists may explicitly state their assumptions or they may imply their beliefs in their work. The more explicitly theorists state their assumptions, the less ambiguity there is in interpreting the theory. Assumptions are not tested; however, they lead to a set of propositions that can be tested. For example, Neuman (1982) assumes that a person is an open system interacting with the environment and responding to stressors.

A *concept* is an abstract word that conveys a mental image of a phenomenon. Concepts are names, labels, or categories for objects, persons, or events derived from one's perceptual experiences. Concepts are the basic building blocks of theory. A concept symbolically represents something, but it is not the object or event per se. Concepts vary in degrees of abstractness: some concepts, like anxiety or pain, are more abstract than medication or procedure. The more general a concept is, the more it transcends time and space, and the greater its abstractness. All concepts are intangible, descriptive terms that persons interpret according to their perceptions and experiences. Concepts must be specifically defined because people have different meanings for them. Alone, concepts are meaningless; they are judged according to their use in statements, such as propositions.

## Conceptual Model

In the literature on theory, nursing continues to address the question of what is the difference between theory, theoretical frameworks, and conceptual models. What one person considers a theory, another person may call a conceptual model. Without clear definitions and criteria for each, the argument is arbitrary and inconclusive. In this book, the following definitions and descriptions are accepted.

A conceptual model is a group of concepts or ideas that are related, but the relationship is not explicit. Models are an abstract perspective or framework representing reality. They use concepts to symbolize meanings, but they are not the real world. Conceptual models have a "set of concepts"; however, the relational statements, explaining the connection between the concepts, are obscure, and therefore are not amenable to testing.

Models are more abstract with fewer specifically defined concepts than theories, and models do not explain how or why phenomena occur.

Some examples of conceptual models in nursing are: Orem's self-care model (1980), Roy's adaptation model (1984), and Johnson's behavioral system model for nursing (1980). The nursing process may also be considered a model because it is a group of related concepts.

## Theoretical Framework

Theoretical frameworks consist of a set of defined concepts and relational statements; however, the relationship between some concepts is loosely described. A theoretical framework needs further explication of the specific relationships among *all* the major concepts to provide a systematic view of the phenomena. Although explicit relational statements in a theoretical framework may be tested, it is not considered a theory because the framework lacks a *set* of interrelated statements.

A *relational statement* is a proposition: it describes a specific relationship between two or more concepts. Relational statements are classified into two groups: associational and causal. *Associational propositions* show which concepts occur together and designate a positive, negative, or no relationship between two concepts. *Causal propositions* describe a cause and effect relationship; a change in one concept causes a change in another. Examples of these two types of statements are shown below:

Associational:   As anxiety increases, tension increases.
                 As anxiety increases, perception decreases.

Causal:   High levels of anxiety cause decreased perception.

A theory contains two or more propositions, a set, which links the concepts and makes the interrelationship among the concepts explicit. The relationship between concepts in the proposition can be tested.

Some nurses believe that King's (1981) work in *A Theory for Nursing: Systems, Concepts, Process* is an example of a theoretical framework. Also, the work of Parse (1981) in *Man-Living-Health: A Theory of Nursing* is considered a theoretical framework, because the interrelationships of the concepts are explicit and each concept is defined.

## Theory

Theory is a highly complex term with arbitrary meanings. For some, theory may include ideas or hunches, whereas others believe that a theory must stand up to rigorous tests. Although there is a lack of consensus among the disciplines as to what a theory is, there is general agreement that theory consists of a set of defined concepts and a systematic, logical network of relational statements or propositions. The statements link the concepts and are amenable to testing. A theory symbolically represents reality but is not reality in itself. Theory is abstract and tentative; it varies in the degree of abstractness of the concepts and statements in the theory. Differences among models, frameworks, and theory are related to their levels of abstraction, degree of explication, and the level of theory development. All theories are models because they claim to represent some aspect of reality; however, all models are not necessarily theories. Conceptual models and theoretical frameworks usually precede and coexist with theory.

Some authors classify theories as descriptive, explanatory, and predictive (Stevens, 1983), as shown in Table 1-3. *Descriptive theory* identifies and describes the major concepts of phenomena, but does not explain how or why the concepts are related. This is the first level of theory development. For example, descriptive nursing theory would provide definitions of concepts such as client, health, and nursing, as in Peplau's work (1952).

*Explanatory theory*, the next level of theory development, attempts to describe how or why the concepts are related. It specifies the associations or relationships among some concepts, but further explication of the logical and empirical adequacy of these relationships is necessary. The theoretical frameworks or models by Johnson, King, Orem, and Roy are examples of explanatory theory.

*Predictive theory* is achieved when the conditions under which concepts are related are stated and the relational statements are able to describe future outcomes consistently. Selye's (1956) theory of stress and the general adaptation syndrome may be considered a predictive theory because it has been repeatedly tested and supported. In nursing and the social sciences, it is generally accepted that predictive and prescriptive (controlling) theories are actively being pursued, but presently do not exist.

In their book, Chinn and Jacobs (1983:70) definition of theory is offered. They state that theory is

A set of concepts, definitions, and propositions that projects a systematic view of phenomena by designating specific interrelationships among concepts for purposes of describing, explaining, predicting, and/or controlling (prescribing) phenomena.

Using this definition, concepts, definitions, and propositions are required in a theory. The terms *set* and *interrelationships* are also key elements in this definition. Set means that a theory must contain two or more propositions, which link the concepts, and the interrelationships among all the concepts must be explicit in the propositions.

Within different disciplines, theories may be found at various stages of development. Some theories are specifically developed as explanations of phenomena, whereas others serve the purpose of prediction, with or without control of phenomena. Depending on one's viewpoint, theory serves several different purposes. Some believe that the purpose of theory is to describe, explain, predict, and control outcomes, whereas others believe theory increases understanding and knowledge. Theory is very useful in guiding education, research, and practice.

## Functional Components

The functional components of any theory are the major concepts and their definitions. These concepts are the focus of the theory or model. In the 1970s, the nursing profession generally agreed that four major concepts are addressed in nursing models: the client, the nature of nursing (role/actions), the meaning of health, and the environment in which client-nurse interactions occur. However, each nursing model provides a different view, or definition of these four major concepts. Nurses who use nursing models must understand the different ways each nursing model defines these concepts.

1. *Who is the client?* The client is usually the recipient of nursing care and may be defined as an individual, family, or community. Theorists may define a client as a person with a need, an impaired health status, a self-care deficit, or an adaptive person capable of change. Some theorists identify only individuals with health problems as the clients, whereas other theorists view any individual or family within the scope of nursing as care recipients.

2. *What is the nature of nursing: the nurse's role?* Nursing models generally describe nursing as a helping discipline, which may involve cognitive acts, behavioral tasks, or interpersonal relationships between the client and the nurse. The nurse may act on the client's behalf or mutually with the client, or may teach the client how to carry out certain activities. One nursing model defines the nurse's role as a self-care agent, another model views the nurse as reducing the client's stressors. The nurse's role in each model should be clearly understood by nurses who use any model.

3. *What is the meaning of health?* Some theorists

describe a health-illness continuum, whereas others refer only to ill health or the presence of health problems. Recently, some theorists have described health as more than the absence of disease. They see health as a dynamic process that changes over time and varies with circumstances. Other theorists view health as interdependent with the changing environment, or as a process that the person has some control over. It is important to identify which view of health a theorist adheres to and whether that viewpoint is congruent with one's own view.

4. *Where do client-nurse interactions occur?* What settings or environment are deemed appropriate for nursing? The *environment* may be defined as the central arena of nursing or the area of interchange with the client in the health setting. Some theorists limit the scope of nursing practice to hospital settings and/or outpatient clinics, whereas others include community concepts and some place no restrictions or limits on this concept.

## GENERAL PERSPECTIVES OF NURSING MODELS

The scope of nursing practice varies widely because of the multiple practice settings, the complexity of the client's health status and situation, and the role of the nurse. Nursing models each present a unique perspective on how to assist clients to attain optimal health. Models of nursing also vary in their levels of development, degree of abstractness, and clarity of concept definitions and relational statements. Most nursing models describe the four major concepts cited previously, and some subconcepts. However, each model describes the major concepts and their interrelationships in a unique way. Also, some models are more applicable to a family or group, such as the models of Neuman and King, whereas other models, such as those of Roy and Johnson, focus on individual clients.

There are three typical approaches used in nursing models: developmental, systems, and interactional. *Developmental models* focus on the client's development through an orderly sequence to attain optimal health and greater degrees of self-responsibility. This approach is illustrated in Orem's and Rogers' models in which the nurse's role is to promote the client's restoration and growth. *Systems models* view clients as interrelated biological, psychological, and social systems. When an imbalance occurs in one system, it disrupts other systems. The nurse's role is to restore equilibrium or facili-

tate adaptation. Roy, Neuman, and Johnson use this approach in their nursing models. *Interactional models* emphasize the client-nurse interactions and the development of a relationship between the client and nurse to work toward the client's goal attainment. Examples of nursing models with this approach are the different models of Orlando, Peplau, and King. All nursing models contain some aspects of each of the three approaches; however, each model emphasizes one approach over the others.

Models and theories serve as the link between nursing practice, research, and education. Ideas for nursing theory may develop in practice, may be tested through research, and then may serve to guide or explain practice. Conceptual models can guide nursing practice. Models are tools for systematic examination of client situations. They assist nurses to organize their thinking, observing, and interpreting. Therefore, models are goal directed and lead to more efficient and effective nursing practice. They also serve as the basis for nursing research, both to test relational statements of the models and to support various studies. In nursing education, nursing models may guide the curriculum and be applied throughout the nursing process.

Currently, some nurse theorists, such as King, Roy, and Parse, continue to develop and refine their models in nursing, whereas others, like Orlando, Levine, and Orem, have developed their work as far as they had planned. In the future, nursing models must clearly differentiate activities that are unique to nursing and different from other health disciplines. Nursing must distinguish either a separate body of knowledge or a distinct manner of applying shared knowledge. Future nursing theories will strive to describe, explain, predict, and control client outcomes. Theories will facilitate the prevention of illness, and the maintenance, promotion, and restoration of the client's optimum health potential.

## APPLICATION OF MODELS IN THE NURSING PROCESS

Nursing models provide a broad framework to interrelate various aspects of the client's complex health situation. Professional nursing practice is based on the knowledge and understanding of various theories, models, and principles from the scientific, behavioral, and humanistic disciplines. With increasing clinical experience, nurse practitioners synthesize theoretical and clinical knowledge and have a broader base to make clinical decisions. Because individual, family, and community clients each present unique health situations, the nurse uses this broad knowledge base to select the model that is most congruent with the client's health situation. The major nursing models each are based on different assumptions and have a unique way of describing the four major concepts—client, nursing, health, and environment—and their relationships. Selection of an appropriate nursing model for a specific client situation requires both in-depth knowledge of nursing models and information about major variables affecting the client situation.

When working with a new client, the nurse gathers preliminary information about the client's health concerns, age, lifestyle and activities of daily living. The purpose is to identify and understand the unique and common variables in the client's situation. The client's health concerns are identified and often redefined. This information is sifted through a set of accepted assumptions and beliefs that the nurse holds about

What constitutes *health* for this client?

What *prevents* this client from achieving health?

What can *nursing* do to facilitate the clients health?

*Health* is the nurse's view of what constitutes health for this person. Health may range from a utopian view of human potential to a more limited view with a chronic illness.

What does the nurse believe *prevents* the client from achieving optimum health? Many explanations are possible such as lack of information, genetic predisposition, multiple stressors, and a combination of any of these factors.

The nurse's view of appropriate *nursing* actions or strategies is based on the legal scope of nursing, knowledge, and experience with similar clients. The range of nursing actions may vary greatly. For example, the nurse may teach or counsel the client, provide comfort measures, or refer the client to a specialist.

For example, if the nurse believes that the client's health is compromised because of hypertension and obesity and that overeating and work pressures are preventing the client from achieving optimal health, then nursing may be viewed as teaching stress management strategies and proper nutrition or referring the client to a dietitian.

The nurse synthesizes the preliminary client information through the preceding questions, along with a broad knowledge base, intuition, and experience, and constructs a theoretical perspective of the client situation. This perspective serves to

1. Direct and prioritize further inquiry
2. Organize data into patterns
3. Identify appropriate health concerns

4. Determine which nursing model is most congruent with the nurse's beliefs and the client situation

Next, the nurse considers the possible models, their underlying assumptions, concept definitions, and the relationships among the concepts. The models are examined to determine acceptance by the nurse and their appropriateness for the client. Each model is different, and the nurse must understand these differences to choose the model that best represents both the nurse's view of health and nursing, and the client's health concern. Some models are more applicable to individual clients with a chronic illness, whereas others are more applicable to a family crisis. Also, some models describe nursing as providing assistance, whereas others facilitate the client's self-care. The nurse examines each model by asking the following questions:

1. *What are the major concepts of the model and how are they defined?* For example, does the model include the nurse and the client, or is it a family developmental model or a crisis model? Aguilera's (1982) crisis model is appropriate for a rape victim, whereas Duvall's (1977) family development model is more appropriate for an expectant couple.

    Is the *client* an open system, a set of interacting parts, an adaptive system, a person in disequilibrium, or someone with a self-care deficit? Is the client an active participant or a passive recipient of nursing care? Can the client be a well individual or family? What is the nurse's view of the client?

    Is the *nurse* a change-agent, a teacher, someone who interacts with the client, changes the environment, or reduces stressors?

    Is *health* a state of system equilibrium, the ability to maintain self-care, an adaptive system, or a dynamic evolving process?

    It is important that the model fit the client situation and that the nurse's view of nursing, client, and health agrees with the way each concept is defined.

2. *What are the relationships among the concepts?* Are these relationships explicit or implicit? Does the model explain how the nurse interacts with the client to facilitate health? In some models, the nurse alters the client's environment to promote adaptation, whereas in other models the nurse interacts with the client to facilitate self-care. If the nurse believes that clients should actively participate in their health care and that health is an

evolving, dynamic process, the nurse would choose a model that most closely represents that view.

3. *What is the focus of the model?* Is the focus the client, the nursing actions, or the nurse-client relationship? For example, Peplau's (1952) model emphasizes the nurse-patient relationship, whereas Neuman's (1982) health care system model focuses on the patient's response to stressors and provides a systems framework to guide health care professionals. The client's situation and the nurse's beliefs about health and the nursing role determine the central focus needed in an appropriate model. For example, when working with an acute psychotic patient, the nurse-client relationship is of primary importance. However, in a child abuse case, a systems approach involving multiple team members may be appropriate.

4. *What are the underlying assumptions of the model?* The assumptions are the theorist's basic premises, accepted truths upon which the model is founded. These assumptions may or may not be stated, but usually can be inferred from their work. Nurses should consider whether they accept and agree with the theorist's underlying assumptions and whether the assumptions represent reality. For example, Roy (1984:37) identifies some basic assumptions, such as "to respond positively to environmental changes, the person must adapt." If a nurse believes that the environment could be adapted, rather than the person, this assumption may not be acceptable.

5. *Will the model direct a plan of action that is appropriate for the client's health status?* In other words, does the model support the main focus of change and provide direction for appropriate nursing actions? For example, Roy's (1984) adaptation model provides a guide for various nursing actions that can assist the individual client with physiological alterations, while a systems model can assist with change for a community client. Selection of the most congruent model, the one that best fits the client situation, facilitates application of the model throughout the nursing process.

The nurse should have a thorough knowledge of each model to respond to these five questions and should be able to compare the client's health situation with each model. Practice in applying models comes with clinical experience. The nurse considers the range of possible models that best fit the client's situation and the nurse's beliefs and chooses the model that is most congruent with both and that includes appropriate nursing actions.

The chosen model has a major influence on nursing practice and each component of the nursing process. Data collection is guided by the major concepts and subconcepts in the model. For example, using Roy's model, the nurse would collect data about the client's physiological needs, self-concept, role mastery, and interdependence, along with related stimuli. Next, the model is used to organize and categorize the client data and to identify behavioral patterns. The nurse using Johnson's model would organize the data in the seven subsystem categories and identify behavioral responses. The model also provides the structure for analyzing and interpreting the data. The nurse using Orem's model would identify universal and developmental self-care requisites and deficits. Health concerns are stated as nursing diagnoses. The plans, which consist of goals, objectives, strategies, and orders, evolve from the chosen model. The model guides the selection of strategies and may serve as the rationale. The nurse using Johnson's model would consider nurturance, protection, or stimulation strategies, whereas Neuman's model would suggest reducing stressors within the three levels of prevention. The model also serves as the basis for nursing implementation. Evaluation of the client's progress is based on the established goals and objectives, which were derived from the chosen model.

This book describes how different models are applied in each component of the nursing process. Chapter 2 provides an overview of various nursing models, developmental models, family models, and broad general models. Readers will find it helpful to review these models before reading succeeding chapters. Section II describes the components of the nursing process. These chapters should be read in sequence as each provides the basis for subsequent chapters. Each component of the nursing process is fully described and illustrated, with the application of different models. The chapters in Sections I and II provide the foundation for understanding the case studies in Section III. These case studies illustrate the complete nursing process applied to a specific client situation, using a selected nursing model.

## SUMMARY

Professional nursing has evolved into a scientific discipline that supports the integration of theory, research, and practice. The nursing process, the core of practice, was legitimized in the *Standards of Nursing Practice* and is tested by the state board exams. The five components of the nursing process are assessment, diagnosis, planning, implementation, and evaluation. With the development of nursing models, nurses are learning to apply these models in the nursing process.

Presently there are many nursing models, some of which continue to be tested and refined by theorists and others. These models are valuable in professional nursing practice and are applied in each component of the nursing process. Models provide a broader understanding of a client's complex situation and are useful as a frame of reference for collecting, organizing, and interpreting data about the client. Models guide the nursing diagnoses, plans, implementation, and evaluation. They provide a logical basis for explaining how nurses assist clients toward optimum health. Today, professional nurses use models as the means to justify each component in the nursing process and to demonstrate the nurse's accountability to the client, the health team, and the agency.

## REFERENCES AND READINGS

Aggleton P and Chalmers H: Models of nursing, nursing practice, and nursing education, J Adv Nurs 12:573, 1987.

Aguilera DC and Messick JM: Crisis intervention: theory and methodology, ed 6, St Louis, 1990, The CV Mosby Co.

Alfaro R: Application of nursing process: a step-by-step guide, Philadelphia, 1986, JB Lippincott.

American Nurses' Association: Standards of nursing practice, Kansas City, Mo, 1973, American Nurses' Association.

Barnum BJ: Holistic nursing and nursing process, Holistic Nurs Pract 1:27, 1987.

Becker PH: Advocacy in nursing: perils and possibilities, Holistic Nurs Pract 1:54, 1986.

Benner P: From novice to expert, Menlo Park, Calif, 1984, Addison-Wesley Co.

Benner P and Tanner C: How expert nurses use intuition, Am J Nurs 87:23, 1987.

Buchanan BF: Conceptual models: an assessment framework, J Nurs Adm 17:22, 1987.

Capers CF: Some basic facts about models, nursing conceptualizations, and nursing theories, J Cont Ed Nurs 16:149, 1986.

Carper BA: Fundamental patterns of knowing in nursing, Adv Nurs Sci 1:13, 1978.

Chance KS: Nursing models: a requisite for professional accountability, Adv Nurs Sci 4:57, 1982.

Chinn PL: Advances in nursing theory development, Rockville, Md, 1983, Aspen Systems Corp.

Chinn PL: Debunking myths in nursing theory and research, Image 17:45, 1985.

Chinn PL and Jacobs MK: Theory and nursing: a systematic approach, ed 2, St Louis, 1987, The CV Mosby Co.

Clark J: Development of models and theories on the concept of nursing, J Adv Nurs 7:129, 1982.

Craig SL: Theory development and its relevance for nursing, J Adv Nurs 5:349, 1980.

Dickoff J, James, P, and Weidenbach E: Theory in a practice discipline. I. Practice oriented theory, Nurs Res 17:415, 1968.

Donnelly GF: The promise of nursing process: an evaluation, Holistic Nurs Pract 1:1, 1987.

Duvall EM: Marriage and family development, ed 5, Philadelphia, 1977, JB Lippincott Co.

Erikson E: Childhood and society, ed 2, New York, 1963, WW Norton & Co, Inc.

Fawcett J: The relationship between theory and research: a double helix, Adv Nurs Sci 1:49, 1978.

Fawcett J: Analysis and evaluation of conceptual models, Philadelphia, 1984, FA Davis Co.

Field PA: The impact of nursing theory on the clinical decision making process, J Adv Nurs 12:563, 1987.

Fitzpatrick JJ: Use of existing nursing models, J Gerontol Nurs 13:8, 1987.

Fitzpatrick JJ and Whall A: Conceptual models of nursing: analysis and application, Bowie, Md, 1983, Robert J Brady Co.

Gerrity PL: Perception in nursing: the value of intuition, Holistic Nurs Pract 1:63, 1987.

Henderson V: Nursing process—a critique, Holistic Nurs Pract 1:7, 1987.

Iyer PW, et al: Nursing process and nursing diagnosis, Philadelphia, 1986, WB Saunders Co.

Johnson DE: Professional practice in nursing. In The shifting scene: directions for practice, NLN Pub. No. 15-1252, New York, 1967, National League for Nursing.

Johnson DE: The behavioral system model for nursing. In Reihl JP and Roy C Sr, editors: Conceptual models for nursing practice, ed 2, New York, 1980, Appleton-Century-Crofts.

Kelly K: Clinical inference in nursing, Nurs Res 15:23, 1966.

King IM: A Theory for nursing: systems, concepts, process, New York, 1981, John Wiley & Sons, Inc.

Knowles LN: Decision making in nursing: a necessity for doing, ANA Clinical Sessions 1966, New York, 1967, Appleton-Century-Crofts.

Krieger D: Foundations of holistic health nursing practice, Philadelphia, 1981, JB Lippincott Co.

Kristjanson LJ, Tamblyn R, and Kuypers JA: A model to guide development and application of multiple nursing theories, J Adv Nurs 12:523, 1987.

Leddy S and Pepper JM: Conceptual bases of professional nursing, Philadelphia, 1984, JB Lippincott Co.

Maslow A: Motivation and personality, ed 2, New York, 1970, Harper & Row, Publishers, Inc.

McHugh M: Nursing process: musings on the method, Holistic Nurs Pract 1:21, 1986.

Meleis AI: Theoretical nursing: development and process, Philadelphia, 1985, JB Lippincott Co.

National League for Nursing: Theory development: what, why and how, New York, 1978, Pub. # 15-1708, National League for Nursing.

Neuman B: The Neuman systems model, New York, 1982, Appleton-Century-Crofts.

Orem DE: Nursing: concepts of practice, ed 2, New York, 1980, McGraw-Hill Book Co.

Orlando IJ: The dynamic nurse-patient relationship: function, process and principles, New York, 1961, GP Putnam's Sons.

Parse RR: Man-living-health: a theory of nursing, Philadelphia, 1981, John Wiley & Sons, Inc.

Parse RR: Nursing science: major paradigms, theories, and critiques, Philadelphia, 1987, WB Saunders Co.

Peplau H: Interpersonal relations in nursing, New York, 1952, GP Putnam's Sons.

Pinnell NN and deMeneses M: The nursing process: theory, application, and related processes, Norwalk, Conn, 1986, Appleton-Century-Crofts.

Rew L and Barrow EM: Intuition: a neglected hallmark of nursing knowledge, Adv Nurs Sci 10:49, 1987.

Rogers ME: The theoretical basis of nursing, Philadelphia, 1970, FA Davis Co.

Roy Sr C: Introduction to nursing: an adaptation model, ed 2, Englewood Cliffs, NJ, 1984, Prentice-Hall, Inc.

Ruffing-Rahal MA: Personal documents and nursing theory development, Adv Nurs Sci 8:50, 1986.

Selye H: The stress of life, New York, 1956, McGraw-Hill Book Co.

Silva MC: Research testing nursing theory: state of the art, Adv Nurs Sci 9:1, 1986.

Stevens BJ: Nursing theory: analysis, application, evaluation, ed 2, Boston, 1983, Little, Brown & Co.

Walker KO and Avant K: Strategies for theory construction in nursing, New York, 1983, Appleton-Century-Crofts.

Young CE: Intuition and nursing process, Holistic Nurs Pract 1:52, 1987.

Yura H and Walsh MB: The nursing process: assessing, planning, implementing, evaluating, New York, 1967, Appleton-Century-Crofts.

Yura H and Walsh MB: The nursing process: assessing, planning, implementing, evaluating, ed 4, New York, 1983, Appleton-Century-Crofts.

CHAPTER

2

# Overview of Selected Models

JANET W. KENNEY

This chapter presents an overview of selected models commonly used in the nursing process. Generally these models are well known, and the major concepts are defined. Some models have been tested in research studies. The chapter is organized into three categories of models: general, nursing, and family models. The major concepts of each model are defined, and the basic structure and essence are described and illustrated. This chapter will familiarize readers with various models that will be applied in the nursing process components in the following chapters. However, readers are strongly encouraged to review primary sources in the literature to fully understand any model prior to applying it in the nursing process. This chapter presents the following models in the order listed below:

### General Models
Maslow's hierarchy of needs
Erikson's eight stages of man
General systems
Aguilera and Messick's crisis intervention

### Nursing Models
Johnson's behavioral systems model
King's theory of goal attainment
Leininger's transcultural nursing model
Neuman's health-care systems model
Orem's self-care nursing model
Parse's man-living-health model
Peplau's interpersonal model
Rogers' science of unitary human beings
Roy's adaptation model

### Family Models
Duvall
Stevenson
Satir
Friedman
Calgary

First, four general models are described; these may be familiar to the reader. Next, nine nursing models are presented, beginning with each theorist's definition of the four major concepts. Each of the theorists' unique concepts and subconcepts is defined and their interrelationships are illustrated. Some nursing models are developed for individual clients; others can be applied to a family or community. The strengths, limitations, and applications in the nursing process are discussed. Three of the five family models presented here were developed by nurses. Models that can be applied to a community are the general systems model and Neuman's health-care systems Model. (A third community model developed by Goeppinger and Schuster is presented in Chapter 6.) Application of these models in each component of the nursing process is shown in Sections II and III.

## GENERAL MODELS
### Maslow's Hierarchy of Needs

Advocates of human needs theory view individuals as integrated, whole beings who are motivated by internal and external needs that create tension. To reduce this tension, an individual seeks to meet specific needs through goal-directed behavior. Abraham Maslow (1970) classified human needs into five categories of predominance and placed them in a hierarchy. This hierarchy of human needs begins with basic fundamental needs of the individual that must be satisfied before proceeding to the next higher level. Throughout life the individual strives to satisfy needs at each level, but at different periods needs within one or more categories may be predominant. The desire to gratify human needs at each level motivates the individual and strengthens goal-directed behaviors. Generally, basic physiological needs and safety needs must be relatively satisfied in the individual before he or she can strive for higher level needs (Fig. 2-1).

### Physiological Needs

A variety of fundamental physical needs have been identified, including air, food, sleep, sex, fluids, exercise, elimination, and stimulation. For survival and satisfactory functioning, every individual must have these basic physiological needs met. The extent or degree to which each of these needs is met varies with the individual. Some people require more sleep or food than others, but individuals must satisfy these needs at their own specific levels.

### Safety

When basic physical needs are relatively satisfied, safety needs emerge; these include security, stability, order, physical safety, freedom from fear, protection, and sometimes dependency. These needs reflect self-protection through the establishment of structure, law, order, and limits.

Needs for safety and protection from harm may become more prominent when the individual is threatened by bodily harm, as in physical illness or potential injury. Safety needs involve both imminent danger or concerns and potential loss, such as loss of the security of a spouse or an occupational position.

### Love and Belonging

As physical and safety needs are reasonably satisfied, the need for love and belonging emerges. Within this category are needs for affectionate relationships, identification within various groups (family, church, and work), and companionship. These needs may be expressed through contact with significant others, tenderness, affection, and intimacy in sharing time spent together. Love and belonging needs may include contact with and affection for family members, friends, and associates of all age groups and both sexes. When love and belonging needs remain unsatisfied, the individual may feel alone, alienated, estranged, and distant from friends and relatives. The need for love encompasses both giving and receiving mutually.

### Esteem and Recognition

When the needs just mentioned have been gratified, the individual's need for esteem and recognition arise. These needs include self-respect, self-esteem, prestige, respect, and esteem from others.

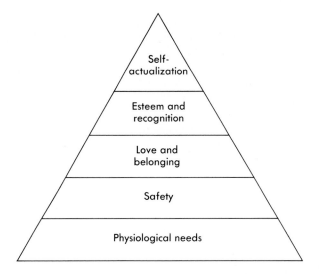

**Fig. 2-1.** Maslow's hierarchy of needs.

An individual may be motivated by the desire to achieve fame, recognition, strength, competency, independence, or an outstanding reputation. This desire for esteem and recognition motivates individuals toward goal-directed behaviors to achieve or gratify these needs in their own unique way. As this need is relatively satisfied, the individual experiences a sense of adequacy, self-worth, self-fulfillment, and contentment.

### Self-Actualization

When the lower needs in the hierarchy have been relatively satisfied, an individual strives toward self-actualization. Young people may grow toward self-actualization, but must usually reach maturity before they have a sense of self-actualization. Self-actualization means that the individual is relatively satisfied with most aspects of life. This includes what the person thinks of self and the level of achievement reached or the ability to fulfill that designated purpose in life. Some adults continue working toward self-actualization all their lives; others arrive at a sense of fulfillment or accomplishment in midlife. The individual feels a sense of having achieved a purpose in life and having developed capabilities to the fullest.

Maslow's hierarchy of needs is a broad model, which can be applied to all components of the nursing process, especially to assessment and to prioritization of nursing diagnoses. It is applicable to individual and family clients. Although the nurse can assist clients to meet the first four needs, the fifth need, self-actualization, is generally left to the client to meet after other needs are met.

## Erikson's Developmental Model

Erik Erikson (1963) is a lay psychoanalyst who extended Freud's theories on man. He emphasized the influence of sociocultural and biophysical dimensions on the individual's development. In Erikson's model, human development is interrelated with cultural and physical growth over eight distinctive stages. Each stage represents a developmental task: a foundation for the next stage as shown in Table 2-1. Each task is never fully resolved, and it may resurface in later years. The critical task at each stage holds a zenith position at that period of development; it becomes less dominant later but may arise again. If the specific task is not accomplished during the critical period, Erikson notes the consequences in the development of undesirable behaviors.

### Erikson's Eight Stages of Man

**Trust versus mistrust.** In infancy the central task is to develop a sense of trust that basic needs will be adequately met. As these needs are met, the infant learns that the world is a safe place to live in. Others' behaviors result in a predictable pattern that can be trusted. Mistrust in the safety and predictability of life occurs when the infant's needs are not satisfactorily met.

**Autonomy versus shame and doubt.** The toddler who has learned to trust begins to test the environment, determining the extent to which the environment can be manipulated. Autonomy develops as the toddler explores and learns control of self and the environment. If independent actions are thwarted or are unacceptable to others, the toddler experiences shame. When attempts to manipulate the environment are ineffectual, the toddler may develop doubt.

**Initiative versus guilt.** As the preschooler tries to be assertive during interactions with others and the environment, approval from others fosters initiative. When the preschooler's actions are not permitted or are disapproved of by others, the child develops a sense of guilt.

**Industry versus inferiority.** The school-age child directs energy toward learning knowledge and skills applicable in the real world. The child who receives satisfaction from those efforts continues to be industrious. The child who has difficulty and whose efforts go unrewarded may feel inferior and inadequate.

**Identity versus role diffusion.** During adolescence the individual searches for current and future identities. This is an attempt to integrate life experiences into a sense of self. To master identity the adolescent must feel an internally consistent self-

**Table 2-1**  Erikson's Stages of Development

| Stages of Development | Age Level |
| --- | --- |
| Trust versus mistrust | Infancy |
| Autonomy versus shame and doubt | Toddler |
| Initiative versus guilt | Preschool |
| Industry versus inferiority | School age |
| Identity versus role diffusion | Adolescence |
| Intimacy versus isolation | Young adult |
| Generativity versus stagnation | Adulthood |
| Integrity versus despair | Older adult |

image. It must agree with others' views. The adolescent who is unable to integrate life experiences and self-image into a consistent identity experiences role diffusion. Feelings of being lost or confused may occur.

**Intimacy versus isolation.** The young adult seeks relationships with others to acquire a sense of sharing, caring, and intimacy. An individual who is unable to share close relationships and feel comfortable in intimate relationships may have a sense of isolation from friends or family members.

**Generativity versus stagnation.** In adulthood the primary task is satisfaction with productivity. This includes work, family, home, and citizenship. These activities and a sense of accomplishment provide the individual with intrinsic rewards, but the adult who is dissatisfied in these areas may feel stagnation. With lack of productivity, the adult may indulge in self-absorption and develop derogatory attitudes toward others.

**Integrity versus despair.** The older adult, satisfied with life and its meaning, who believes that life is fulfilling and successful, has integrity. A sense of despair develops when the adult fears death and finds failure with self and others.

Erikson's developmental model depicts eight psychosocial stages in the life cycle. It identifies critical developmental tasks at each stage and the consequences when a critical task remains unaccomplished. Although each task is age-appropriate, the tasks are never completely resolved and may arise at any time in the life cycle. This developmental model has limited use in the nursing process. Each client should be assessed and analyzed according to the age-appropriate developmental level. The model is used in conjunction with other, broader models that include biopsychosocial concepts.

## General Systems Theory

General systems theory serves as a model for viewing man as interacting with the environment.

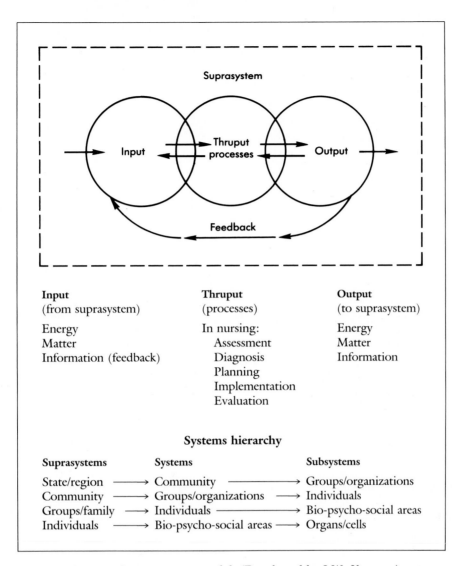

Fig. 2-2. Open systems model. (Developed by J.W. Kenney.)

One of the first theorists to develop systems theory was Ludwig von Bertalanffy (1968), who synthesized the following abstract laws in systems theory development:

1. Systems are organized complexities in which behavior is determined by interaction among various components.
2. No system repeats its interaction, but continuous interaction among variables produces uniquely dynamic situations infinitely.
3. Evolution proceeds from a less to a more differentiated state; dynamic interaction between individuals and the environment results in increasing complexity for both.
4. Regular changes are found in the evolution of all systems as they move toward higher states of order, differentiation, and probability.
5. People are living, open (metabolizing) systems, exhibiting self-differentiation, pro-

viding energy, and having a stored information system (genetic code) to steer the process.

A *system* consists of a set of interacting components within a boundary that filters the type and rate of exchange with the environment. Systems are composed of both structural and functional components. Structure refers to the arrangements of the parts at a given time; function is the process of continuous change in the system as matter, energy, and information are exchanged with the environment.

All living systems are *open* in that there is continual exchange of matter, energy, and information (Fig. 2-2). In open systems there are varying degrees of interaction with the environment from which the system receives input and gives back output in the form of matter, energy, and information. Theoretically, no closed systems exist, as they would be totally isolated from interacting with the environment.

The universe consists of a *hierarchy of systems* (numerous suprasystems, systems, and subsystems), and each system may be viewed as having one or more suprasystems and subsystems. For example, the individual as a system belongs to suprasystems in a family, community, and region. An individual's subsystems are composed of organ systems or biopsychosocial components.

Each system has discrete, definable *boundaries* that filter and regulate the flow of input and output exchange with the environment. Boundaries may consist of physical or abstract lines of demarcation that separate the system from the surrounding environment. The boundary filter may be very permeable or fairly impermeable, depending on the component it is screening in or out of the system.

For survival, all systems must receive varying types and amounts of matter, energy, and information from the environment. Through the process of selection, the system regulates the type and amount of *input* received.

The system uses the input through self-regulation to maintain the system's equilibrium or homeostasis. Some types of inputs are used immediately in their original state, whereas others require complex transformation *(throughput)* for use. Matter, energy, and information are continuously processed through the system and released as outputs.

After processing input, the system returns *output* (matter, energy, and information) to the environment in an altered state, affecting the environment.

The system continuously monitors itself and the environment for information to guide its operation. This *feedback* information of environmental responses to the system's output is utilized by the system in adjustment, correction, and accommodation to the interaction with the environment. Feedback may be positive, negative, or neutral.

Substances that occupy space and can be exchanged between the system and environment are considered *matter*.

The ability to perform, carry out tasks, and overcome resistance, in a physical and emotional sense, may be considered *energy*.

Through dynamic interaction with the environment, the system exchanges *information* in different forms, such as verbal and behavioral communication, visual media, taste, smell, and touch. Information is used by the system in the process of selection and decision making.

For survival, a system must achieve a balance internally and externally. *Equilibrium* depends on the ability of the system to regulate input and output with the environment to achieve a balanced relationship of the interacting parts. Because balance is continually changing, a self-regulating mechanism within the system monitors the interaction of inputs and outputs with the environment by using information from feedback. Through interactions with the environment, the system uses various *adaptation* mechanisms to maintain equilibrium. Adaptation may occur through accepting or rejecting the matter, energy, or information and by accommodating the input and modifying the system's responses to maintain or regain equilibrium.

Systems theory is applicable in the nursing process of the individual, family, and community client. It is frequently used to assess and analyze a community. However, because it is so broad, supplemental models are often required to delineate input, throughput, and output.

## Aguilera and Messick's Crisis Intervention Model

Donna Aguilera and Janice Messick (1990) synthesized the views of several behaviorists in their crisis intervention model. They consider crisis a stressful event or change in the individual's life, involving loss or threat of loss that disrupts the individual's equilibrium. Crises are categorized as maturational or situational. Maturational crises are those events that occur routinely. They include marriage, pregnancy, going away to school, and the death of a friend or spouse. Situational crises are unexpected events, such as failing an examination, losing a job, receiving a promotion, and sustaining an injury.

These authors describe three balancing factors. Each factor must be present in a threatening situation to avert a crisis. These factors reduce the risk of a crisis and help the individual maintain equilibrium. The three factors are realistic perception of the event, adequate situational supports, and adequate coping mechanisms, as shown in Fig. 2-3.

### Realistic Perception of the Event

The meaning an individual attaches to an event influences the perception of it. Sometimes past experiences evoke feelings unrelated to the event; these feelings may distort the individual's perception and magnify the consequences of the event. When an individual attaches great significance to an event, a distorted perception is likely. The individual's feelings and emotions may create an unrealistic picture of the present and future, which hinders effective decision-making and may lead to crisis. Those with a realistic perception of the event are able to view the situation in perspective. This

**Situational or maturational events**

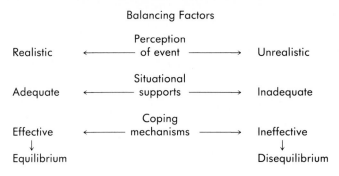

Fig. 2-3. Aguilera and Messick's crises intervention model.

reduces the chance that their emotions will cloud decision-making. A realistic perception of the event may avert a crisis.

### Adequate Situational Supports

Individuals rely on others to assist them in times of need. Significant others reflect an appraisal of the individual's self-worth and the meaning of the event. When faced with a loss or threat of loss, individuals share the meaning of the event with significant others. This sharing helps the individual place the event in perspective. Situational supports are considered adequate when individuals feel they can share the concern with and receive support from significant others. Sometimes an individual cannot share the concern with others for fear of losing respect or esteem. When individuals lack others with whom to share events or concerns, their situational supports are inadequate. This may cause disequilibrium and lead to a crisis.

### Adequate Coping Mechanisms

From life experiences, individuals learn a repertoire of coping responses or patterns. These patterns assist individuals in reducing tension, in adapting to daily stressful events, and in maintaining equilibrium. Occasionally, a stressful event occurs that overwhelms the individual. It may be an unfamiliar situation, the magnitude of the concern, or several concerns occurring simultaneously. When usual coping responses are ineffective, disequilibrium and crisis may occur.

Aguilera and Messick's crisis intervention model describes three balancing factors: realistic perception of the event, situational supports, and coping mechanisms. Each factor must be adequately present to maintain equilibrium and avoid a crisis. In crisis intervention, each factor is assessed, and if one factor is missing or inadequate, means are sought to enhance or develop that factor. This cri-

sis model is excellent for individuals or families experiencing situational or maturational crises, such as unwanted pregnancy, loss of a family member, rape or abuse, or a chronic health problem.

## NURSING MODELS

Nine nursing models were selected for presentation in alphabetical order. For purposes of comparison, a brief description of each theorist's four major concepts is shown in Table 2-2. In the table the term *nursing* refers to the nurse's role or actions; *client* is the recipient of nursing care or one who qualifies for nursing care; *health* refers to the theorist's view of what constitutes health; and *environment* is the setting in which nursing occurs.

### Johnson's Behavioral System Model

Dorothy Johnson's (1980) model is a synthesis of theories and concepts from the behavioral and biological sciences, integrated into a systems framework. Stress and adaptation theories are emphasized in this model.

Each person is viewed as a behavioral system composed of seven subsystems. The subsystems interact and are interdependent. Each person strives to achieve balance and stability both internally and externally and to function effectively by adjusting and adapting to environmental forces through learned patterns of response. When these forces are too great, and the person is unable to adapt or achieve optimum functioning, behavioral instability develops in one or more of the subsystems. This reduces functional capacity and efficiency and depletes energy.

Nurses assist any person threatened or potentially threatened by behavioral system imbalance to maintain efficient and effective functioning. They regulate external forces to preserve the client's be-

---

### Johnson's Beliefs

*Nursing:* regulation of external forces to stabilize client's behavioral system and restore, maintain, or attain balance

*Client:* a behavioral system (person) threatened or potentially threatened by illness (imbalance) and/or hospitalization

*Health:* an efficient and effectively functioning behavioral system (person) who maintains balance/stability by adapting/adjusting to outside forces

*Environment:* no specific setting is identified

**Table 2-2**   Major Concepts of Nine Nursing Theorists

| Theorist | Nursing | Client | Health | Environment |
|---|---|---|---|---|
| Johnson's behavioral system model | Regulation of external forces to stabilize client's behavioral system and restore, maintain, or attain balance | A behavioral system (person) threatened or potentially threatened by illness (imbalance) and/or hospitalization | An efficient and effectively functioning behavioral system (person) who maintains balance/stability by adapting/adjusting to outside forces | No specific setting is identified |
| King's theory of goal attainment | An interaction process between client and nurse whereby during perceiving, setting goals, and acting on them, transactions occur and goals are achieved | An individual (personal system) or group (interpersonal system) unable to cope with an event or a health problem while interacting with the environment | An ability to perform the activities of daily living in one's usual social roles; a dynamic life experience of continuous adjustment to environmental stressors through optimum use of resources | Any social system in society; social systems are dynamic forces that influence social behavior integration, perception, and health, such as hospitals, clinics, community agencies, schools, and industry |
| Leininger's transcultural nursing model | A humanistic and scientific mode of helping a client, through specific cultural caring processes (cultural values, beliefs, and practices) to improve or maintain a health condition | An individual, family, group, society, or community with possible physical, psychological, or social needs, within the context of their culture, who is a recipient of nursing care | Defined by specific culture and the local people's viewpoint; technology-dependent cultures view health and health care differently from non-technology–dependent societies | Any culture or society worldwide where ethnocaring is practiced by nurses assisting clients |
| Neuman's health-care systems model | Assisting clients to reduce stress factors and adverse conditions that affect optimum functioning | Individual, family, or group with an identified or suspected stressor that may disrupt harmony and balance | Level of wellness in which all needs are met and more energy is built and stored than is expended | Internal and external forces surrounding the client at the time; nurse-client settings are not described |
| Orem's self-care model | A service of deliberately selected and performed actions to assist individuals or groups to maintain self-care, including structural integrity, functioning, and development | Individual or group unable to continuously maintain self-care in sustaining life and health, in recovering from disease or injury, or in coping with their effects | Individual or group's ability to meet self-care demands that contribute to maintenance and promotion of structural integrity, functioning, and development | Any setting in which a client has unmet self-care needs/requisites and in which a nurse is present is implied but not specified |
| Parse's man-living-health model | Guiding individuals and families to share and uncover the personal meaning of their | Any person or family concerned with their quality of life situation; man is viewed as an open | Process of lived experiences, unfolding, continually changing, including a synthesis of | Undefined setting, but any health-related setting is implied |

**Table 2-2**  Major Concepts of Nine Nursing Theorists—cont'd

| Theorist | Nursing | Client | Health | Environment |
|---|---|---|---|---|
| | living-health situation | whole being, influenced by past and present lived experiences, who interacts with the environment through choices and responsibility for those choices | values and way of living | |
| Peplau's interpersonal model | Goal-directed interpersonal process to promote clients' forward movement of their personality and personal living | Any individual who feels or recognizes unmet needs | Ability to accomplish interpersonal activities and developmental tasks within a productive level of anxiety | Any health-related setting is implied, but not defined |
| Rogers' science of unitary human beings | Science and art to facilitate and promote symphonic interaction between human beings and their environment | Any human being or individual and his or her environment | Expression of the life process characterized by behaviors emerging from mutual, simultaneous interaction between human beings and their environment; a continuum based on value judgments | Four-dimensional negentropic energy field identified by pattern and organization and encompassing all that is outside any given human field; any setting worldwide where nurse and client meet |
| Roy's adaptation model | Promotion of the client's adaptation in the four modes to enhance health using the nursing process | Person, family, group, or community with unusual stresses or ineffective coping mechanisms | State and process of being and becoming an integrated and whole person | All conditions, circumstances, and influences surrounding and affecting the development and behavior of persons or groups; any health-related situation is implied as the setting |

havioral (biopsychosocial) system at an optimum level by imposing external regulations or controls, changing structural elements in desirable directions, or fulfilling functional requirements of the subsystems.

Johnson's model is based on the interaction of the person's behavioral system and subsystems with the environment, as shown in Figs. 2-4 and 2-5.

### Behavioral System

In systems theory, a system is a whole with interdependent parts. The parts have a structure and a process, or pattern of behavior. Systems are characterized by organization, interaction, interdependence, and integration of the parts. Through interaction both within the subsystems and with the external forces acting on it, the system strives to maintain balance and stability by adjusting and adapting.

### Subsystems

There are seven interdependent subsystems. A disturbance in one may affect the others. Each subsystem has a unique function or special task neces-

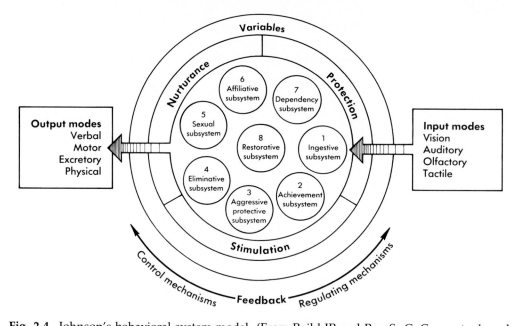

**Fig. 2-4.** Johnson's behavioral system model. (From Reihl JP and Roy Sr C: Conceptual models for nursing, ed 2, New York, 1980, Appleton-Century-Crofts, p 227.)

sary for an integrated performance of all the subsystems, and each has both structure and function. Four structural elements influence each subsystem. First is the *goal* or *drive*, defined as the purpose of the behavior and the consequences achieved. In general, the goal of each subsystem is universal, but individual variations exist. Second, an individual's subsystem *set* reflects the "person's predisposition to act with reference to the goal." Set distinguishes the range of behaviors available to the individual to achieve a particular goal. Preferred behaviors are developed through learning, maturation, and experience. Third, each subsystem has a *choice* of alternative behaviors to achieve specific goals. The goal is achieved by the individual's subsystem *behavior*, which is the only observable aspect of each subsystem. This behavior is examined for its efficiency in achieving the goal.

Each subsystem has an established set of behav-

ioral responses or tendencies toward a common goal or drive. These responses are developed through maturation, experience, and learning. They are influenced by biopsychosocial factors. Over time, responses may be modified, but an observable recurrent pattern of responses continues.

Each of the seven subsystems has a unique goal:
1. Ingestive—to take in from the environment needed resources to maintain integrity, achieve pleasure, and internalize the external environment (Grubbs, 1980)
2. Achievement—to master or control self or environment through seeking some standard of excellence, such as physical, social, or creative skills
3. Aggressive—to protect self and others from potentially threatening objects, persons, or ideas; serves as a self-preservation mechanism

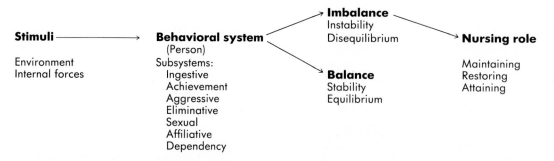

**Fig. 2-5.** Responses of behavioral system to stimuli. (Adapted from Fitzpatrick JJ and Whall AI: Conceptual models in nursing: analysis and application, Bowie, Md, 1983, Robert Brady Co, p 121.)

4. Eliminative—to expel biological waste from the system
5. Sexual—to procreate and gratify feeling attractive to and cared about by others
6. Affiliative or attachment—to relate to or belong to something or someone. Its purpose is to achieve social inclusion, intimacy, and strong social bonds for security and ultimately for survival
7. Dependency—to obtain resources needed for assistance, attention, reassurance, and security; aids in gaining approval, attention, trust, and reliance

### System Requirements

Each subsystem requires that functional needs be met and regulating mechanisms be intact to maintain stability and balance. Functional requirements are met through the individual's own efforts or through assistance from the environment. These requirements include protection, nurturance, and stimulation. *Protection* refers to safeguarding the individual from noxious influences with which the system cannot cope, defending the individual from unnecessary threats and coping with a threat on the individual's behalf (Grubbs, 1980). *Nurturance* means supporting the individual's adequate adaptive behaviors through nourishment, training, and conditions that support appropriate behaviors. *Stimulation* promotes continued growth and development. Different forms of stimulation are used for different purposes to maintain or enhance behavioral stability.

Individuals use a variety of *regulating and controlling mechanisms* to evaluate and choose desirable behavior. These mechanisms are learned through experience in childhood and are usually internalized by adulthood. The three major types of regulating and controlling mechanisms that individuals use are biophysiological, psychological, and sociocultural. These mechanisms provide a monitor and feedback to the system. They guide behavioral alterations and coordination among the subsystems.

### Behavioral Patterns

Each system and subsystem develops patterned, repetitive, and purposeful responses to form an organized and integrated functional unit. These patterned responses determine the interaction of the subsystems, the system, and the environment. The behavioral patterns establish the relationship of the system or person to objects, events, and situations in the environment. These patterns are orderly, purposeful, and predictable. They maintain efficient functioning of the system.

In Johnson's view, the goal of nursing is to maintain, restore, or attain a balance of stability in the client's behavioral system. When the person's system cannot adapt or adjust to external environmental forces, the nurse acts as an external regulatory force to modify or change the structure or guide functional requirements to restore stability.

This model applies only to an individual whose behavioral system is threatened or potentially threatened with instability. The model is useful in the nursing process for ill individuals. It includes biopsychosocial aspects of health; however, a developmental model may also be required for a complete nursing assessment and analysis. Johnson's model does not specify the environmental setting in which nursing occurs, nor does it address a person's health maintenance and promotion requirements.

### King's Theory of Goal Attainment

In 1971, Imogene King introduced a conceptual model consisting of three interacting systems. Over the next 10 years she further refined and developed her model (King, 1981). King's latest model of nursing incorporates three dynamic interaction systems: personal, interpersonal, and social, which lead to development of a theory of goal attainment.

According to this theory, individuals (personal systems) form groups (interpersonal systems) and groups compose a society (social systems). The major characteristics of these three concepts and King's theory are shown in Table 2-3; the subconcepts are described later.

---

## King's Beliefs

*Nursing:* an interaction process between client and nurse whereby during perceiving, setting goals, and acting on them, transactions occur and goals are achieved

*Client:* an individual (personal system) or group (interpersonal system) unable to cope with an event or a health problem while interacting with the environment

*Health:* an ability to perform the activities of daily living in one's usual social roles; a dynamic life experience of continuous adjustment to environmental stressors through optimum use of resources

*Environment:* any social system in society; social systems are dynamic forces that influence social behavior, interaction, perception, and health, such as hospitals, clinics, community agencies, schools, and industry

**Table 2-3**  Characteristics of King's Concepts

**Personal system**

| | |
|---|---|
| Perception | Growth and development |
| Self | Time |
| Body image | Space |

**Interpersonal system**

| | |
|---|---|
| Role | Communication |
| Human interaction | Transactions |
| | Stress |

In King's view, nurses and individuals are personal systems who interact when the individual (or group/interpersonal system) is unable to cope with an event or a health problem. These personal systems enter the health care system (social system) or request services from a health professional and interactions occur, leading to transactions and goal attainment for the individual or group. Interactions between the nurse and the client include assessment, analysis, and interpretation for planning, which may or may not be purposeful and systematic and lead to goal attainment. However, when transactions occur, such as nurse or client goal-directed behaviors, then goals are achieved.

The major concepts in King's model and theory of goal attainment are described here:

*Personal systems* are *individuals/clients* viewed as open, interacting, and exchanging matter, energy, and information with the environment. Individuals are social, sentient, rational, reacting, perceiving, controlling, purposeful, action oriented, and time oriented, with rights and responsibilities. The personal system is understood by examining the interaction of six concepts: perception, self, body image, growth and development, time and space.

*Interpersonal systems* are two or more individuals or groups interacting. These interactions are understood by exploring such concepts as role, interaction, communication, transaction, and stress.

*Social systems* are dynamic forces and compose *society* and the *environment*. They influence social behavior, interaction, perception, and health. Health delivery organizations are a form of social system and can be understood by examining such concepts as: organization; power, authority, and status; and decision-making.

King's theory of goal attainment was primarily derived from the interpersonal system, which interacts with the personal and social systems. In this

theory, King (1981:145-148) defines her subconcepts as:

*Interaction*—process of perception and communication between person and environment and between person and person, represented by verbal and nonverbal behaviors that are goal-directed

*Perception*—each person's representation of reality; it involves (1) taking energy from the environment organized by information, (2) changing energy, (3) processing of information, (4) storing of information, and (5) giving information in overt behaviors

*Communication*—process whereby information is given from one person to another, either directly in face-to-face meetings or indirectly through telephone, television, or the written word

*Transaction*—observable behavior of human beings interacting with their environment

*Role*—set of behaviors expected of persons occupying a position in a social system; rules that define rights and obligations in a position; relationship with one or more individuals interacting in a specific situation for a purpose

*Stress*—dynamic state whereby a human being interacts with the environment to maintain balance for growth, development, and performance

*Growth and development*—continuous changes in individuals at the cellular, molecular, and behavioral levels of activities

*Time*—continuous flow of events in successive order that implies change, a past, and a future

*Self*—personal system that is a complex, unified whole, who perceives, thinks, desires, imagines, decides, identifies goals, and selects means to achieve them

*Space*—physical area called territory, existing in all directions, defined by the behavior of individuals with boundaries that identify personal space

In her theory of goal attainment, King (1981:149) provides the following propositions, which show the relationships between her major concepts:

1. If perceptual accuracy is present in nurse-client interactions, transactions will occur.
2. If nurse and client make transactions, goals will be attained.
3. If goals are attained, satisfactions will occur.
4. If goals are attained, effective nursing care will occur.
5. If transactions are made in nurse-client interactions, growth and development will be enhanced.
6. If role expectations and role performance as

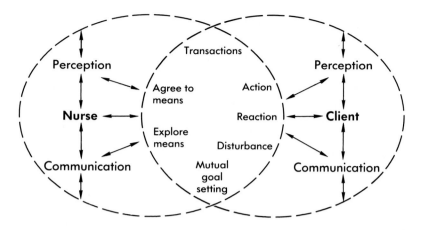

**Fig. 2-6.** Schema of King's theory of goal attainment. (From King IM: A theory for nursing: systems, concepts, process, New York, 1981, John Wiley & Sons, Inc, p 157.)

perceived by nurse and client are congruent, transactions will occur.

7. If role conflict is experienced by nurse or client or both, stress in nurse-client interactions will occur.
8. If nurses with special knowledge and skills communicate appropriate information to clients, mutual goal setting and goal attainment will occur.

King's model views nurses as interacting with clients, who are unable to cope with environmental stressors, through perception and communication to achieve transactions. The nurse and client establish mutual goals and explore and agree on means to achieve the goals. When transactions occur, goals are achieved, as shown in Fig. 2-6.

The focus of King's model is the nurse-client interaction within a systems approach. Strengths of this model include active client participation in mutual goal setting, decision-making, and interactions to achieve the client's goals. Also, the model can be applied in numerous health care settings and includes the importance of collaboration among health professionals. This model can be applied to individuals, families, or groups; major psychological, sociocultural, and interpersonal concepts are addressed. However, an individual's physiological status also needs to be considered for a holistic approach. This model may not be useful for clients who cannot communicate appropriately, such as small children and comatose or psychotic clients, other than for use with their families.

### Leininger's Transcultural Nursing

Madeleine Leininger initially described transcultural nursing in the 1970s, and in 1978 she presented a theory-generating model for the study of transcultural nursing theory and practice. She defines transcultural nursing as

a subfield of nursing which focuses upon a comparative study and analysis of different cultures and subcultures . . . with respect to their caring behavior; nursing care; and health-illness values, beliefs and patterns of behavior with the goal of developing a scientific and humanistic body of knowledge . . . to provide culture-specific and culture-universal nursing care practices (1978:8).

More recently, Leininger (1981) has shifted her emphasis to describing care, transcultural and ethnocaring. The major focus of her work is the "humanistic and scientific study of all people from different cultures . . . [in] ways the nurse can assist people with their daily health and living needs" (1981:8).

In Leininger's view, nursing is synonymous with "caring," which she believes is the central focus. She has classified 28 ethnocaring and nursing care constructs, as shown in Fig. 2-7, which are re-

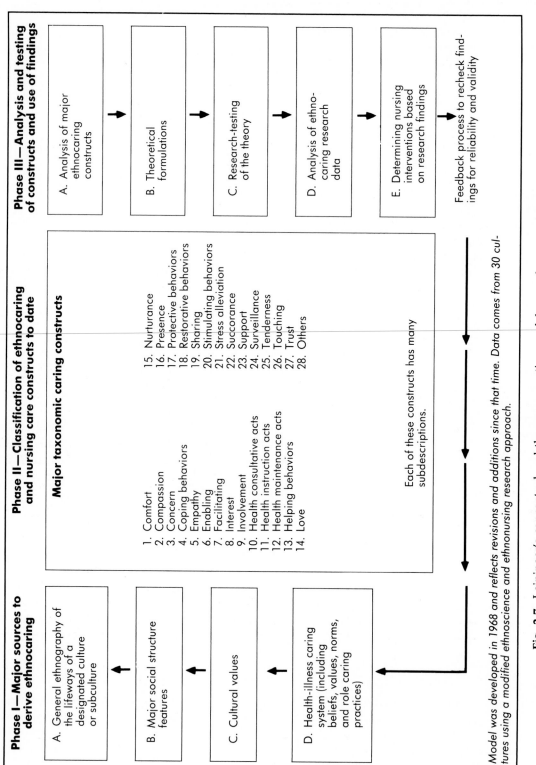

**Fig. 2-7.** Leininger's conceptual and theory-generating model to study transcultural and ethnocaring constructs. (From Leininger M: Caring: an essential human need, Thorofare, NJ, 1981, Charles B Slack, Inc.)

**Phase I—Major sources to derive ethnocaring**

A. General ethnography of the lifeways of a designated culture or subculture

B. Major social structure features

C. Cultural values

D. Health-illness caring system (including beliefs, values, norms, and role caring practices)

**Phase II—Classification of ethnocaring and nursing care constructs to date**

**Major taxonomic caring constructs**

1. Comfort
2. Compassion
3. Concern
4. Coping behaviors
5. Empathy
6. Enabling
7. Facilitating
8. Interest
9. Involvement
10. Health consultative acts
11. Health instruction acts
12. Health maintenance acts
13. Helping behaviors
14. Love

15. Nurturance
16. Presence
17. Protective behaviors
18. Restorative behaviors
19. Sharing
20. Stimulating behaviors
21. Stress alleviation
22. Succorance
23. Support
24. Surveillance
25. Tenderness
26. Touching
27. Trust
28. Others

Each of these constructs has many subdescriptions.

**Phase III—Analysis and testing of constructs and use of findings**

A. Analysis of major ethnocaring constructs

B. Theoretical formulations

C. Research-testing of the theory

D. Analysis of ethnocaring research data

E. Determining nursing interventions based on research findings

Feedback process to recheck findings for reliability and validity

*Model was developed in 1968 and reflects revisions and additions since that time. Data comes from 30 cultures using a modified ethnoscience and ethnonursing research approach.*

lated to caring behaviors, processes, needs, consequences, conflicts, and gaps.

*Ethnocaring* is defined as "the systematic study and classification of nursing care beliefs, values, and practices as cognitively perceived by a designated culture through their local language, experiences, beliefs, and value system" (Leininger, 1978:15). *Ethnonursing* is the use of knowledge about the local cultural or subcultural group's values, beliefs, and practices related to health and nursing.

*Nursing* is the humanistic and scientific application of knowledge in "caring" for individuals, families, and communities, with emphasis on their unique cultural values, beliefs, and health practices. Leininger (1981:13) lists 28 caring constructs, which are applicable to all health professionals, including comfort, compassion, coping behaviors, empathy, involvement, love, protective and restorative behaviors, support, and trust. Nurses assist individuals and groups to improve or maintain human conditions by applying knowledge of culturally sanctioned caring modes of intervention. *Transcultural nursing* involves integrating cultural views, knowledge, and experiences in planning and implementing care specific for individuals of a culture.

Leininger's work is unique for nursing because it is considered a theory-generating model, rather than a model to guide nursing practice. The 28 care constructs are applicable in nursing, but also can be used by any health professional. The model emphasizes a world view, with consideration for cultural differences. It is useful for nurses working with individuals, groups, families, or communities with unique cultural beliefs, values, and practices. Transcultural nursing involves integrating cultural views, knowledge, and experiences in all areas of the nursing process; however, this model does not provide a specific guide to assess clients—individuals, groups, or communities—nor does it guide nursing diagnoses, planning, or intervention. The model provides a guide to generate theories for nursing practice in specific cultures.

### Neuman's Health-Care Systems Model

Betty Neuman first described her model in 1974 and refined it in later publications and in her 1982 book. This is a complex systems model, with a focus on stress reactions and stress reduction. The model was developed for use by any health profession, not just nursing.

This comprehensive model, as shown in Fig. 2-8, depicts the client as a core circle with several protective layers. The client is continuously ex-

---

## Neuman's Beliefs

*Nursing:* assisting clients to reduce stress factors and adverse conditions that affect optimum functioning

*Client:* individual, family, or group with an identified or suspected stressor that may disrupt harmony and balance

*Health:* level of wellness in which all needs are met and more energy is built and stored than is expended

*Environment:* internal and external forces surrounding the client at the time; nurse-client settings are not described.

---

posed to internal and external *stressors,* which require *lines of defense* and *reactions.* Nursing *interventions* can occur before or after stressors and at three levels of *prevention.*

The *person* is viewed as an open system interacting with the environment through interpersonal and extrapersonal factors. Each individual is a dynamic composite of physiological, psychological, sociocultural, and developmental variables that influence the state of wellness or illness. Individuals are continuously exposed to various stressors in the environment, both beneficial and noxious, and respond by adjusting to the environment or adjusting the environment. Through interactions and adjustments, the individual maintains system harmony and balance, internally and externally.

The individual is composed of a central core or basic structure with three protective layers. The central core consists of normal temperature range, organ strength, weakness, ego structure, and knowns or commonalities. The three surrounding layers protect the individual from stressors. First, a "flexible line of defense," the outer layer, acts as a dynamic, rapidly changing buffer of stressors, but is highly vulnerable to internal factors such as loss of sleep or hunger. The second layer, or "normal line of defense," evolves over time to maintain a steady state. It consists of coping patterns, lifestyle, and the individual's usual ways of handling stress. The innermost layer, "lines of resistance," consists of internal factors that attempt to stabilize the individual and restore the normal line of defense when a stressor breaks through.

*Wellness-illness* is viewed as a continuum of health, and is reflected in the harmony or balance of the individual's interaction and adjustment to the environment. Health is a level of wellness in

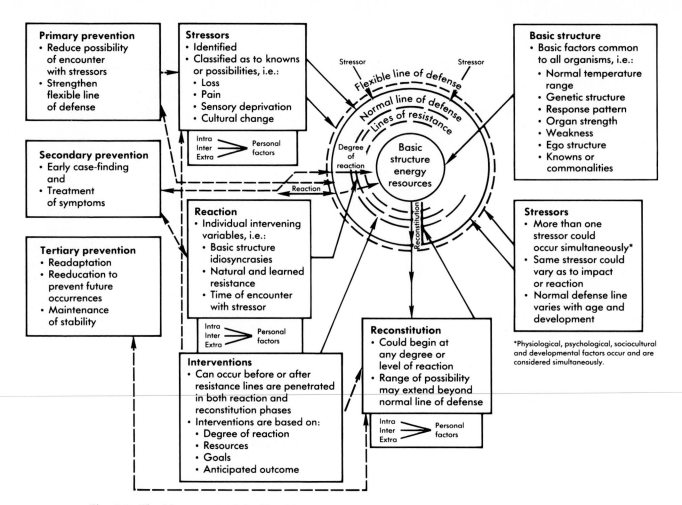

**Fig. 2-8.** The Neuman model of health care systems. (From Neuman B, editor: The Neuman systems model: application to nursing education and practice, Norwalk, Conn, 1982, Appleton-Century-Crofts.)

which all needs are met and more energy is built and stored than is expended. Wellness is shown by an individual's homeostasis, and is defined as

a state of balance requiring energy exchanges whereby man is able to adequately cope with his stressors and/or regain his optimal state of health following a reaction to a stressor and thus preserve his system integrity (1982:9).

Illness occurs in varying degrees when needs are not sufficiently satisfied and more energy is needed and expended than is available.

*Stressors* are noxious or beneficial stimuli that produce tension and have the potential to disrupt system stability and harmony. Stressors are categorized as intrapersonal—forces operating within the individual; interpersonal—forces operating between the individual and others; and extrapersonal—forces outside the individual. Stressors vary in nature, timing, degree, and potential for change, and require energy to cope and to return to stability. They are considered to be any situa-

tion, condition, force, or potential source that is capable of creating instability within the individual or reducing the individual's lines of defense or resistance.

*Nursing* is concerned with the client's reactions or possible reactions to stressors. The goals of nursing actions are to attain or maintain the client's system balance and conserve energy by vigorously controlling variables affecting the client. Nursing intervention is initiated when a stressor is suspected or identified. Interventions are based on four factors: the client's degree of reaction, resources, goals, and anticipated outcomes. Neuman describes nursing interventions as three levels of prevention: primary, secondary, and tertiary. *Primary prevention* consists of interventions initiated before or after an encounter with a stressor; it includes decreasing the possibility of encounter with stressors and strengthening the flexible lines of defense in the presence of stressors. *Secondary prevention* consists of interventions initiated after encounter with a stressor: it includes early case finding and treatment of symptoms following a reaction to a stressor. *Tertiary prevention* consists of interventions generally initiated after treatment; it focuses on readaptation, reeducation to prevent future occurrences, and maintenance of stability.

Neuman's model is applicable in all components of the nursing process. It is especially useful for individuals and families because it views the client as a composite of physiological, psychological, sociocultural, and developmental variables. It is a holistic approach because each system or subsystem cannot be isolated; rather the influence of each system on the whole must be considered. The three levels of prevention are useful guides for planning nursing interventions. The model can also be applied across all clinical areas.

### Orem's Self-Care Nursing Model

Dorothea Orem first published her concepts of nursing in 1959, then further developed and refined the model in 1980 and 1985. Originally, she designed her model for nursing curricula to differentiate nursing actions. This model focuses on identifying client's self-care requisites or needs and nursing actions to meet the client's requisites.

Orem's model is based on three major constructs: self-care requisites, self-care and nursing systems (see Table 2-4). Central to Orem's model is the belief that individuals function and maintain life, health, and well-being by caring for themselves. When an individual or group is unable to meet their needs (self-care requisites), self-care deficits occur, and therapeutic self-care demands arise, which lead to nursing assistance. The three *self-care*

**Table 2-4**  Orem's Major Concepts

| Self-care requisites | Self-care | Nursing systems |
|---|---|---|
| Universal self-care | Demands | Wholly compensatory |
| Developmental self-care | Capabilities | Partly compensatory |
| Health deviation self-care | Deficits | Supportive-educative |

*requisites* are universal, developmental, and health-deviation. Orem defined three *nursing systems* according to the degree of nursing assistance required by the client: wholly compensatory, partly compensatory, and supportive-educative.

#### Self-Care Requisites

Self-care activities are behaviors that the individual or guardian personally initiates and performs to maintain life, health, and well-being. These requisites describe the individual's purpose for self-care.

*Universal self-care requisites* are those activities necessary to meet the basic needs of daily living. They are common to everyone throughout life and are adjusted for age, developmental stage, environment, and other factors. They are associated with maintaining life processes, structural integrity, and functioning. Individuals who are able to meet their universal self-care needs are at one end of the continuum, and those who require total assistance are at the other end. Orem's universal self-care requisites are

1. Maintenance of sufficient air, water, and food
2. Balance between activity and rest
3. Balance between solitude and social interaction
4. Provision of care associated with elimination processes and excrements
5. Prevention of hazards to human life, functioning, and well-being
6. Promotion of human functioning and development within social groups

*Developmental self-care requisites* are associated with developmental processes and conditions occurring during the life cycle. There are two categories of developmental self-care. The first is maintaining conditions that support life processes and promote development; the second is the prevention of harmful effects on human development and the provision of care to overcome these effects.

*Health-deviation self-care requisites* are associated with individuals who are ill or injured or have a pathological condition and are receiving medical

### Orem's Beliefs

*Nursing:* a service of deliberately selected and performed actions to assist individuals or groups to maintain self-care, including structural integrity, functioning, and development

*Client:* individual or group unable to continuously maintain self-care in sustaining life and health, in recovering from disease or injury, or in coping with their effects

*Health:* individual or group's ability to meet self-care demands that contribute to the maintenance and promotion of structural integrity, functioning, and development

*Environment:* any setting in which a client has unmet self-care needs/requisites and in which a nurse is present is implied but not specified care. Orem identified six requisites for individuals with health deviations:

1. Seeking and securing appropriate medical assistance
2. Recognizing and taking care of these conditions
3. Implementing prescribed diagnostic, therapeutic, and rehabilitative measures
4. Recognizing and regulating the effects of treatment
5. Modifying the self-concept and acceptance of the condition
6. Learning to live with the condition in a lifestyle that promotes continued development

### Self-Care

When the self-care *demands* exceed an individual's self-care *capabilities*, then self-care *deficits* occur, which may require nursing intervention. Therapeutic self-care demands are those universal and developmental requisites, and possibly health-deviation self-care requisites necessary for life, health, and well-being. Capabilities refers to the individual's ability to acquire knowledge for action, and to act on that knowledge to meet one's self-care requisites. Self-care deficits occur when an individual is unable to perform the necessary actions to meet one's self-care requisites.

### Nursing Systems

Nursing is a human service consisting of "actions deliberately selected and performed . . . to help individuals or groups under their care to maintain or change conditions in themselves or their environments" (Orem, 1980:5). Nurses assist individuals with self-care activities that they are unable to perform for themselves; the goal is guiding patients to perform their own self-care.

To determine which nursing system would be appropriate, the nurse first calculates the therapeutic self-care demands of the individual or group by examining each universal, developmental, and health-deviation self-care requisite. The nurse also considers factors affecting these requisites and the interrelationships among the requisites. Based on the type of self-care deficits the patient cannot meet, the nurse determines which nursing system would be most effective. Orem described three nursing systems.

The *wholly compensatory nursing system* is used with patients who are unable to engage in any form of deliberate action, who cannot or should not perform actions, or who are unable to attend to themselves and make rational decisions about self-care. The nursing actions consist of performing the patients' therapeutic self-care, compensating for

their inability, and supporting and protecting the patients.

The *partly compensatory nursing system* is for patients who are unable to perform some self-care activities, such as those with actual or medically prescribed limitations, inadequate scientific or technical knowledge or skills, or impaired readiness to learn or perform special activities. The nurse may perform some self-care activities to compensate for patient limitations or may assist the patient as required.

The *supportive-educative nursing system* assists patients who are able or can learn to perform therapeutic self-care, yet require assistance in decision-making, behavior control, or acquiring knowledge or skills. The nurse may assist the patient through guidance, support, teaching, or environmental change.

Orem's model is widely used in nursing education and practice. It is a comprehensive model for assessment and analysis of an individual, especially in the physiological, social, and developmental areas. Also, the nursing systems are excellent guides to plan and implement nursing care. The model is very useful for chronically ill clients in the hospital or in other settings. It can easily be adapted to groups with similar self-care deficits, but the model is not appropriate for families. Also, this model limits the nurse's role to working only with clients who are unable to provide their own self-care requisites, which does not include health maintenance and prevention of illness.

## Parse's Man-Living-Health Model

Rosemary Parse first described her existential-phenomenological view of man and health in 1981. Her work is based on Martha Rogers' (1970) view of unitary man as more than the sum of parts, and on Rogers' principles of nursing science: helicy, complementarity, and resonancy. Parse also incorporates Rogers' concepts of energy field, openness, pattern and organization, and four-dimensionality in her work. These principles and concepts are synthesized with the existential and phenomenological views of Kierkegaard, Sartre, Dubos, and others in Parse's concepts, principles, and theoretical structures (Figs. 2-9 and 2-10).

*Man* is viewed as an open, whole being, coexisting and participating with the environment while continuously coconstituting patterns of relating. As an open being, man freely chooses situations, attaches meaning to those situations, and bears the responsibility for decisions. Man is involved in becoming and reaching beyond self to achieve potentials and possibilities. Through coparticipating with the environment and freely choosing to live certain

**Principle 1:** Structuring meaning multidimensionally is cocreating reality through the languaging of valuing and imaging.

**Principle 2:** Cocreating rhythmical patterns of relating is living the paradoxical unity of revealing-concealing and enabling-limiting while connecting-separating.

**Principle 3:** Cotranscending with the possibles is powering unique ways of originating in the process of transforming.

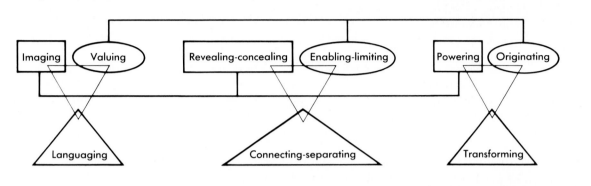

Relationship of the concepts in the **squares:**
Relationship of the concepts in the **ovals:**
Relationship of the concepts in the **triangles:**

**Powering** is a way of **revealing and concealing imaging.**
**Originating** is a manifestation of **enabling and limiting valuing.**
**Transforming** unfolds in the **languaging of connecting and separating.**

**Fig. 2-9.** Relationship of principles, concepts, and theoretical structures of man-living-health. (From Parse RR: Man-living-health: a theory of nursing, New York, 1981, John Wiley & Sons, Inc, p 69.)

## Parse's Beliefs

*Nursing:* guiding individuals and families to share and uncover the personal meaning of their living-health situation

*Client:* any person or family concerned with their quality of life situation; man is viewed as an open whole being, influenced by past and present lived experiences, who interacts with the environment through choices and responsibility for those choices

*Health:* process of lived experiences, unfolding, continually changing, including a synthesis of values and way of living

*Environment:* undefined setting, but any health-related setting is implied

values, man coconstitutes by creating meaning with others and the world and cocreates self in becoming. Man lives with predecessors, contemporaries, and successors all at once in coexistence, which gives meaning to becoming.

*Health* is viewed as an open process of becoming through rhythmically unfolding in the man-environment relationship. It is an incarnation of man's choosing and man's patterns of relating value priorities. Health is a continuously changing process of interacting with the environment, transcending with the possibilities, and reaching beyond in a negentropic unfolding. Man is viewed as a composite of more than the sum of parts, a wholeness of biological, social, psychological and spiritual aspects within the context of the environment and lived experiences. Health is *not* good, bad, more or less, nor is health adapting, coping, or a steady state.

The theory of man-living-health is derived from these views and is reflected in three principles:

*Principle 1:* Structuring meaning multidimensionally is cocreating reality through the language of valuing and imaging. This principle asserts that reality is continuously cocreated by assigning meaning based on past, present, and future and is expressed through language by means of values and images or symbols.

*Principle 2:* Cocreating rhythmic patterns of relating is living the paradoxical unity of revealing-concealing and enabling-limiting while connecting-separating. This principle means that man continually has an unfolding cadence of coconstituting patterns of interacting with the

---

**Assumptions**

1. Man is coexisting while coconstituting rhythmical patterns with the environment.
2. Man is an open being, freely choosing meaning in situation, bearing responsibility for decisions.
3. Man is a living unity continuously coconstituting patterns of relating.
4. Man is transcending multidimensionally with the possibles.

5. Health is an open process of becoming, experienced by man.
6. Health is a rhythmically coconstituting process of the man-environment interrelationship.
7. Health is man's patterns of relating value priorities.
8. Health is an intersubjective process of transcending with the possibles.
9. Health is unitary man's negentropic unfolding.

**Man-Living-Health**

| **Principles** | Structuring meaning multidimensionally | Cocreating rhythmical patterns of relating | Cotranscending with the possibles |
|---|---|---|---|
| **Concepts** | Imaging Valuing Languaging | Revealing-concealing Enabling-limiting Connecting-separating | Powering Originating Transforming |

**Theoretical structures**
**Powering** is a way of **revealing and concealing imaging.**
**Originating** is a manifestation of **enabling and limiting valuing.**
**Transforming** unfolds in the **languaging of connecting and separating.**

**Fig. 2-10.** Parse's theory of man-living-health. (From Parse RR: Man-living-health: a theory of nursing, New York, 1981, John Wiley & Sons, Inc, p 73.)

world, including revealing-concealing (simultaneously disclosing some aspects of self while hiding others), enabling-limiting (as man moves in one direction, man is limited in movement in another), and connecting-separating (as man links with one phenomenon, man unlinks with another, leading to greater complexity).

*Principle 3:* Cotranscending with the possibles is powering unique ways of originating in the process of transforming. This principle asserts that man goes beyond the actual in interrelationships with others and propels into the future by incarnating intentions and actions in moving toward possibilities. Transforming occurs through originating and powering, a process of man-environment-energy interchange with recognition of continuous affirmation of self.

Nursing focuses on guiding individuals and families in sharing the meaning of the changing health process and in making choices. The goal of nursing is to enhance the quality of life as perceived by the individual and the family. Parse describes three dimensions of health: illuminating

meaning, synchronizing rhythms, and mobilizing transcendence.

*Illuminating meaning* occurs as the nurse guides the client and the family to relate the personal meaning of the health situation from their viewpoint through explicating. *Synchronizing rhythms* of the client and the family occurs as the nurse "dwells with" them, moves with their rhythm, and leads them to recognize the harmony of the lived experience in context. *Mobilizing transcendence* occurs as the nurse guides the client to visualize the future possibilities and to move beyond and plan for changing the lived health patterns.

In Parse's view, nursing is not offering professional advice, nor assisting the client to adapt to or change the health situation. It is the interpersonal interrelationship of the client and nurse to promote health and quality of life by moving beyond present health patterns.

Parse's model is complex and existential, which may make it difficult for a novice to understand and apply. Parse states that her model is not congruent with the commonly accepted form of the nursing process, which assumes that the nurse is an authority on health (Parse, 1987). Although the model is difficult to apply in the nursing process and probably more appropriate for the "expert" clinician, because it does not provide specific guidelines or rules, it is a model that can guide the nurse. The model emphasizes understanding the client and family's perception of the personal meaning of their health situation and guiding them to recognize and act on future possibilities for changing their lived health situation. The model could be applied to any family and to any individual who is coherent and able to communicate.

## Peplau's Interpersonal Model

In 1952, Dr. Hildegard Peplau described her major concepts of nursing. In later publications, she modified some of these concepts. Peplau views the *individual* as a developing self-system with unique biochemical, physiological, and socio-psychological characteristics and needs. Throughout life, individuals encounter anxiety-producing experiences, which create tension and can be transformed into either health-promoting or health-debilitating behaviors. Peplau believes that an individual's behaviors are purposeful and directed toward self-maintenance, reduction of anxiety arising from unmet needs, and achievement of higher needs. When unmet needs are felt or recognized, individuals may seek professional assistance.

*Health* is viewed as a continuum with varying degrees of anxiety. Peplau defines health as "forward movement of personality and other ongoing human processes in the direction of creative, constructive, productive, personal, and community living" (1952:12). Health is the relief of anxiety and tension, and the redirecting of energy to facilitate need satisfaction, self-awareness, and the integration of meaningful life experiences.

*Nursing* is "a significant, therapeutic, interpersonal process; . . . an educative instrument, a maturing force, that aims to promote forward movement of [the] personality" (1952:16). This process is initiated when a person expresses a felt need. The nurse-patient relationship facilitates the patient's identification and resolution of unmet needs, while simultaneously promoting growth and development of both, within the therapeutic relationship. Peplau identifies six roles that nurses may assume while working with patients: teacher, resource, counselor, leader, technical expert, and surrogate. These roles are used in the four phases of the goal-directed interpersonal relationship to assist patients to (1) examine their interpersonal relationships, felt needs, and problems and (2) define, understand, and productively resolve those problems. During the relationship, the attitudes toward the patient

---

### Peplau's Beliefs

*Nursing:* goal-directed interpersonal process to promote clients' forward movement of their personality and personal living

*Client:* any individual who feels or recognizes unmet needs

*Health:* ability to accomplish interpersonal activities and developmental tasks within a productive level of anxiety

*Environment:* any health-related setting is implied, but not defined.

---

and the relationship are also examined by the nurse to understand their interpersonal dynamics and develop therapeutic use of self. Nurses use communication techniques, unconditional acceptance, and empathy. These skills promote a trusting relationship, the patient's self-reliance, and independent decision-making. The four phases in the nurse-patient relationship are described below.

*Orientation* refers to the initiation of the relationship when the patient recognizes a felt need or difficulty and seeks professional assistance. Upon mutual agreement, the nurse defines the nature of the reciprocal relationship and its purposes. The nurse explains that the collaborative role is to identify, examine, and find ways to resolve the patient's problem.

*Identification* begins the working phase. The nurse-patient relationship develops and strengthens as initial attitudes of the patient and nurse are explored. Their perceptions and expectations of each other are clarified. A trusting relationship may develop if they openly share their thoughts and feelings. During this phase, they work to identify the patient's problems or difficulties.

*Exploitation* refers to the discussion of solutions after mutual identification and understanding of the patient's problems. The patient's and nurse's roles and responsibilities in resolving the problem are clarified. The patient gradually assumes responsibility for control of the problem and decision-making. There is progressive independence and self-reliance. During this phase the patient may test the relationship and experience dependent and independent feelings, which need to be discussed.

*Resolution* refers to the final phase, when the patient and nurse collaborate to resolve the problem; they also must work through their psychological dependency needs. They should discuss termination before the last meeting, because this prepares them for the final separation. Successful resolution occurs when both summarize the relationship, its meaning, and accomplishments. This promotes the growth and maturity of both individuals.

Peplau's model describes nursing as a therapeutic, growth-producing relationship. It proceeds through the four phases just mentioned. The nurse and patient explore their relationship, the patient's problems, and potential solutions. This model is a useful guide to plan implementation strategies or to cite as scientific rationale. It also may serve as a supporting approach to assess and analyze the nurse-client relationships and can be applied to both individual and family clients.

### Rogers' Science of Unitary Human Beings

Martha Rogers first described her science of unitary man in 1970. This model was designed to stimulate development of nursing theories, rather than to be used for direct application in practice. Rogers' conceptual system focuses on understanding the interaction between human beings and their environment. She views this interaction as the central focus of nursing, as shown in Fig. 2-11. Since 1970, Rogers has further refined her model and pre-

sented it at numerous conferences and in various journals.

In Rogers' model, unitary human beings and environment are interrelated and continually and simultaneously evolving. Both human beings and

---

## Rogers' Beliefs

*Nursing:* science and art to facilitate and promote symphonic interaction between human beings and their environment

*Client:* human being or individual and his or her environment

*Health:* expression of the life process characterized by behaviors emerging from mutual, simultaneous interaction between human beings and their environment; a continuum based on value judgments

*Environment:* four-dimensional negentropic energy field identified by pattern and organization and encompassing all that is outside any given human field; any setting worldwide where nurse and client meet

---

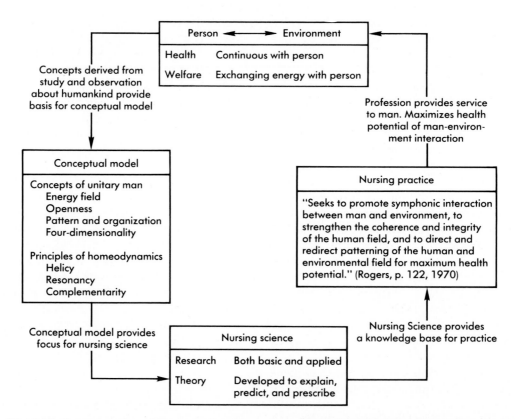

**Fig. 2-11.** Interpretation of Rogers' view of nursing, showing interrelationship among man, environment, health, and nursing. (From Fitzpatrick JJ and Whall AL: Conceptual models in nursing: analysis and application, Bowie, Md, 1983, Robert J Brady Co, p 250.)

environment have four major concepts: energy fields, open system, pattern, and four-dimensionality. The nature and direction of the relationship between human beings and their environment are shown through three principles: resonancy, helicy, and integrality.

*Unitary human beings* are irreducible wholes, different from the sum of their parts, and cannot be understood by reducing them to their parts. Human beings are four-dimensional energy fields characterized by pattern, integral with their own unique environmental fields, and they continuously evolve creatively.

*Environment* is an irreducible, four-dimensional energy field with pattern and characteristics different from those of its parts. An environmental field is unique to its specific human field; yet both fields continuously change and creatively evolve together.

*Energy fields* are the fundamental units of humans and the environment. Both humans and the environment are infinite, irreducible fields that evolve together. Energy refers to the dynamic nature, and field is the unifying concept. Human beings and environment *are* energy fields that cannot be examined separately; they are irreducible, continuously open, and integral to each other.

*Open system* refers to the continuous, infinite, unbounded exchange between human beings and environmental energy fields. The closed system model of equilibrium, adaptation, and homeostasis is no longer acceptable; causality is invalid in a theory of accelerating evolution.

*Pattern* is the distinguishing characteristic of the energy fields. Human and environmental energy fields are single wave patterns, with changing rhythms and intensity. Each human energy field pattern is unique yet integral with its own unique environmental energy field, with evolving diversity and complexity.

*Four-dimensionality* refers to "a non-linear domain without spatial or temporal attributes" (1984). The "relative present" or the "infinite now" for an individual represents the four-dimensional human field.

*Nursing* is a learned profession based on application of a science ("an organized body of abstract knowledge derived from scientific research and logical analysis") and an art ("the imaginative and creative use of this knowledge in human service") (1984). The focus of nursing's concern is unitary human beings as a synergistic phenomenon interacting with their environment. Rogers views nursing as concerned with "the nature and direction of unitary human development integral with the environment" (1980:330), to promote symphonic inter-

action and integrity of the human energy field. Nurses recognize and assist human beings to establish patterns associated with their maximum health potential. *Health* is viewed as a continuous interchange and repatterning toward maximum health potential, with the emphasis on promotion.

Three principles of homeodynamics were postulated by Rogers to describe the nature and direction of change, as derived from the conceptual system just described:

*Principle of resonancy:* continuous change from lower to higher frequency wave patterns in human and environmental fields

*Principle of helicy:* continuous, innovative, probabilistic increasing diversity of human and environmental field patterns characterized by nonrepeating rhythmicities

*Principle of integrality:* continuous mutual human field and environmental field process (formerly titled complementarity)

Rogers' concepts and principles are unique to her conceptual system of unitary human beings, although other nurse theorists have adopted some of them. This conceptual system is brought together in Rogers' statement that, "Unitary man (human being) and . . . environment are in continuous, mutual, and simultaneous interaction, evolving toward increased differentiation and diversity of field pattern. . . . Change is always innovative. There is no going back, no repetition. Causality is contraindicated" (1980:333). Application of Rogers' conceptual system in the nursing process requires advanced knowledge and study of the meaning and interrelationship of her concepts and principles.

### Roy's Adaptation Model

Sister Callista Roy first published her conceptual model of adaptation in the 1970s and has continued to refine and further develop her model in subsequent publications. Roy's model is based on general systems theory as applied to the individual and Helson's view of adaptation as related to focal, contextual, and residual stimuli.

The focus of Roy's model is the set of processes by which a person adapts to environmental stressors. Each person is a unified biopsychosocial system in constant interaction with a changing environment. When the demands of environmental stimuli are too great or the person's adaptive mechanisms are too low, the person's behavioral responses are ineffective for coping.

Roy (1984) views the *person* as an adaptive system that functions as a whole through interdependence of its parts. The system consists of input, control processes, output, and feedback. Input are

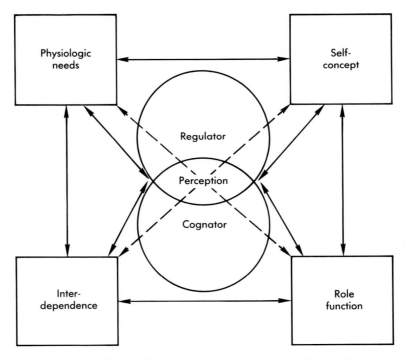

**Fig. 2-12.** Interpretation of Roy's adaptation model, showing relationships among the subsystems of the person. There is direct interaction between all of the adaptive modes and between each adaptive mode and the regulator and the cognator. (From Fitzpatrick JJ and Whall AL: Conceptual models in nursing: analysis and application, Bowie, Md, 1983, Robert J Brady Co, p 166.)

---

### Roy's Beliefs

*Nursing:* promotion of the client's adaptation in the four modes to enhance health using the nursing process

*Client:* person, family, group, or community with unusual stresses or ineffective coping mechanisms

*Health:* state and process of being and becoming an integrated and whole person

*Environment:* all conditions, circumstances, and influences surrounding and affecting the development and behavior of persons or groups; any health-related situation is implied as the setting

---

stimuli from the external environment and the internal self, including information (stimuli) from the cognator and regulator mechanisms. The control processes include both biological and psychological coping mechanisms of the person, as well as cognator and regulator responses. Output is the adaptive and ineffective behavioral responses of the person. Feedback is information regarding the behavioral responses that is conveyed as input in the system (Figs. 2-12 and 2-13).

Each person is affected by stressors, called stimuli. The *focal stimuli* are a change immediately confronting the person; these require an adaptive response. *Contextual stimuli* (all other stimuli present in the person or environment) and *residual stimuli* (those beliefs, attitudes, or traits that affect the person's present situation) mediate and contribute to the effect of the focal stimuli/stressor and determine the level of stress or adaptation.

Each person's ability to adapt to changing stimuli is determined by the person's *adaptation level,* which is a constantly changing point determined by the collective effect of the focal, contextual, and residual range of stimuli that can be tolerated at a given point in time. Roy describes two basic internal processes used in adapting, the *regulator subsystem* and the *cognator subsystem.* The regulator subsystem receives and processes changing stimuli from the external environment and the internal self through neural-chemical-endocrine channels. It produces automatic, unconscious reactions on target organs or tissues, which then effect body responses that serve as feedback (additional stimuli) for input. The cognator subsystem receives varying internal and external stimuli involving psychological and social factors. Physical and physiological factors, including bodily responses from the system are also included. These changing stimuli are pro-

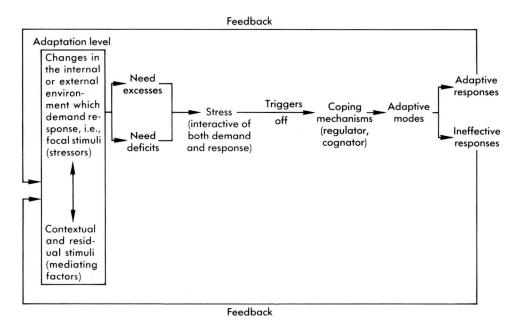

**Fig. 2-13.** Interpretation of Roy's process of stress adaptation. (From Fitzpatrick JJ and Whall AL: Conceptual models in nursing: analysis and application, Bowie, Md, 1983, Robert J Brady Co, p 167.)

cessed/controlled through various cognitive/emotive pathways, which include perception/information processing, learning, judgment, and emotion. The regulator and cognator subsystems produce behavioral responses in four effector modes: physiological, self-concept, role function, and interdependence. The person's behavioral responses in these four modes determine whether the adaptation is an effective or ineffective response to stimuli. Adaptive responses promote the integrity of the individual by conserving energy and promoting the survival, growth, reproduction, and mastery of the human system.

*Health* is defined as "a state or a process of being and becoming an integrated and whole person" (1984:39). Through adaptation, the person's energy is freed from ineffective coping attempts and can be used to promote integrity, healing, and enhance health. Integrity implies soundness leading to completeness or unity.

*Nursing* is considered the science and practice of promoting adaptation for holistic functioning of persons through application of the nursing process to affect health positively. Nursing aims to increase the person's adaptive responses by decreasing the energy needed to cope in a given situation so there is more energy for other human processes. Nursing promotes adaptation in the four modes, which contribute to health, quality of life, and dying with dignity.

Using the nursing process with Roy's model, there are two levels of assessment. In *first-level as-*

*sessment* the nurse assesses the person's adaptive and ineffective behaviors in each of the four modes. The *physiological* mode includes oxygenation, nutrition, elimination, activity and rest, skin integrity, the senses, fluids and electrolyes, and neurological and endocrine function. There are three psychosocial adaptive modes: self-concept, role function, and interdependence. The *self-concept* mode consists of the individual's feelings and beliefs at a given point in time that influence behavior. This mode includes psychic integrity, physical self, personal self, self-consistency, self-ideal/self expectancy, moral-ethical-spiritual self, learning, inner self-concept, and self-esteem. The third mode, *role function,* includes role, position, role performance, role mastery, social integrity, primary role, secondary role, tertiary role, and instrumental and expressive behaviors. *Interdependence,* the fourth mode, addresses the ability to love, respect, and value others and to respond to others in a similar manner. This mode includes affectional adequacy, nurturing, significant others, support systems, receptive behaviors, and contributing behaviors.

Each of these four modes has specific problems that may be identified. After assessing the adaptive and ineffective behaviors in each mode, the nurse proceeds to the *second-level of assessment* by determining the focal, contextual, and residual stimuli that contribute to each ineffective behavior or adaptive behavior needing reinforcement. The *focal stimuli* are those immediately confronting the person.

*Contextual stimuli* are all other stimuli present within the person or from the environment. *Residual stimuli* are beliefs, attitudes, or traits that have an effect on the person's present situation.

The nursing diagnosis, derived from the two assessment levels, is a statement of the behaviors and stimuli that are ineffective or require reinforcement. Nursing goals are identification of those adaptive behavioral outcomes that are mutually agreed on by the person and the nurse. Nursing interventions to accomplish the goals aim to manage the focal, contextual, or residual stimuli by removing, increasing, decreasing, or altering these stimuli so that they fall within the person's "adaptation level." Evaluation is a reassessment of attainment of the goal of adaptive behavior.

*Environment* is defined as internal and external stimuli, including focal, contextual, and residual, which collectively constitute the person's "adaptation level" or zone of coping ability. Environmental stimuli include all the conditions, circumstances, and influences surrounding and affecting the development and behavior of the person or group. The person's stage of development, family, and culture are significant stimuli affecting all human adaptation.

Roy's model views the person as an adaptive system that responds to internal and external environmental stimuli in four adaptive modes, namely physiological, self-concept, role function, and interdependence. The person's adaptation level is determined by the intensity and variety of focal, contextual, and residual stimuli. Nursing promotes the person's adaptation level by manipulating the environmental stimuli to reduce ineffective responses or to reinforce adaptive behaviors. Roy's model includes biopsychosocial factors and is broad enough to use with individuals in all components of the nursing process. It is an excellent tool for assessing and analyzing the client's health patterns and for identifying nursing diagnoses. When nursing implementation strategies are directed at changing focal, contextual, or residual stimuli, Roy's model can serve as a useful theoretical approach.

## FAMILY MODELS

The use of a specific family model provides a perspective or focus for understanding the family. Family models have been categorized according to their basic focus as developmental, interactional, structural-functional, and systems models. First, two family developmental models, Duvall's and Stevenson's, are presented. Next, Satir's Family Interactional Model is described. Friedman's Structural-Functional Family Model illustrates the structural-functional focus, as does Calgary's Family Model, which also includes the systems approach. There are many other family models available and relevant in nursing; however, these models serve as a reference and guide for application in the nursing process as described in this book. Application of these models in the nursing process is shown in Sections II and III.

### Duvall's Family Developmental Model

Evelyn Duvall's (1977) family developmental framework provides a guide to examine and analyze the basic changes and developmental tasks common to most families during their life cycle. Although each family has unique characteristics, normative patterns of sequential development have been described by Duvall. These stages and developmental tasks (see Table 2-5) illustrate common family behaviors that may be expected at specific times in the family life cycle. The stages of family development are marked by the age of the oldest child, although there is some overlapping of stages when there are several children in the family.

Stage I (*beginning families*) begins with the married couple as they establish a mutually satisfying relationship. The couple's tasks center on forming an intimate relationship and balance in their lives together, family planning, and establishing a harmonious relationship with in-laws and new friends. Adjusting to pregnancy and planning for parenthood are also critical tasks during this stage.

Stage II (*early childbearing*) begins when the first child is between birth and 30 months; at this time the family tasks involve adjusting to the critical needs and demands of an infant while continuing to establish a satisfying home environment.

**Table 2-5**  Duvall's Family Developmental Stages and Tasks

| Stages of development | Basic family tasks |
| --- | --- |
| I Beginning families | Physical maintenance |
| II Early childbearing | Allocation of resources |
| III Families with pre-schoolers | Division of labor |
| IV Families with school children | Socialization of members |
| V Families with teenagers | Reproduction, recruitment, and release of members |
| VI Launching center families | Maintenance of order |
| VII Middle-aged families | Placement of members in the larger society |
| VIII Aging families | Maintenance of motivation and morale |

Changes in roles and responsibilities with parenthood are critical tasks.

Stage III *(families with preschoolers)* begins as the parents adapt to the challenging needs and interests of the preschool child in a way to promote the child's growth. In adapting to the preschooler's needs, the parents may find their energy and privacy reduced. With the addition of another infant, parents may experience increased child-rearing responsibilities and the need for more living space in the home and more personal time to maintain intimacy and communication.

Stage IV *(families with school children)* begins as the oldest child enters school; the family tasks revolve around adjusting to community activities involving the child, encouraging the child's educational achievement, and maintaining a satisfying marital relationship. Critical tasks include balancing time and energy to meet the demands of work, the children's needs and activities, adult social interests, and the requirements of open communication and harmony in the marital and in-law relationships.

Stage V *(families with teenagers)* begins when the oldest child becomes a teenager; a gradual emancipation commences as the child develops increasing independence and autonomy. Families with teenagers must adapt to balancing freedom for growth with meeting family responsibilities. Critical tasks during this period are maintaining open communication between parents and teenagers, continuing intimacy in the marital relationship, and establishing outside interests and careers as teenagers leave the home.

Stage VI *(launching center families)* begins when the first child leaves the home and lasts until the last child has left. Parents must both prepare their children to live independently and accept the departure of the children. After the children have left, the parents must reorganize to reestablish the family unit. Husband and wife roles and responsibilities will shift during this period if the wife returns to work. With the birth of grandchildren, parental roles and self-images require some family accommodation.

Stage VII *(middle-aged families)* begins after the children have left the home, when middle-aged parents have more time and freedom to cultivate their social and leisure interests. This may also be a period for rebuilding the marriage and maintaining satisfying relationships both with aging parents and with the children and their families. Planning for retirement while maintaining physical and emotional health and careers are major family concerns.

Stage VIII *(aging families)* begins with the retirement of one or both spouses and continues until the deaths of both marital partners. Critical tasks focus on finding sufficient energy and motivation to seek and engage in pleasurable leisure activities within financial and health limitations. Major tasks are adjusting to retirement with changing lifestyles and accepting the deaths of friends and spouse. Within this period the family may also close the home and move into a retirement community, thus having to establish ties with new friends in a new community and to find new leisure activities.

Within each of the successive stages of family development, Duvall identified eight basic tasks, as shown in Table 2-5, that lead to successful family life within society. These tasks promote family adjustment and adaptation of the individual members. When families fail to accomplish these tasks, the family collectively or its members individually may experience unhappiness, societal disapproval, and difficulty in achieving harmony and self-actualization. The family tasks involve responsibilities to satisfy the biological, cultural, and personal needs and aspirations of the members at each stage of family development. These eight basic tasks include the following:

1. *Physical maintenance*—The family is responsible for providing shelter, appropriate clothing, sufficient nourishing food, and adequate health care.
2. *Allocation of resources*—Resources include finances, personal time, energy, and relationships. Family members' needs are met through division of cost and labor to provide material goods, space, and facilities, and through interpersonal relations to share authority, respect, and affection.
3. *Division of labor*—Family members decide who will assume what responsibilities, such as providing income, managing the household tasks, maintaining the home and car, caring for young, old, or incapacited family members, and other designated tasks.
4. *Socialization of family members*—The family assumes responsibility for guiding development of mature and acceptable patterns of socially acceptable behavior in eating, elimination, sleeping, sexuality, aggression, and interaction with others.
5. *Reproduction, recruitment, and release of family members*—Childbearing, adoption, and rearing of children are family responsibilities, along with incorporating new members through marriage. Policies are established for including others in the family, such as in-

laws, relatives, step-parents, guests, and friends.

6. *Maintenance of order*—Order is maintained by the communication of acceptable behavior. The types of intensity of interactions, patterns of affection, and sexual expression are sanctioned by parental behavior to ensure acceptance in society.

7. *Placement of members in the larger society*—Family members establish roots in society through relationships in the church, school, political and economic system, and other organizations. The family also assumes responsibility for protecting family members from undesirable outside influences and may prohibit membership in objectionable groups.

8. *Maintenance of motivation and morale*—Family members reward each other for their achievements and provide for an individual's needs of acceptance, encouragement, and affection. The family develops a philosophy of life and sense of family unity and loyalty, thereby enabling members to adapt to both personal and family crises.

Duvall's developmental model is an excellent guide for assessing, analyzing, and planning around basic family tasks at a specific developmental stage. The nurse must first determine the family's stage of development, then examine the tasks that are appropriate for the respective stage.

However, this model does not include the family structure or physiological aspects, which should be considered for a comprehensive view of the family. The model is applicable for nuclear families with growing children, and families who are experiencing health-related problems.

## Stevenson's Family Developmental Model

Joanne Stevenson (1977) describes the basic tasks and responsibilities of families in four stages:

Emerging family (from marriage for 7 to 10 years)

Crystallizing family (with teenage children)

Interacting family (children grown and small grandchildren)

Actualizing family (aging couple alone again)

She views family tasks as maintaining a common household, rearing children, and finding satisfying work and leisure. These tasks also include sustaining appropriate health patterns and providing mutual support and acculturation of family members. The four stages are delineated by the number of years the couple are married and their approximate age. Tasks for each stage are in the following text.

### The Emerging Family

There are two major family tasks in the first 7 to 10 years of marriage. First, the couple strives for independence from their parents. Second, they develop a sense of responsibility for family life. This includes economic, emotional, and sociocultural responsibilities. Independence and responsibility are accomplished in the following ways:

Advancing self-development and the enactment of appropriate roles and positions in society

Initiating the development of a personal style of life

Adjusting to a heterosexual marital relationship or to a variant companionship style

Developing parenting behaviors for biological offspring or in the broader framework of social parenting

Integrating personal values with career development and socioeconomic constraints (Stevenson, 1977:15)

### The Crystallizing Family

When families reach the early middle years with teenage children, different responsibilities emerge. The family assumes responsibility for growth and development of individual members and outside organizations. The parents provide assistance to both the younger and older generations without exerting control over them. These tasks are accomplished by the following:

Developing socioeconomic consolidation

Evaluating one's occupation or career in light of a personal value system

Helping younger persons become integrated human beings

Enhancing or redeveloping intimacy with spouse or significant other

Assuming responsible positions in occupational, social, and civic activities, organizations, and communities

Maintaining and improving the home or other forms of property

Using leisure time in satisfying and creative ways

Adjusting to biological or personal system changes that occur (Stevenson, 1977:18)

### The Interacting Family

In the later middle years, most of the children leave the home but return periodically with their own children. The older family members absorb the small children into the home. Relationships between work and leisure change. The older family now assumes responsibility for "continued survival and enhancement of the nation." To accomplish these responsibilities, the adult members are involved in

Maintaining flexible views in occupational, civic, political, religious, and social positions

Keeping current on relevant scientific, political, and cultural changes

Developing mutually supportive (interdependent) relationships with grown offspring and other members of the younger generations

Reevaluating and enhancing the relationship with spouse or significant other or adjusting to their loss

Helping aged parents or other relatives progress through the last stage of life

Deriving satisfaction from increased availability of leisure time

Preparing for retirement and planning another career when feasible

Adapting self and behavior to signals of accelerated aging processes (Stevenson, 1977:25).

### The Actualizing Family

In late adulthood, the aging couple are engaged in discovering meaning in their lives. They accept the process of grief and dying. They "assume responsibility for sharing the wisdom of age, reviewing life, and putting [their] affairs in order." This task is accomplished by

Pursuing a second or third career, new interests, hobbies, or community activities

Learning new skills that are well removed from previous learnings

Sharing wisdom accrued from the past with individuals, groups, communities, and nations

Evaluating the totality of past life and putting successes and failures into perspective

Progressing through the stages of grief, death, and dying with significant others and with self (Stevenson, 1977:29)

Stevenson's developmental model describes family tasks and responsibilities over four stages. The stages encompass child-rearing, spouse relationships, and interaction with community organizations. The model is useful with nuclear families because it examines psychosocial patterns at a specific stage of development. However, the model does not include family structure, nor does it address health promotion and health-related concerns that the family may face.

## Satir's Interactional Family Model

Virginia Satir (1972) believes that the family's interactional health depends on its ability to share and understand the members' feelings, needs, and behavior patterns. She thinks that healthy, nurturing families help their members know themselves through communication of everyday events. This communication promotes each individual's self-confidence and self-worth. Satir views the healthy family as hopeful, trusting of others, and curious about what society has to offer. The family operates on a growth-producing, reality-oriented basis. This promotes intimacy among its members. Family rules about money, chores, and power are explicit and understood by everyone. Also, the healthy family establishes links with society. These links are established through membership in various groups.

Satir's model of the healthy family consists of four concepts: self-worth, communication, rules, and links to society.

Each member and the family unit demonstrate feelings of high esteem and *self-worth*. These attitudes are conveyed by behaviors showing integrity, honesty, responsibility, compassion, and love. These attitudes flow outward from each individual, and a sense of trust radiates from all members. They accept their own strengths and inadequacies as well as those of others. Without self-worth, family members build walls of distrust, isolation, and loneliness. They fear others will cheat them, use them, or step on them. This leads to unhealthy family interaction.

*Communication* directly influences the relationships among family members. Patterns of communication include body movements, posture, tone of voice, and spoken words. In healthy families, communication is open, direct, clear, and honest. The members are receptive and encourage open, honest sharing of feelings and needs. They value what others have to say, supporting each member's attempts in both verbal and physical communication. Unhealthy families block communication among members; they may give ambiguous messages or not listen at all. This leads to distrust and low self-worth among the family members.

Each family has a set of *rules* it lives by. These rules may be explicit or implicit. Most families assume that everyone knows and understands the rules, but this is not always true. Families have rules about money, responsibilities, activities, special privileges, privacy, sexual expression, language, territoriality, and authority. In many situations, rules define what actions are appropriate; they may also guide how feelings are expressed and may help achieve goals or impede goal achievement. Some rules may be outdated, unfair, unclear, or inappropriate. In healthy families the rules are known to all members, allow for freedom, and encourage discussion among the members.

Unhealthy families may have implicit rules that restrict family members. These rules may be inflexible and inhibit the growth of the members.

The family unit and individual members have *links to society* through organizations and friends. The organizational links include schools, church, political groups, recreational groups, and clubs. Links with friends are usually formed through common interests. With these links the family and its members keep actively involved in the community and relate to the world around them. Healthy families have many links with society, believing society has much to offer and trusting their selection of groups to be a positive influence and interaction. They believe society offers opportunities for choices and change, growth, and development. These opportunities are welcomed, desirable, and normal. Unhealthy families view society with distrust and fear exposure to others' values. They avoid involvement in organizations, preferring to remain isolated. They do not welcome experiences outside the family.

Satir's interactional family model addresses four major psychosocial concepts considered important in a healthy family. The model is limited because it does not include family structure, functions, and developmental level. The model can be applied to any type of family, but additional models may be necessary for a comprehensive approach in the nursing process.

### Friedman's Structural-Functional Family Model

Friedman's family model was developed from sociological frameworks and systems theory by Marilyn Friedman (1986). The family is the focus of the model, as it interacts with suprasystems in the community and with individual family members in the subsystem. The model is comprised of two components—structural and functional—as shown in Table 2-6. The structural component ex-amines the family unit, how it is organized, and how members relate to one another in terms of their values, communication network, role systems, and power. The functional component refers to the interactional outcomes resulting from the family organizational structure. There are six parts to family functions. The structural-functional components and parts all intimately interrelate and interact: each component and part is affected by the others.

#### Structural Components

*Value systems:* Values develop over time by exposure to and experience with influential groups and individuals, such as parents, culture, religion, and ethnic groups. Values lead to chosen behaviors, which are reinforced by others. Values are expressed by family members' behaviors—how they allocate resources and where time and energy are invested. Some of these values are health care, materialism, education, independence, productivity, and cleanliness.

*Communication patterns:* As families evolve, they develop communication patterns, ways of relating to each other that may be functional or dysfunctional. Communication involves verbal and nonverbal behaviors, including tone, intent, and message. Communication patterns include who talks with whom, who listens, who seeks feedback, and who validates the message. Are family members able to share feelings and needs with others? What are the quality, quantity, and topics of conversation? What topics or types of communication are denied or avoided among the family?

*Role structure:* In a family, members adopt varying roles that may change over time. Roles can be formal or informal, adopted or assigned. What are the formal and informal roles of family members? What roles are expected in the family, and which are assigned or adopted by whom? Are there conflicts between role expectations of others and the roles adopted by members? How flexible are family members in changing roles as needed?

*Power structure:* The family power structure is determined by various influencing factors. Some factors include the social and ethnic class, family communication patterns, interpersonal and financial resources, family coalitions, and implementation of decisions. To identify the family power structure, consider who is really in charge of the family and why. Who makes the major decisions or has the last word? Who is consulted about family plans or changes? Who makes the rules? And who enforces discipline? The family power structure

**Table 2-6**  Friedman's Family Model Components

| Structural components | Functional components |
| --- | --- |
| Family composition | Affective |
| Value systems | Physical necessities and care |
| Communication patterns | |
| Role structure | Economic |
| Power structure | Reproductive |
| | Socialization and social placement |
| | Family coping |

may be authoritarian, democratic, laissez-faire, paternalistic, maternalistic, or egalitarian, or may vary with the issue at hand.

### Functional Components

*Affective:* The social and emotional developmental needs of family members must be recognized and met by family members. These functions include reducing tension, maintaining morale, and conveying esteem and love for family members.

*Physical necessities and care:* The parents are responsible for providing food, clothing, shelter, and health care and for protecting family members from danger.

*Economic:* The adult family members are responsible for obtaining sufficient resources, including financial, space, and material goods, and allocating these resources appropriately to family members. Both family values and power structure have impact on allocation of resources.

*Reproductive:* The adult family members assume responsibility for conception and contraception.

*Socialization and social placement:* The adult family members determine appropriate social roles for children, instill family values and expectations, and confer their socioethnic status on the children. This is accomplished by providing and sharing experiences with others in the family, schools, community organizations, and religious groups.

*Family coping:* For family stability and growth, the members need adaptive patterns and problem-solving abilities to respond to demands and expectations outside the family that create change within the family.

Friedman's structural-functional family model provides a broad framework for examining the interactions among family members and within the community. This model incorporates physical, psychosocial, and cultural aspects of the family along with interacting relationships. The family developmental stage and additional structural aspects could be added. This model is very applicable in the nursing process to any type of family and their health-related problems.

## Calgary's Family Model

Calgary's family model is an integrated conceptual framework of several theorists' work that was adapted for nurses at the University of Calgary. The model is based on three major categories: family structure, function, and development. Each of the three categories is further subdivided, as shown in Table 2-7. Although the family may be examined by looking at specific parts, each part in-

teracts with others and changes the whole family configuration.

### Family Internal Structure

*Family composition* refers to all members living in the home. This definition includes nuclear families, single-parent families, homosexual couples, boarders, grandparents, step-parents, and children. The *family* is defined as the attributes of affection, loyalty, and durability of those residing together.

*Rank order* refers to the children's age and birth order. It is believed that birth order influences levels of motivation and achievement, along with vocational choices.

*Subsystems* in a family are delineated by generation, sex, interests, and function, according to Minuchin (1974). Each family member belongs to several subsystems that differentiate the level of power and skills. Examples include a step-parent who lacks power over the children or acts like a child, while a child may have the power of a parent.

*Boundary* refers to which family member(s) participates in what functions and how. Boundaries protect the family members by obtaining, containing, retaining, and disposing of information, products, or people. For example, a family may prevent members from bringing in drugs or using vulgar language, or it may prevent members from divulg-

**Table 2-7** Calgary Family Model

| Family structure | Family development | Family functions |
|---|---|---|
| **Internal** | | **Instrumental** |
| Family composition | Developmental stage | Daily living activities |
| Rank order of members | Developmental tasks | Allocation of tasks |
| Subsystems in family | Attachments | |
| Boundaries of family | | |
| **External** | | **Expressive** |
| Culture | | Communication |
| Religion | | Problem-solving |
| Social class status and mobility | | Roles |
| Environment | | Control |
| Extended family | | Beliefs |
| | | Alliances/coalitions |

Adapted from Calgary Family Assessment Model. In Wright LM and Leahey M: Nurses and families: a guide to family assessment and intervention, Philadelphia, 1984, FA Davis Co.

ing family information to outsiders. Boundaries can be diffuse, rigid, or permeable and may change over time.

### Family External Structure

*Culture* is the learned and shared behaviors characteristic of the group. It includes ethnic identity, cultural patterns, and adaptation in new geographical areas. Some cultures are highly family-oriented, whereas others maintain a distinct distance.

*Religion* refers to the family values, size, health care practices, and socialization patterns. It includes level of community involvement and maintaining of certain traditions, both religious and hygienic.

*Social class status and mobility* strongly influence the family value system. The adults' educational attainment, income, and occupation usually determine their values, which influence their lifestyles and behavior patterns.

*Environment* refers to both the general neighborhood and the home. The type of neighborhood (commercial or residential) and proximity to stores, transportation, recreation, and health facilities are considered. In the home, the amount of space and privacy, along with access, safety, security, kitchen utilities, and bathrooms, are important factors.

*Extended family* includes grandparents, aunts, uncles, and cousins along with step relatives. These family members may live nearby or far away from those in the household.

### Family Developmental Level

Family developmental level is based on the length of marriage and the child-rearing stages. Theorists, such as Duvall (1977), have identified eight stages, with eight tasks in each stage. Most other developmental theorists identify fewer stages and tasks. In this model, three major areas are defined; these can be further subdivided by referring to other developmental theorists.

*Stages* refers to the length of the marriage and the age of the eldest child. Families move through normal transitions in child-rearing, although with additional children, some stages are overlapping. Ethnic and cultural differences also should be considered.

*Tasks* can be considered either general maintenance types of responsibilities, such as employment, spending, health, education, and socialization (which may be defined in a general way), or specifically defined, depending on the family's developmental stage.

*Attachments* are the unique and relatively enduring emotional ties between two family members. This bond may be between mother and daughter, child and grandparent, or brother and sister. The reciprocal nature of this bond and the quality of the relationship are considered.

### Family Functions

Family functions include the actual behaviors of family members in relation to daily activities and their emotional interactions.

*Activities of daily living* are the patterns of working, eating, sleeping, exercise, recreation, and socialization. What activities do the family do together and which activities are done alone?

*Allocation of tasks* refers to which family members take on or are assigned specific tasks, such as grocery shopping, preparing meals, cleaning house, paying bills, and maintaining health.

*Communication between family members* includes verbal and nonverbal and the range and types of emotions and feelings expressed in the interaction. In verbal communication, the focus is on the meaning of the words; in nonverbal communication, the focus is on the body posture, eye contact, expressions, touch, and gestures. The emotions expressed in communication are reflected in the tone of voice and nonverbal message, such as anger, joy, sadness, and praise. It is also important to note the congruity between the spoken words, the nonverbal behaviors and the emotions expressed.

*Problem-solving* refers to the family's method of identifying and solving problems. Who in the family recognizes and identifies problems? How does the family handle problems? Is one person the decision-maker, or do members share the problems and solutions? Are outside family members, friends, or professionals sought for council or assistance? Is there one pattern of problem-solving in the family, or does the manner of problem-solving depend on the type of problem?

*Roles of family members* are their established patterns of behavior as they interact with another member. Each member has several overlapping roles, which are unique in each dyad, but change over time. For example, a woman may be a wife, mother, daughter, employee, student, sister, and friend. Roles may be assumed or assigned, complementary or conflicting. How each member feels about his or her roles is important.

*Control* refers to the methods that family members use to influence each other's behavior. Parents control their children through rewards, such as praise, special privileges, toys, and hugs, or punishment, such as criticism, spanking, or denial of rewards. Adults often use words, affection, and gifts or the withholding of these to control other adult family members. What are the family members' patterns of controlling other members? Are these behaviors normal and healthy, or are they disruptive and dysfunctional?

*Beliefs* are the attitudes, expectations, values, and priorities that the family hold. Are members expected to achieve, excel, save face, or be honest, trustworthy, and reliable? Some families place importance on materialistic status symbols, whereas others emphasize altruism, the work ethic, and religious beliefs. The family's values and beliefs influence their lifestyle and behavior patterns, along with how their time and money are spent.

*Alliances/coalitions* refers to the direction, balance, and intensity of relationships among family members. These relationships may include two or three family members and may change over time. In healthy families, three-member coalitions provide a flexibility for change in the intensity of the relationship among the members.

The Calgary family model is comprehensive and incorporates three major areas, namely, the structure, function, and development of the family. It is complex, with too many subconcepts for the nurse to fully explore each area. When using this model, the nurse must determine which areas are most important and focus on those, while acquiring some general information in other areas. This is a good model for assessing family data; however, additional knowledge of sociological theories are necessary to analyze and interpret the data and to develop plans for the family. The Calgary family model can be applied to any type of family with any health-related concern.

## SUMMARY

This chapter presented an overview of several general, nursing, and family models that can be applied in the nursing process. Major concepts and subconcepts were described and illustrated. The strengths, limitations, and possible applications of each model were briefly discussed. In any nursing process, a holistic view of the client is desired, however, some models may not include areas that are particularly relevant to the client's health situation. Therefore, it is acceptable for the nurse to include another model or certain aspects of another model to supplement the central model. The synthesis of models is part of the creative art of nursing practice. For example, Roy's Adaptation Model may be very appropriate for a specific client situation, but a developmental viewpoint would also be relevant, so Erikson's Stages of Development could be a supplemental model. In a family nursing process, Friedman's model may be appropriate, but lacks

specific guides for health care. Therefore, Orem's Self-Care Model may provide an appropriate supplement.

Section II describes each component of the nursing process in detail, with examples of how to apply different models in each component. Section III provides case studies for individual, family, and community clients and illustrates application of selected models in a complete nursing process.

## REFERENCES AND READINGS

Aguilera DC and Messick JM: Crisis intervention: theory and methodology, ed 6, St Louis, 1990, The CV Mosby Co.

Capers DF and Kelly R: Neuman nursing process: a model of holistic care, Holistic Nurs Pract 1:19, 1987.

Chinn PL and Jacobs MK: Theory and nursing: a systematic approach, ed 2, St Louis, 1987, The CV Mosby Co.

Clark J: Development of models and theories on the concept of nursing, J Adv Nurs 7:129, 1982.

Clements IM and Roberts FB, (editors): Family health: a theoretical approach to nursing care, New York, 1983, John Wiley & Sons, Inc.

Cuff-Carney D: Holistic family therapy: individuals or families? A therapist's perspective, Holistic Nurs Pract 2:45, 1987.

Duvall EM: Marriage and family development, ed 5, Philadelphia, 1977, JB Lippincott Co.

Erikson E: Childhood and society, ed 2, New York, 1963, WW Norton & Co., Inc.

Fitzpatrick JJ and Whall AL: Conceptual models of nursing: analysis and application, Bowie, Md, 1983, Robert J. Brady Co.

Friedman MM: Family nursing: theories and assessment, ed 2, New York, 1986, Appleton-Century-Crofts.

Johnson DE: The behavioral systems model for nursing. In Reihl JP and Roy C Sr, editors: Conceptual models for nursing practice, ed 2, New York, 1980, Appleton-Century-Crofts.

Kane CF: Family social support: toward a conceptual model, Adv Nurs Sci 10:18, 1988.

King I: Toward a theory for nursing: general concepts of human behavior, New York, 1971, John Wiley & Sons, Inc.

King I: A theory for nursing: systems, concepts, process, New York, 1981, John Wiley & Sons, Inc.

Leininger M: Transcultural nursing: concepts, theories and practices, New York, 1978, John Wiley & Sons, Inc.

Leininger M: Caring: an essential human need, Thorofare, NJ, 1981, Charles B Slack, Inc.

Leininger M: The essence of nursing and health, Thorofare, NJ, 1984, Charles B Slack, Inc.

Maslow A: Motivation and personality, ed 2, New York, 1970, Harper & Row, Publishers, Inc.

Meleis AI: Theoretical nursing: development and progress, Philadelphia, 1985, JB Lippincott Co.

Minuchin S: Families and family therapy, Cambridge, Mass, 1974, Harvard University Press.

Neuman B: The Neuman systems model, New York, 1982, Appleton-Century-Crofts.

Orem DE: Nursing: concepts of practice, ed 2, New York, 1980, McGraw-Hill Book Co.

Orem DE: Nursing: concepts and practice, ed 3, New York, 1985, McGraw-Hill Book Co.

Parse RR: Man-living-health: a theory of nursing, New York, 1981, John Wiley & Sons, Inc.

Parse RR: Nursing science: major paradigms, theories, and critiques, Philadelphia, 1987, WB Saunders.

Peplau HE: Interpersonal relations in nursing, New York, 1952, GP Putnam's Sons.

Riehl J and Roy Sr C, editors: Conceptual models for nursing practice, ed 2, New York, 1980, Appleton-Century-Crofts.

Rogers ME: Theoretical basis of nursing, Philadelphia, 1970, FA Davis Co.

Rogers ME: Science of unitary human man. In Reihl JP and Roy Sr C, editors: Conceptual models for nursing practice, ed 2, New York, 1980, Appleton-Century-Crofts.

Rogers ME: Science of unitary human beings: a paradigm for nursing. Printed material distributed at the Nursing Theorists Conference, Alberta, Canada, May 1984.

Roy Sr C: Introduction to nursing: an adaptation model, ed 2, Englewood Cliffs, NJ, 1984, Prentice-Hall Co.

Roy Sr C and Roberts SL: Theory construction in nursing - an adaptation model, Englewood Cliffs NJ, 1981, Prentice-Hall Co.

Satir V: Peoplemaking, Palo Alto, Calif, 1972, Science and Behavior Books.

Stevenson JS: Issues and crises during middlescence, New York, 1977, Appleton-Century-Crofts.

von Bertalanffy L: General systems theory: foundation, development, and applications, New York, 1968, George Braziller, Inc.

Wright LM and Leahey M: Nurses and families: a guide to family assessment and intervention, Philadelphia, 1984, FA Davis Co.

# Components of the Nursing Process

# Assessment: Overview of Data Collection

PAULA J. CHRISTENSEN

## GENERAL CONSIDERATIONS

Assessment is the foundation of the nursing process. Accurate data collection leads to identification of the client's health status, strengths, and concerns for nursing diagnoses. This provides direction for nursing implementation and alleviation of client concerns. The purpose of assessment is to identify and obtain pertinent data about the client. The American Nurses' Association (1980) states that nursing is the diagnosis and treatment of human responses to actual or potential health problems. Therefore, the main focus of data collection is the client's *response* to health concerns or problems. These responses can be biophysical, sociocultural, psychological, or spiritual in nature. In other words, nurses consider clients in a multifocal way. Individuals, families, and communities have multiple aspects that are interrelated and influence each other. All these aspects or potential response areas are considered to ensure a comprehensive and accurate assessment. To accomplish this, the nurse needs a strong knowledge base in a variety of disciplines. Knowledge of the theories, norms, and standards of behavior and functioning provides a foundation to collect pertinent information from clients and make sound judgments about their health.

This chapter begins with a brief historical overview of data collection. Factors influencing data collection, characteristics of the nurse-client relationship, phases of assessment, and patterns of behavior and functioning are then discussed. Three major methods for data collection and specific examples of each are given. The application of models to data collection is provided. The most important points for assessment are listed below and are summarized at the end of the chapter:

1. A systematic format is used for data collection.
2. The data are comprehensive and multifocal.
3. A variety of sources is used for data collection.
4. Appropriate methods are used for data collection.
5. The data are verifiable.
6. The data reflect updating of information.
7. The data are recorded and communicated appropriately.

The assessment process is applicable to all clients: individuals, families, and communities. Specific examples of data collection for each type of client are provided in the next three chapters.

### Historical Perspectives

Nursing care has frequently included a limited assessment of clients' health-related concerns. Traditionally the nurse depended on medical diagnoses to give direction to nursing care. Nurses also used intuition during contact with their clients, for example, "I just have the feeling that Mr. Polaski is going downhill," or "Something tells me I better check Ms. Armond's blood pressure more frequently." These intuitions were based on an important form of data collection that still exists today—subjective impression—one that cannot be refuted yet also cannot be the sole source of data obtained. Behavioral, social, nursing, and medical sciences have developed to the point of providing certain concrete indicators of health, cited within theories, norms, and standards. These health indicators provide nurses with a basis for collecting data and making judgments.

Nurses have become increasingly accountable and responsible for making sound nursing assessments and clinical judgments on which to base implementation. Medical diagnoses and intuitions now serve as cues for further data collection. Because nursing practice focuses on maintenance, restoration, and promotion of health, the nurse must conduct a comprehensive and valid nursing assessment to meet those goals.

### Factors Influencing Data Collection

Several factors influence the process of data collection—how the data are presented by the client and how they are perceived by the nurse. Both the client and the nurse enter a situation with previous experiences and knowledge that influence their perceptions and interpretations. More specifically, the nurse and the client are influenced by their respective (1) physical, mental, and emotional states and needs; (2) cultural, social, and philosophical backgrounds; (3) number and functional ability of senses; (4) past experiences associated with the present situation; (5) meaning of the event; (6) interests, preoccupations, preconceptions, and motivational levels; (7) knowledge or familarity with the situation; (8) environmental conditions and distractions; and (9) presence, attitudes, and reactions of others.

These factors create a situation in which both client and nurse may automatically assign personal meanings or interpretations to the situation. Difficulty arises when the nurse's perception or interpretation is used as fact. The nurse can develop the ability to differentiate actual data from personal interpretation through an adequate knowledge base, self-awareness, and conscious attention to potential misinterpretations.

The nurse's level of proficiency also plays a role during the assessment of a client's health status. The novice or beginning nurse relies on more structured guidelines for assessment, ensuring that specific data are obtained in a deliberate and conscious manner. Nurses with more experience develop a perceptual awareness that can begin with vague hunches and intuitive assessments. The process for data collection is internalized, and accurate conclusions are made from inadequate information as expert nurses perceive "wholes" rather than "bits and pieces" of information (Rew and Borrow, 1987). Highly proficient nurses learn to trust their intuitive hunches and follow up on them to find confirming data. Their personal knowledge and experience along with their empirical knowledge provide the bases for transformation of their skills and understanding that leads to expert performance (Benner, 1984).

### Nurse-Client Relationship

The nurse-client relationship is the means for applying the nursing process. This relationship is the vehicle by which the nurse works mutually with the client to facilitate the client's optimal level of health. Carl Rogers (1961) identified three aspects that facilitate personal growth in a relationship: (1) genuineness—the ability to be aware of one's own feelings, or being real; (2) respect for the separateness of another—accepting the other unconditionally; and (3) a continuing desire to understand or empathize with the other. These aspects are applicable to all human relationships, especially the nurse-client relationship.

Trust, empathy, caring, autonomy, and mutuality are also important characteristics basic to the development of a nurse-client relationship (Sundeen et al, 1989). These concepts are reciprocal during nurse-client interactions, but the nurse is responsible for their initiation. Therefore, the nurse needs to identify specific actions that communicate trust (consistency, honesty), empathy (touch, sincerity), caring (genuineness, eye contact), autonomy (nonjudgmental, nonthreatening), and mutuality (inclusion of the client in decision-making).

Effective nurse-client relationships can be attained when nurses are willing to look at their own values, beliefs, behaviors, prejudices, strengths, and limitations. Exploration of these aspects of "self" creates an awareness where nurses can consciously use the self during interactions with others. This awareness cannot be achieved through intellectual development alone; nurses must be open to the discovery of their own motivations and feelings through experience and relationships with others.

### Communication

Communication skills are necessary for developing relationships. Knowledge of communication theory is essential for acquiring expertise in the ability to understand and be understood by others. Communication is a two-way process that occurs between individuals or groups of people and consists of verbal and nonverbal messages. Verbal messages are communicated through words in a given language. Words are labels placed on an object or event. Our previous experiences with an object or event influence what we perceive when we hear or see a given word. Therefore, the more abstract the word, the more likely we are to personalize its meaning and misinterpret what another is saying. For example, the word "anxiety" may be interpreted in many different ways, whereas

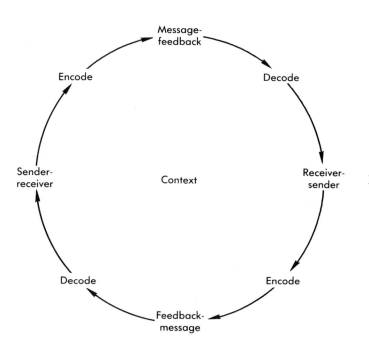

Fig. 3-1. Communication model.

"chair" has a more specific connotation. Nonverbal messages are conveyed through vocal cues, action cues, object cues, use of space, and touch (Stuart and Sundeen, 1987). In many situations nonverbal communication reveals the true, often unacceptable message. These messages may be conscious or unconscious, intended or unintended. The nurse's goal is to communicate verbal and nonverbal messages that are conscious, intended, and congruent. In other words, the verbal and nonverbal messages should be saying the same thing.

Messages are encoded and sent by the sender, and the receiver decodes them. The receiver, in turn, encodes feedback to the sender, and the sender decodes the feedback (Fig. 3-1). The sender and receiver may exchange roles several times during an interaction. This is the dynamic nature of communication: we are always exchanging messages and feedback. Our knowledge of the language, previous experiences, the situation, anxiety levels, and functional ability of senses influence how we encode and decode the messages and feedback.

Communication occurs on two levels: thoughts and feelings. Thoughts consist of ideas, opinions, beliefs, and facts. Feelings are our emotions. The five basic emotions are happiness, sadness, fear, anxiety, and anger. Many people communicate on the thinking level most of the time. Feelings tend to be buried or hidden in order to protect ourselves from being vulnerable. The nurse's role is to help the client communicate on both levels when appropriate. During times of increased stress or crisis, in

**Table 3-1** Facilitative Communication Techniques*

| Verbal | Nonverbal |
|---|---|
| Open-ended statements and questions | Thoughtful silence |
| Related questions | Touch |
| Verbalization of the implied | Active listening |
| Clarification of statements | Watching and eye contact |
| Consensual validation | Open body language |
| Sharing of perceptions | |
| Restatement, repetition of main idea | |
| Reflection of feelings and content | |
| Focus | |
| Summary | |

*Definitions of techniques are in the glossary.

particular, clients need assistance in expressing feelings regarding the situation. When feelings are expressed along with thoughts, the client's anxiety level usually decreases and effective problem solving can occur.

The appropriate and effective use of facilitative communication techniques fosters the development of the nurse-client relationship (Table 3-1). These techniques are useful as enabling methods that should be incorporated naturally into any nurse-client interaction. The techniques chosen are based on the nurse's comfort with them. As with any newly learned skill, the techniques may seem artificial and awkward at first, until they are practiced and mastered. The use of these techniques does not guarantee a meaningful relationship. All aspects of the situation must be taken into account, such as the client's health status, environmental influences, and the nurse's knowledge and use of self.

## PHASES OF ASSESSMENT

The nature and amount of data required and secured for an adequate assessment are determined by the client's health concerns and strengths, type of setting or agency, purpose of the interaction, data sources, nurse's knowledge and skills, and available resources. For example, data that a nurse obtains when caring for a new young mother and child in a walk-in clinic differ greatly in type, depth, and breadth from data obtained when working with an elderly group of clients in a residential facility. In the first situation, the nurse has limited time with the client and focuses the assessment on immediate concerns. When assessing the elderly client group, the nurse has ongoing contact to obtain a greater scope of information. Both approaches are considered comprehensive because the nurse collects data regarding multifocal aspects of clients that influence their health.

The client (individual, family, or community group) is the primary source for data collection. Thus, the data should reflect the client's perception of the health concern or situation as accurately as possible. The nurse determines the reasons why the client is initiating health care, or, if the nurse initiates the contact, what are the client's perceptions of health concerns. In addition, the nurse should ascertain the client's desires, wishes, hopes, and expectations for achieving optimum health.

The first phase of assessment, then, is to gather preliminary information from the client regarding immediate health concerns, demographic information such as age, lifestyle, and activities of daily living. This data base helps the nurse to understand the client's perceptions of health, what factors influence the client's health, and what nursing can do to facilitate the client's achievement of optimum health. Preliminary information is obtained during the initial interview with a client.

The second phase of assessment is to determine which model to use to guide further data collection and provide direction for the remainder of the nursing process components with the client. As indicated in Chapter 1, the nurse considers the major concepts of the model and their interrelationships, the focus and assumptions of the model, and, finally, whether the model gives direction for a plan that is appropriate to the client's health concerns. This examination leads to choosing a model that is congruent with the client's situation and the nurse's view of health and nursing.

The third phase of assessment is either a more focused or a general assessment of the client's health status. If the client expressed a specific health concern related to pain during the preliminary information phase, the nurse then focuses on determining the exact nature of that concern first. Next, if appropriate, the nurse conducts a general assessment of other aspects of the client's life. The breadth of this type of assessment allows for an in-depth understanding of the biophysical, sociocultural, psychological, and spiritual influences on the client's health. Using the chosen model as a guide, the nurse determines the nature and scope of any additional information that is needed to facilitate the identification of concerns and strengths within the context of the situation.

### Patterns of Behavior and Functioning

The process of data collection results in obtaining data pieces that may or may not be significant to the client's health concerns. Judgments about a client's health status cannot be made from isolated pieces of data alone. Therefore, the nurse needs to look for traits or behaviors that relate to each other, occur repeatedly over time, and are pertinent to the client's health status. These reoccurring traits and behaviors are called patterns of data and form the foundation on which the data are analyzed/synthesized, and nursing diagnoses are identified.

All clients have common patterns of behavior and functioning. A *pattern* is viewed as a composite sample of traits or behaviors characterized by rate, rhythm, intensity, duration, and amount. The individual is a combination of biophysical, psychological, sociocultural, and spiritual aspects. The family has a certain definable structure and process. The community is made up of systems and subsystems that influence its functions.

The patterns given in Table 3-2 are examples of similar characteristics each client group possesses.

Theories, norms, and standards describe the healthy aspects of clients' patterns of behavior and functioning. These patterns can serve as guidelines for data collection. All clients possess certain basic patterns; yet each client may exhibit or combine patterns in a different way. Looking for differences and similarities among clients helps the nurse avoid using personal interpretation of data during the data collection process.

**Table 3-2**  Patterns of Behavior and Functioning

| Individual | Family | Community |
|---|---|---|
| Exercise | Communication | Socialization |
| Circulation | Roles | Power |
| Self-concept | Physical maintenance | System linkage |
| Valuing | Decision making | Boundary mainte-<br>nance |

## METHODS FOR DATA COLLECTION

Data are collected by means of three methods: interaction, observation, and measurement. Interaction data are obtained by means of any relevant verbal communication with the client, health care personnel, or significant others. Observation data are gathered by means of the senses, and include written documents. Measurement data are obtained by means of instruments that quantify information. Definitions and examples of these methods are given below.

All the methods of data collection have strengths and limitations. They should not be used in isolation, because valid assessments are rarely made by using one method alone. In some situations, two methods dominate, depending on the age and health status of the client, the nurse's expertise, and the given situation. Generally, nurses use at least two of the three methods for data collection.

Data obtained from all the methods must be accurate, that is, impartial and unbiased by the nurse's personal interpretations of the client's situation. To prevent use of his or her own perceptions, the nurse states or records the information as factually as possible.

### Interaction

Interaction is defined as a mutual or reciprocal exchange of verbal information between the nurse and the client. Interactions serve many purposes throughout the nursing process, such as obtaining information regarding the major health concern, patterns of living, and function of systems; building rapport; assessing learning needs and providing information; establishing mutual plans; giving directions, explanations, support, and encouragement; and evaluating progress. Our focus here is to discuss interactions in the data collection component. The main purposes, then, are to develop rapport and obtain information. Nursing today is often based on a series of intermittent interactions with clients rather than on sustained relationships. The same characteristics discussed previously about growth-producing relationships also apply to isolated nurse-client interactions.

Interviews or transitory relationships between two people can be classified as directive-interrogative, rapport-building, or open-ended (Enelow and Swisher, 1986). The *directive-interrogative interview* involves asking for specific information; the purpose is primarily to get data. The nurse maintains control of the direction of the interview, and the client is a passive participant. This type of interviewing is advantageous when a specific amount of data is needed in a short time. A disadvantage is that the client is passive and may not be able to discuss concerns. History taking is an example of a directive-interrogative interview. The *rapport-building interview* focuses on building a relationship, not on obtaining information. Open, empathic responses are used by the interviewer to facilitate the client's control of the interview. Data emerge and a relationship develops, but rapport building takes time, and specific data may not be obtained. The *open-ended interview* is a combination of the first two types; the goals are to obtain information from the client and to build rapport. The client's concerns emerge through the use of a variety of communication techniques. The interviewer starts with the least amount of authority (open-ended statements and questions) to encourage the client to direct the topics of discussion. Gradually, the interviewer uses increasing authority to provide more specific focus and obtain needed information that has not surfaced.

All three types of interviews have a place in nurse-client interactions. In general, the nurse should use the least amount of authority necessary to obtain the information needed within the time allotted.

The nurse enters each client interview with a purpose. Is the interaction primarily to obtain information? If so, what information? What type of interview will facilitate meeting the purpose? The time allotted also affects the method used. If the purpose is to build rapport, what topics and communication techniques promote rapport with this client? The data obtained will be more relevant and meaningful if the nurse is purposeful during an interaction. The client probably will be more cooperative and open when the nurse provides some direction as well.

Interaction data are obtained through effective communication and interviewing skills. The outcome of interactions is data that reflect what the client said and what the nurse observed. Statements by the client should be noted as direct quotations. Paraphrasing what someone says tends to increase

**Table 3-3**  Accurate Statements of Interaction
Data versus Personal Interpretations

| Accurate interaction data | Personal interpretations |
| --- | --- |
| **Individual client** | |
| "I'd rather be left alone now." | Client is angry |
| "I'm afraid of what they will find during surgery." | Client is afraid of surgery |
| **Family client** | |
| "My mother is hardly ever at home." | Mother does not care about time spent with child |
| "I'm expected to do all the housework around here with no help." | Family expects mother/wife to do all the work around the home |
| **Community client** | |
| "The city council meets once a month." | City council meetings are held infrequently |
| "A lot of teenagers in this part of town are pregnant." | Teenage pregnancies are epidemic |

the probability of interpreting or placing one's own meaning to the data. Table 3-3 provides examples of accurate statements of interaction data versus personal interpretations of them.

These personal interpretations may or may not be accurate. Insufficient data is given to be able to make conclusive judgments. The interpretations need to be used as cues for further data collection. Through the use of communication techniques such as reflection, validation, and clarification, the nurse determines the most accurate meaning of the data presented.

### Observation

Observation is a process of noting pieces of information or cues through the use of the senses (sight, touch, hearing, smell, and taste). Nurses use these senses in a variety of ways to observe the client's (1) characteristics of appearance and function, (2) content and process of interactions and relationships, and (3) environment. Each sense is discussed in relation to these three categories.

The sense of sight is used to identify visual cues that clients and data sources project. Examples of data collected through the use of *sight* are as follows:

1. Characteristics of appearance and function: posture, gait, balance; dress; color, shape, amount, approximate size of visible elements; prostheses; data from written records about characteristics (such as nurses' notes).
2. Content and process of interactions: nonver-

bal communication such as body movements, gestures, eye contact, personal space, use of touch, seating arrangements, patterns of communication.
3. Environment: client's room (home or agency), personal belongings present, space available, cleanliness, and furniture; neighborhood characteristics, such as number of houses and cleanliness; data from written sources about client's environment.

The sense of *touch* is used to determine qualities of an object or person. Through simple touch or the use of palpation* and percussion* the following data can be obtained:

1. Characteristics of appearance and function: texture, moisture, temperature, density, and muscle and skin tone.
2. Content and process of interactions: not applicable.
3. Environment: temperature of air, moisture (humidity), and furniture.

*Hearing* is primarily used to actively listen to clients' verbal messages or to note interaction data. Other important uses of hearing are:

1. Characteristics of appearance and function: auscultation* of lung, heart, and bowel sounds; percussion (along with touch) of tissue; ability to speak
2. Content and process of interactions: amount of interacting with others, tone of voice(s), interruptions in conversations, and specific content of what is said
3. Environment: client's room (home or agency), auditory stimuli; house/neighborhood noise levels; usual sounds in home or community

The senses of *smell* and *taste* are used less frequently. The odors of the client, room, home, and environment are detected through smell. Local foods and, in some environments, chemicals in the air can be detected through taste.

Maintaining accuracy in observing clients is an important element of data collection. Examples of observation data that are accurate versus notations of personal interpretations are given in Table 3-4. Recording specifically what is seen, felt, heard, smelled, or tasted is more accurate than recording an interpretation of it.

### Measurement

Measurement is a form of observation. The method is considered separately to indicate that certain data are conducive to more precise observa-

---

*The terms *palpation, percussion,* and *auscultation* are specific to the individual client. Refer to physical examination texts for an in-depth explanation of these concepts.

**Table 3-4**  Accurate Observation Data versus Personal Interpretations

| Accurate observation data | Personal interpretations |
| --- | --- |
| **Individual client** | |
| Shoulder-length, dark brown hair with dull sheen | Long, dirty brown hair |
| Smiles frequently | Appears to be happy |
| Nail beds pink, rapid capillary refill of toes and fingers | Good circulation of extremities |
| **Family client** | |
| Mother does not look at son when he speaks | Mother angry at son |
| Parents laugh when speaking about sexual history | Parents pleased with sex life |
| Articles of clothing lying on floor and furniture | Messy house |
| **Community client** | |
| Sounds of two local factories present | Noisy environment |
| Garbage cans standing upright with lids on | Neat neighborhood |
| All board members present at meeting | Active and interested people on board |

**Table 3-5**  Accurate Measurement Data versus Personal Interpretations

| Accurate measurement data | Personal interpretations |
| --- | --- |
| **Individual client** | |
| Blood pressure 130/76 | Normal blood pressure |
| Smoked 10 cigarettes in 1-hour interview | Smokes a lot |
| Height 5'4", weight 120 lb | Average height and weight |
| **Family client** | |
| Four rooms in house with six family members | Inadequate space for family |
| Sister interrupted brother five times in 30 minutes | Sister doesn't respect brother's right to talk |
| Mother's age, 40 yr; father's age, 40 yr; child's age, 2 yr | Late starting childbearing; didn't want child earlier or infertility problem |
| **Community client** | |
| Fifteen homes located in one city block | Crowded neighborhood |
| Population 3000 | Small town |

tion. Measurement is used to ascertain the extent, dimensions, rate, rhythm, quantity, or size, frequently through the use of instruments in addition to the senses. Some forms of measurement data are laboratory values, vital signs, and height and weight for the individual client; number and ages of family members and number of rooms in dwelling for the family client; and population, number of blocks in a district, and epidemiological data for the community client. General observation data that can be quantified are also considered measurement date (for example, observation datum: smoked cigarettes during interview; measurement datum: smoked five cigarettes during 30-minute interview). Table 3-5 gives examples of accurate measurement data in contrast to personal interpretations of measurement data.

Again, stating or recording data precisely is more accurate than recording a personal interpretation. Only after data are clustered, validated, and analyzed (compared with theories, norms, and standards) should inferences be made.

## USE OF MODELS FOR DATA COLLECTION

Nursing and related models provide systematic direction for data collection. The definitions of the major concepts either directly or indirectly suggest ways to obtain relevant information and the data that should be collected. The concepts also help the nurse to organize pertinent clinical data meaningfully. Typically, no single model is sufficiently comprehensive to use in isolation; others may be needed to supplement an individualized and multifocal assessment of the client situation. Some specific examples of models relevant to data collection of individual, family, and community clients are given in subsequent chapters.

## DOCUMENTING DATA

The recording of interaction, observation, and measurement data is facilitated by the use of a columnar approach for educational purposes. This format allows the nurse to note the sequence and methods used to collect data. Depending on the client situation, two of the three methods are used predominantly. The width of the data collection columns can vary accordingly. For example, an infant client can provide minimal, if any, verbal data. Some interaction data may be obtained from the parent or staff; therefore, the interaction column would be the smallest.

When recording data in the client's record, the nurse notes appropriate data from all three methods of data collection. The data may be organized in a variety of ways. The initial entries are made on the nursing data base, health history, or client assessment forms designated by the agency, institution, or practice. Subsequent data entries are made according to the expected documentation procedure. The data may be clustered according to major concepts of a model; nursing diagnoses; problems; goals; or systems. A combination of approaches also could be used.

## Example

| Interaction | Observation | Measurement |
| --- | --- | --- |
| Statements from client/parent/staff | Observations of client/record | Measurements of client |

## GUIDELINES FOR DATA COLLECTION

The American Nurses' Association (1973) standards for nursing practice are the basis for most of the following guidelines for data collection. These guidelines are appropriate for data collection regarding all clients.

1. *A systematic format is used for data collection.* Data collection is systematic. Specific nursing and related models provide guides for data collection. Other, more eclectic approaches are useful as well. The nurse begins data collection by assessing the client's major concern first, including multifocal influences related to the concern. Next, a more general assessment of the client's health status is included, if appropriate, based on the selected model, the client situation, and the practice setting.

2. *The data are comprehensive and multifocal.* The data reflect the life experiences of the client. Whatever the client group (individual, family, or community), the nurse considers socioeconomic, political, biophysical, developmental, cultural, psychological, and spiritual influences. Given the amount of potential data that can be obtained from or about any client, a totally comprehensive data collection is unlikely. Yet the data must represent a variety of factors that influence the client's patterns of living. The nurse uses judgment in focusing data collection on areas most pertinent to the client's health situation.

3. *A variety of sources is used for data collection.* The client is usually the primary source for data collection, but inasmuch as perceptions of events and circumstances vary, other sources are also necessary. Validation of data through a variety of sources strengthens the nurse's assessment. Specific examples of sources are given in the following chapters on data collection from individual, family, and community clients. Some general examples of data sources include the client, family, and signifi-

cant others; health care personnel; printed information concerning client; and written records.

4. *Appropriate methods are used for data collection.* At least two data collection methods are used to ensure validity of data obtained. The appropriateness of the methods depends on the client's age, health status, and sources used.

5. *The data are verifiable.* The data gathered through the use of interaction, observation, and measurement can be substantiated. The nurse's personal interpretations or perceptions of a situation may lead to further data collection but should not be stated as data themselves. Data are confirmed by obtaining additional information from the client or other sources. Interaction, observation, and measurement skills are used to validate and clarify the client's (or other's) statements, nurse's observations, and any incongruencies in the data.

6. *The data reflect updating of information.* Data collection is continuous. The data reflect appropriate updating of information from the variety of sources used. As new data are obtained, any changes in the health concerns or status of the client also should be noted.

7. *The data are recorded and communicated appropriately.* Data collection is virtually useless unless it is communicated appropriately in the client's record. To increase nurses' accountability and responsibility for data collection, information is written and kept in a retrievable record-keeping system.

## SUMMARY

A variety of factors influencing the process of data collection are discussed, along with the importance of the nurse-client relationship. Interaction, observation, and measurement are the three methods used for data collection. General guidelines are identified to facilitate application and an accurate assessment of the client's health status, strengths, and concerns. Chapters 4 through 6 provide specific examples of these guidelines as applied to data collection for the individual, family, and community client.

## REFERENCES AND READINGS

American Nurses' Association: Standards: nursing practice, Kansas City, Mo, 1973, The Association.

American Nurses' Association: Nursing: a social policy statement, Kansas City, Mo, 1980, The Association.

Arnold E and Boggs K: Interpersonal relationships: professional communication skills for nurses, Philadelphia, 1989, WB Saunders Co.

Atkinson LD and Murray ME: Understanding the nursing process, ed 3, New York, 1986, Macmillan, Inc.

Bates B: A guide to physical examination, ed 4, Philadelphia, 1987, JB Lippincott Co.

Benner P: From novice to expert: excellence and power in clinical nursing practice, Menlo Park, Calif, 1984, Addison-Wesley Co.

Carnevali D: Nursing care planning: diagnosis and management, ed 3, Philadelphia, 1983, JB Lippincott Co.

Enelow AJ and Swisher SN: Interviewing and patient care, ed 3, New York, 1986, Oxford University Press.

Malasanos L, Barkauskas V, Moss M, and Stoltenberg-Allen K: Health assessment, ed 5, St Louis, 1990, The CV Mosby Co.

Marriner A: The nursing process: a scientific approach to nursing care, ed 3, St Louis, 1983, The CV Mosby Co.

Murray RB and Zentner JP: Nursing assessment and health promotion strategies through the life span, ed 4, Englewood Cliffs, NJ, 1988, Prentice-Hall, Inc.

Rew L and Borrow EM: Intuition: a neglected hallmark of nursing knowledge, Adv Nurs Sci 10:49, 1987.

Rogers C: On becoming a person, Boston, 1961, Houghton Mifflin Co.

Sierra-Franco MH: Therapeutic communication in nursing, New York, 1978, McGraw-Hill Book Co.

Stuart GW and Sundeen SJ: Principles and practice of psychiatric nursing, ed 3, St Louis, 1987, The CV Mosby Co.

Sundeen SJ, Stuart GW, Rankin ED, and Cohen SA: Nurse-client interaction: implementing the nursing process, ed 4, St Louis, 1989, The CV Mosby Co.

Watson AB and Mayers MG: Assessment and documentation: nursing theories in action, Thorofare, NJ, 1981, Charles B Slack, Inc.

CHAPTER

4

# Assessment: Data Collection for the Individual Client

PAULA J. CHRISTENSEN

## GENERAL CONSIDERATIONS

Historically, the individual client has been the main focus of nursing care. Nurses now realize that caring for the individual involves working with more than the client and his or her isolated health concerns. The client's family and significant others, beliefs, and background all influence the client and subsequent care. A *nursing data base* is essential to identify the client's responses to health concerns. Thus the way in which nurses collect and organize data is important so that appropriate nursing diagnoses may be generated. The *client's perceptions* of health concerns and related responses, reasons for seeking health care, and expectations for achieving optimum health are essential data in the nursing assessment. Data reflecting the client's biographical status and biophysical, psychological, sociocultural, and spiritual health are needed to ensure a multifocal approach to care. All three methods for data collection— interaction, observation, and measurement—are used to obtain a comprehensive and accurate set of data.

Nurses use their empirical and personal knowledge, experience, and clinical judgment for determining the type of data to obtain during the assessment. Data should be collected that are relevant to generating nursing diagnoses for independent nursing actions (health promotion, maintenance, and restoration or referral) as well as collaborative biomedical health concerns (pathological condition or medical treatment). Ongoing assessment and monitoring of both the nursing and biomedical domains are important to the practicing professional nurse.

This chapter describes the phases of assessment applied to the individual client. A discussion of the types of biographical data needed and the sources of information is included. Examples of selected models used to guide data collection for the individual client are also provided. Some sample methods and questions are given to facilitate the nurse's use of models during assessment.

### Preliminary Information

Preliminary biographical information is obtained during the initial interview with the client. Most agencies have a specific form indicating what information is needed. The box on p. 65 provides an example of important biographical data. A directive-interrogative interview approach is frequently used to complete the data form. Ideally, much of the information could be obtained during an open-ended discussion.

Other preliminary information for the individual client includes a brief assessment of the client's health concerns and strengths. Many health care agencies provide a guideline, such as a nursing history form, for obtaining these data. Often, the forms are organized according to patterns of biophysical health such as nutrition, elimination, rest/ sleep, activity/exercise, and hygiene; psychological health such as coping, interaction, and self-concept; sociocultural health such as cultural practices, recreation, and significant relationships; and spiritual health such as religious beliefs and values. Figure 4-1 is an example of a nursing history form. Modifications of this type of form are made to individualize data collection for clients from different age groups (children, elderly) or for clients experi-

---

### Biographical Data

Name _____
Address _____
Age _____
Date of birth _____
Place of birth _____
Gender _____
Ethnic group _____
Religious preference _____
Primary language spoken _____
Marital status _____
Education _____
Occupation _____
Health insurance _____
Income _____

---

encing similar health concerns (pregnancy, chronic illness).

It is important for the nurse to ascertain the client's responses to the health concern and how the concern affects the client's lifestyle. Additional data are obtained to ensure a multifocal and comprehensive data base after the nursing model is chosen to guide further data collection.

### Sources of Data

The individual client is usually the primary source of data. Other sources used to collect data are

Family and significant others
Survey of client's physical environment
Medical records
Social service records
Developmental records
Results of diagnostic tests
Nursing care conferences

Nursing notes
Nursing rounds
Change of shift reports
Progress notes
Kardex
Health team members

### MODELS FOR DATA COLLECTION

Models provide useful approaches to data collection. They give direction to obtaining systematic and purposeful data. The nurse decides which model or combination of models is appropriate for the client's age, health status, and situation. The nurse's knowledge of various models and the client situation determine the choice. For example, if a nurse is working in an emergency room or on a telephone hotline, a crisis-oriented model is most appropriate. If the client population requires long-term care, a model addressing promotion of self-care and optimum independence is the choice. The

chosen format is considered a *general guide* for data collection, not a rigid tool.

Initial data collection focuses on the client's primary expressed concerns and how the concerns affect or are affected by other patterns of living. Additional data are obtained using the major concepts of the chosen nursing model, along with any other supplemental concepts that facilitate a multifocal view of the client's health situation. For example, if the client's expressed concern is psychological, related to coping with stress, the nurse begins by assessing psychological coping and health. To obtain multifocal data, the nurse uses the nursing model and related psychological concepts to determine the nature and scope of additional information needed as to how the client's stress affects or is affected by other patterns of living.

### Nursing Model

A number of nursing models assist with systematic data collection of individuals. Chapter 2 provides examples of current nursing models. Also, several nursing textbooks provide an overview of nursing models, for example, Roy and Reihl (1980) and Fitzpatrick and Whall (1983). The ensuing discussion focuses on the use of one nursing model, developed by Sr. Callista Roy (1984) as a systematic format for data collection.

Roy provides a multifocal approach in her first-level assessment of the client's four modes of adaptation. The adaptive or effector modes are identified as physiological, self-concept, role function, and interdependence. The *physiological mode* includes activity and rest, nutrition, elimination, oxygenation, fluids and electrolytes, endocrine function, skin integrity, the senses, and neurological function. The *self-concept mode* incorporates the physical self and personal self. *Role function* involves role performance and role mastery as well as primary, secondary, and tertiary roles. The need for affectional adequacy and support systems of family, friends, and community are all parts of the *interdependence mode*.

During first-level assessment, the nurse determines the client's adaptive and ineffective behaviors in each of the four modes. Examples of methods (and questions) for data collection using this model are shown in Table 4-1. The methods are arranged according to interactions, observations, and measurements. After the first-level assessment, the nurse then determines the focal, contextual, and residual stimuli that contribute to each ineffective or adaptive behavior needing reinforcement. This second-level assessment focuses on the factors that influence the behaviors of concern. They are di-

*Text continued on p. 72.*

# ROCKFORD MEMORIAL HOSPITAL ADMISSION/ASSESSMENT RECORD

## GENERAL INFORMATION

Date _____ Time _____ Mode of Entry _____ From _____ To Room _____

Accompanied by: Name _____ Phone _____

Person to Contact _____

Disposition of: Clothes _____ Money/Jewelry _____ Meds _____

Oriented to: Bed _____ Bathroom _____ Intercom _____ Call Light _____

Personal electrical equipment inspected: (list) _____

Vitals: Temp ____ P ____ R ____ BP ____ HT ____ WT ____

PROCEDURES/TREATMENTS/NOTES *Documentation for Same-Day admission surgical patients*

_____
_____
_____
_____
_____
_____

Signature _____

## HEALTH AND ILLNESS PERCEPTION          STRENGTH _____ CONCERN _____

*Remainder of this page omitted due to completion of pre-admission history ☐*

Reason for this admission as stated by patient: (Describe symptoms)

Patient's understanding of problem: ☐ Excellent ☐ Good ☐ More explanation needed

Describe previous general health: _____

## HEALTH HISTORY

| Medical: | Surgical | Allergies and Transfusions: (describe reaction) |
|---|---|---|
| | | |

## HEALTH MAINTENANCE          Strength _____ Concern _____

Menstruation _____ Self Breast Exam _____ Pap Smear _____ Last Period _____

Contraceptives _____ Testicular check/Prostate _____

Smoking _____ Pack/Day _____ Caffeine _____ Alcohol _____ Recreational Drugs _____

Last Meal _____

## FAMILY HISTORY

Diabetes _____ Arthritis _____
Cancer _____ TB _____
Hypertension _____ Seizures _____
Cardiac _____ Anemia _____
Renal _____
Other _____

| MED/DOSE | TIMES | LAST DOSE | MED/DOSE | TIMES | LAST DOSE |
|---|---|---|---|---|---|
| | | | | | |
| | | | | | |
| | | | | | |
| | | | | | |
| | | | | | |
| | | | | | |

Have you had problems maintaining your medication schedule: _____

## ACTIVITY–EXERCISE–SELF CARE          *(Please circle any positive findings)*          STRENGTH _____ CONCERN _____

Exercise/Work Pattern/Energy Level: _____

Self-Care Abilities:

Grade ADL by 0 = Independent; 1 = Needs Equipment; 2 = Needs Person; 3 = Equipment & Person; 4 = Dependent

Personal Hygiene: ____ Dressing: ____ Feeding: ____ Ambulating/Transfers: ____

Disabilities: ____ Prosthesis: ____ Equipment: ____

CARDIAC

Apical/radial strong and regular, chest pain, neck vein distention, pacemaker, palpitations, fainting, orthopnea, vertigo

PULMONARY

Normal/Abnormal breath sounds, coughing, asthma, hemoptysis, sputum, dyspnea, cyanosis

PERIPHERAL VASCULAR

Peripheral pulses present, varicosities, claudication, vascular access: (Describe)

NEURO-MUSCULAR-ORTHO

Orientation: _____
Sensation: _____
Movement: _____
Gait: _____

66

ROCKFORD MEMORIAL HOSPITAL **ADMISSION/ASSESSMENT RECORD**

| NUTRITIONAL & METABOLIC | STRENGTH _____ CONCERN _____ |

Special diet/Weight loss diet _____
Supplements _____ Intolerance _____
Weight gain or loss within last six months _____
Appetite _____
Poor swallowing, nausea and vomiting, poor dentition, change of taste _____

| INTEGUMENTARY | STRENGTH _____ CONCERN _____ |

Warm and dry, rash, lesions, petechiae, jaundice, discoloration _____
Number identified areas and describe: _____

| MUCOUS MEMBRANES/MOUTH | STRENGTH _____ CONCERN _____ |

Pink and moist _____
Teeth: _____ Dentures _____ Upper _____ Lower _____ Partial Plate _____
Hair: Distribution, texture, loss _____
Nails: Changes in color, texture _____

| ELIMINATION | STRENGTH _____ CONCERN _____ |

BOWEL: Pattern: _____ Last Bowel Movement: _____ Bowel Sounds: _____
Bowel Management _____
Constipation, diarrhea, hemorrhoids, bleeding, incontinence, ostomy: _____
Change in appearance of stools: _____
URINE: Clear, incontinence, dribbling, retention, dysuria, urgency, frequency, hesitancy, nocturia, discharge, urinary diversion _____
Changes in appearance of urine: _____
Urinary Devices: _____
ABDOMEN: Soft, tender, distended, rigid _____

| COGNITIVE & PERCEPTUAL | STRENGTH _____ CONCERN _____ |

Vision: _____ Visual Aids: _____
Hearing: _____ Hearing Aids: _____
Communication Barriers: _____
Thought Process Disturbances: Describe changes in memory, learning abilities, decision making: _____

| PAIN | STRENGTH _____ CONCERN _____ |

Location: _____
Description: _____
Intensity (0-10): _____ Precipitating Factors: _____
Relieving Factors: _____

| SLEEP - REST |

STRENGTH _____
CONCERN _____
Sleep Pattern: _____
Hrs/Night: _____ Times: _____
Naps: _____ Aids/Rituals: _____
Problems getting to sleep, waking early, dreams, nightmares, confusion at night: _____

| HOME MAINTENANCE | STRENGTH _____ CONCERN _____ |

1. Prior to this admission lived: Alone, With Family or other person, in Long Term Care Facility ( _____ Name of Facility).
2. Prior to this admission, required assistance for activities of daily living: Never, _____ days/month.
3. If support services were used at home, who provided them: _____
4. Considering the current reason for admission and recent history, what level of service is likely to be needed at discharge: None _____ Home Services _____ Long-Term Care _____

| VALUES - BELIEFS | STRENGTH _____ CONCERN _____ |

Spiritual Needs: _____ Referral to Pastoral Services: _____

| GROWTH AND DEVELOPMENT-ROLE RELATIONSHIP-COPING | STRENGTH _____ CONCERN _____ |

Who lives with you: _____
Occupation: _____ Who or what helps you handle stress: _____
Have you had any major life changes? _____

| SAFETY |

LEVEL I _____ Inability to understand/follow directions
_____ No problems noted at this time _____ History of falls prior to this admission (within 6 months)
LEVEL II _____
_____ Age over 70 LEVEL IV
_____ Hypotension, including orthostatic _____ Disoriented and restless
_____ Incontinence - bowel or bladder _____ One occurrence of falling during hospitalization
_____ Uncompensated Sensory Impairment - visual, auditory, or tactile _____ Triad of ambulation difficulty, bowel/bladder incontinence or urgency, and inability to follow directions.
_____ Dizziness/balance problems
LEVEL III _____
_____ Disorientation or history of intermittent confusion

Level Assignment _____ Safety brochure discussed _____
Level Reassignment _____
Primary Nurse: _____
Signature: _____ Date _____
Signature: _____ Date _____

**Fig. 4-1.** Example nursing history form. (Used with permission from Rockford Memorial Hospital, Rockford, IL.)

**Table 4-1**   Data Collection of Individual Client Based on Roy's Model

| Area of data collection | Interactions | Observations | Measurements |
|---|---|---|---|
| **A. Physiological mode*** | | | |
| 1. Activity and rest | What kinds of physical activity do you engage in? How long has it been since you've exercised?<br>What type of work do you do for a living?<br>Are you satisfied with the amount of exercise you get each week? | What is the tone of the client's muscles?<br>Are height and weight proportional?<br>Is any atrophy present?<br>Observe motor function:<br>  Muscle masses<br>  Joint mobility<br>  Posture and gait<br>  Coordination | Frequency and regularity of exercise<br>Duration of physical exercise<br>Length of time since client has exercised<br>Height and weight |
| | How much sleep and rest do you get each 24 hours?<br>Do you take naps?<br>Do you feel rested with the amount of sleep you get?<br>What helps you sleep (e.g., backrubs, music)?<br>How often do you wake up during the night? | What is the client's non-verbal language?<br>  Yawning<br>  Circles under eyes<br>  Concentration on discussion | Usual number of hours of sleep and rest<br>Number of hours sleep and rest needed to feel rested<br>Medications and dose used for sleep |
| 2. Nutrition | How many meals do you eat per day?<br>How much and what types of liquid do you drink each day?<br>What is your knowledge of the four basic food groups?<br>With whom do you eat?<br>Where do you eat your meals?<br>How often do you eat at home? In restaurants?<br>Do you take daily vitamins? With iron? With minerals?<br>Any recent changes in diet or weight?<br>Any increase or decrease in appetite?<br>What kind of foods can and do you eat? | What are the tone, texture, and coloring of skin and mucous membranes?<br>Are height and weight proportional?<br><br>What is the texture of hair? Condition of scalp?<br>What is the condition of nails? | Three-day recall: specific food and fluid intake for 3 days<br>Height and weight<br>Fat caliper reading<br>Lab results: CBC, electrolytes |
| 3. Elimination | How often do you urinate and have a bowel movement?<br>What do your bowel movements look like (consistency, color)?<br>What does your urine look like (clarity, color)?<br>Do you have any burning or foul smell of your urine? | What are the color and odor of the urine?<br>What are the consistency and color of stools? | Frequency and amount of urination<br>Frequency of bowel movement<br>Amount and kind of laxative, bulk agent, or enemas<br>Lab results: urine and feces |

*Physical examination: inspection, auscultation, palpation, and percussion of all physiological patterns.

**Table 4-1** Data Collection of Individual Client Based on Roy's Model—cont'd

| Area of data collection | Interactions | Observations | Measurements |
|---|---|---|---|
| | Do you need laxatives to have a bowel movement? Enemas? | | |
| | Do you experience any pain during a bowel movement? | | |
| 4. Oxygenation | Do you smoke cigarettes? Cigars? A pipe? | What are the color and temperature of extremities? Face? | Number of cigarettes, cigars, or pipes smoked per day |
| | Do you inhale the smoke? | Note characteristics of respirations, use of accessory muscles, cough. | Number of seconds it takes for capillary refill |
| | What do you understand about the effects of smoking? | Is there rapid capillary refill when toenails and fingernails are pinched? | Blood pressure, pulses, respirations, temperature |
| | Are your arms or legs unusually cool to the touch? | | ECG |
| | Do you have any bleeding problems? | What is the color of mucous membranes? | Lab results: CBC, prothrombin time |
| | Do you have high blood pressure? | Are pedal pulses palpable? | |
| | Do you experience chest pains, shortness of breath, or "fluttering" in your chest? Any cough? | | |
| 5. Fluid and electrolytes | How much fluid do you drink per day? | What is the client's skin turgor? | Amount of fluid drunk per day |
| | Are you unusually thirsty? | What is the condition of the mucous membranes? | Blood pressure, pulse, respiration, temperature |
| | Do you have a history of high blood pressure? | Is dependent edema present? | Medication and dose |
| | Are you receiving any medication to regulate your blood pressure or "water" in your body? | Note signs of fatigue, restlessness, level of consciousness. | Measurement of ankles |
| | Do you add salt to food while cooking? At the table? | | ECG |
| | Do you take any potassium supplements? | | Lab results: CBC, electrolytes, urinalysis |
| 6. Endocrine function | Are you cold or hot most of the time? | Are height and weight proportional? | Temperature |
| | Do you have a history of diabetes? Thyroid problems? If so, what medications are you taking? | What are the texture and appearance of body hair? Skin? | Names and doses of medications |
| | Women: | | Blood pressure, pulse, respirations, temperature |
| | Have you ever had any difficulty with hormones? | | Lab results: thyroid function, hormone levels |
| | When was onset of secondary sex characteristics? | | |
| | Are you taking birth control pills? | | |

*Continued.*

**Table 4-1**   Data Collection of Individual Client Based on Roy's Model—cont'd

| Area of data collection | Interactions | Observations | Measurements |
|---|---|---|---|
| | How old were you when your first period started?<br>When was your last period?<br>How often do you get your period?<br>Do you know how to examine your breasts?<br>Do you have regular Pap smears? | | Date of last menstrual period<br>Number of days in usual cycle<br>Frequency of self-examination of breasts |
| 7. Skin integrity | Describe your skin condition. Is it dry, oily, itchy?<br>Do you have any rashes or cuts?<br>Are you able to sense pain and change in temperature? | What is the condition of the skin?<br>Temperature<br>Turgor<br>Pigmentation<br>Character<br>Perspiration | Size of areas affected by dryness, rash<br>Length of break in integument |
| 8. Senses | Do you have difficulty with your sight? Hearing? Touch? Taste? Smell?<br>How long have you had the difficulty?<br>How has this affected your lifestyle?<br>What have you done to compensate for this change?<br>Are you experiencing any pain? When did it start? Is it constant, or does it come and go? Describe the pain. | Are there any physical defects in the client's eyes, ears, nose, tongue, hands, or skin?<br><br>Note nonverbal indications of sensory impairment:<br>Difficulty seeing or hearing<br>Pain | Number of impairments<br>Duration of time affected by the difficulty |
| 9. Neurological function | Have you noticed any changes in your attention span? Alertness? Memory?<br>Do you have any difficulty swallowing? Eating? Walking?<br>Have you ever experienced a seizure? When? How many?<br>Do you have tremors? Where? How long? | Note level of consciousness, orientation, gait.<br>Look for changes in facial, mouth, and neck function (cranial nerves).<br>Check for:<br>Pupil reactivity<br>Strength and equality of grip and foot push<br>Sense of pain and light touch | Reflex function<br>EEG<br>Lab results: blood gases, electrolytes<br>Blood pressure, pulse, respiration, temperature |
| B. Self-concept mode<br>  1. Physical self | What is your highest and lowest weight?<br>Have you had any physical alterations of your body?<br>Was or is it difficult for you to accept those changes? | What is the nature of the client's clothes? Tight or loose-fitting?<br>Does the client shield or avoid touching or looking at certain areas of the body?<br>What is the nature of | Height and weight |

**Table 4-1**  Data Collection of Individual Client Based on Roy's Model—cont'd

| Area of data collection | Interactions | Observations | Measurements |
|---|---|---|---|
| | How have those changes affected your relationship with others?<br>How do you feel about your weight and appearance? | scars, deformed body parts, and alterations in function?<br>Whom does the client interact with?<br>What is the client's affect? | |
| 2. Personal self | What religion and values were you raised with? Do you practice them now?<br>What kind of involvement do you have with your church? Are you comfortable with that?<br>How do you usually express your feelings and thoughts to others? Are there some times when you don't? When are they?<br>Describe some characteristics of the type of person you'd most like to be. Do you see yourself as that person? Is your description realistic to you?<br>What do you do when you have a problem?<br>How do you see yourself in relation to other people? Better than? Equal to? Less than equal to? | Note nonverbal communication:<br>Body language<br>Eye contact<br>Gestures<br>Affect<br>Tone of voice<br>How is the client groomed?<br>Hair<br>Clothes<br>Nails<br>Teeth<br>Skin | Frequency of attendance at church-related or spiritual activities |
| C. Role function mode | What is your family's expectations of you? Significant others' expectations of you?<br>Are these people clear in expressing their expectations? Are they expressed verbally, through actions, or hints?<br>What do you think others expect of you?<br>What are your expectations of yourself? How do they fit with what others expect of you?<br>What do you do for a living? Are you meeting your own and others' expectations at work? Are they compatible? If | Note activities of the client:<br>Parenting<br>Studying<br>Reading<br>Cooking<br>Cleaning<br>Leisure<br>Being sick<br>Occupation<br>Gender | How much time per day or week the client spends in various activities listed<br>Age |

*Continued.*

**Table 4-1**   Data Collection of Individual Client Based on Roy's Model—cont'd

| Area of data collection | Interactions | Observations | Measurements |
|---|---|---|---|
| | not, do you talk with those concerned?<br>Do you feel overextended? Underachieving? | | |
| D. Interdependence mode | Who are the people in your family? To whom do you feel closest? For what reasons?<br>Who are other people important to you?<br>Who do you socialize with other than your family? How often? Are you satisfied with this contact?<br>What activities in and outside the home are you involved with?<br>How do you see yourself fitting into your family? Your group of friends?<br>Do you feel in competition with family or friends (for example, material goods or status)?<br>What do you do to show affection and caring for others?<br>How do others show affection and love toward you?<br>Are you satisfied with the amount of affection you show others? They show you?<br>Do you have any pets? What are their names? | Note nonverbal signs while interacting with others (such as family, friends, interviewer, pets).<br>Observe nurturing behaviors: care and attention, protection, recognition, offering help, signs of love/respect/value, touch.<br>Observe client's ability to receive nurturing from others. | How often the client interacts with family<br>Number of people or activities the client interacts with outside work and family<br>Number of pets |

rectly related to the etiological clause in the nursing diagnosis statement.

## Eclectic Data Collection Models
### General Eclectic Model

Specific assessment data to determine patterns of health can be obtained using a variety of general concepts in an eclectic multifocal model. Viewing the individual client as a bio-psycho-socio-spiritual being provides a basis for data collection. The concepts within this model are compatible with most nursing models. The eclectic model is particularly useful in combination with a nursing model because many nursing models are limited in their scope. Therefore, the nurse can use these concepts as a guide for a nursing data base along with the major concepts of a nursing model to obtain comprehensive and multifocal data. The box on p. 73 shows a format based on this model. The sequence of these concepts and patterns listed provides an order that the nurse may use throughout the interview and examination process. This order provides a systematic and purposeful approach to data collection. The nature and amount of data obtained vary, depending on the client's health status, type of setting, purpose of interaction, data sources, the

## Format for Data Collection Using Biopsychosociospiritual Model

Informant _____
Major concern _____
History of major concern _____
Current health status
   Biophysical health
      Mental status _____
      Daily activity patterns
         Nutrition _____
         Elimination _____
         Exercise _____
         Hygiene _____
         Substance use _____
         Sleep and rest _____
         Sexual activity _____
      Past biophysical health
         Restorative interventions _____
         Allergies _____
         Immunizations _____
         Growth and development _____
         Foreign travel _____
         Family health history _____
   Psychological health
      Coping patterns _____
      Interaction patterns _____
      Cognitive patterns _____
      Self-concept _____
      Emotional patterns _____
      Sexuality _____
      Family coping patterns _____
   Sociocultural health
      Cultural patterns _____
      Significant relationships _____
      Recreation/leisure patterns _____
      Environment _____
      Economic _____
   Spiritual health
      Religious beliefs and practices _____
      Values and valuing practices _____
Review of systems
Physical examination

nurse's skills and knowledge, and the resources available.

The nurse begins with discussion of the *major concern* and *history of the major concern*. This allows the client to express the primary issues that initiated the need for health care services. By doing this, the nurse has reinforced interest in the client's individual situation.

The *current health status* is addressed next. Most of these data are obtained through interaction and observation. Because the *biophysical health* of the in-

dividual includes numerous facets, assessing each is an overwhelming task. There are, however, some general patterns of biophysical health that serve as a starting point for data collection. Assessing the client's mental status is usually done within the context of the interview. Observations regarding the client's appearance and behavior; speech and language; mood; thought processes, thought content, and perceptions; and cognitive functions (Bates, 1987) are elicited as the nurse interacts with the client. More specific mental status examinations are indicated for clients exhibiting alterations in this function. Daily patterns of nutrition, elimination, exercise, hygiene, substance use, sleep and rest, and sexual activity provide an understanding of the client's biophysical capabilities and limitations. Anatomy and physiology texts as well as sources on health maintenance and promotion give norms of physical appearance and function to guide data collection. Past biophysical health data are important to gain a perspective on the client's current health status. Restorative interventions, such as surgeries and major treatments as well as allergies and immunizations, should be known. Important past health data also include the presence or absence of alterations in growth and development, foreign travel, and family health history, including genetic and familial physical and emotional illnesses.

*Psychological health* is assessed through data collection related to patterns of interaction, cognition, emotions, coping, self-concept, sexuality, and family coping. Texts on mental health, psychology, family theory, sexuality, and communication provide norms of psychological health that guide data collection.

*Sociocultural health* patterns that are important to assess are cultural background, significant relationships, and recreation. Data concerning the client's environment and economic situation also are included. Social patterns are found in sources describing specific cultures, social influences, leisure theory, personal space, and interpersonal relationships, and provide a base for data collection regarding sociological health.

*Spiritual health* includes religious beliefs and practices and values and valuing practices. The congruence of beliefs, values, and their practices is often important in maintaining spiritual health. References that deal with the "meaning of life" issues, specific religious practices, and valuing help the nurse collect data about spiritual health patterns.

Table 4-2 provides a general eclectic model and examples of methods that can be used for data collection regarding biophysical, psychological, sociocultural, and spiritual health patterns.

The *review of systems* data are obtained primarily through the interaction method. The nurse interviews the client regarding the function and suspected dysfunction of the major systems of the body. Some systems are addressed in the aforementioned daily activity patterns of biophysical health, and there is no need to repeat them. The focus is on other systems, such as skin, eyes, cardiac, respiratory, and musculoskeletal. Refer to

texts regarding health history and physical assessment for in-depth guidance in obtaining these data.

A *physical examination* or assessment is needed to validate data obtained during interviews and to obtain new data. Whether the nurse conducts the initial complete physical examination is determined by the accepted procedure of the agency, institution, or practice. Ongoing physical assessment is done by the nurse to assess the client's functional abilities and behaviors, to monitor the client's condition to detect changes or trends, and to determine need for consultation or referral to other health care professionals. Observation and measurement methods are used through the skills of inspection, auscultation, palpation, and percussion to perform physical assessments. The nature and amount of physical assessment data obtained is dependent on the situation. Whatever the scope of data, a systematic approach should be used. In general, a cephalocaudal/regional format is usually appropriate. Components of a complete physical examination include observation and pertinent measurement of the major body systems and functions. Physical examination and health assessment texts provide norms for the anatomy and physiology of systems and functions, and techniques of examination.

### Gordon's Framework

Gordon (1987) presents an eclectic multifocal model for data collection based on 11 functional health patterns. This assessment structure can be applied to many of the nursing models as well. She recommends that the nurse obtain the history of the patterns during the interview and then examine the client for indicators of patterns. The functional health patterns identified by Gordon (1987:93) are (1) health perception-health management, (2) nutritional-metabolic, (3) elimination, (4) activity-exercise, (5) cognitive-perceptual, (6) sleep-rest, (7) self-perception–self-concept, (8) role-relationship, (9) sexuality-reproductive, (10) coping-stress tolerance, and (11) value-belief.

In her work, Gordon defines each pattern and gives questions and direction to guide the nursing history and client examination.

### Other Models

Models from other disciplines are useful in providing a systematic approach to data collection. A more general or multifocal model is Maslow's (1968) work on hierarchy of needs.

Developmental models are more specific and limited in scope. Erikson (1963) discusses psychosocial development throughout the life span for

*Text continued on p. 85.*

**Table 4-2**  Data Collection of Individual Client Based on Eclectic Assessment Model

| Area of data collection | Interactions | Observations | Measurements |
|---|---|---|---|
| I.  Current Health Status | | | |
| A.  Biophysical health* | | | |
| 1.  Mental status | | | |
| a.  Appearance and behavior | | What is the client wearing? Is it appropriate for the environment? Any visible alterations in function? Note steadiness of gait, movements, posture. Is the client awake and alert? Does the client respond appropriately to questions? How is the hygiene and grooming? Hair Clothes Teeth Skin Nails | |
| b.  Speech and language | | Note characteristics of speech (quantity, rate, volume, fluency). Is the client able to express self with language? | |
| c.  Mood | How do you feel about the health concerns you are experiencing? | Note nonverbal communications: body language, eye contact, gestures, affect, facial expressions. | |
| d.  Thought processes, thought content, and perceptions | | Note logical progression of client's speech and explanations. Are the client's statements relevant to the situation? Do the client's perceptions of the situation seem grounded in reality? | |
| e.  Cognitive functions | | Is the client oriented to time, place, and person? Note the client's ability to maintain attention on conversation. | |
| 2.  Daily activity patterns | | | |
| a.  Nutrition | What kind of foods can and do you eat? How many meals do you eat per day? | What are the tone, texture, and coloring of skin and mucous membranes? | Three-day recall: specific food and fluid intake for 3 days Height and weight |

*Physical examination: inspection, auscultation, palpation, and percussion of all physiological patterns.            *Continued.*

**Table 4-2**   Data Collection of Individual Client Based on Eclectic Assessment Model—cont'd

| Area of data collection | Interactions | Observations | Measurements |
|---|---|---|---|
| | What is your knowledge of the four basic food groups? Whom do you eat with? Where do you eat your meals? How often do you eat at home? In restaurants? Do you take daily vitamins? With iron? With minerals? Any recent changes in diet or weight? Any increase or decrease in appetite? | Are height and weight proportional? What is the texture of hair? Condition of scalp? What is the condition of nails? Gums? Teeth? | Lab results: CBC, electrolytes |
| b. Elimination | How often do you urinate and have bowel movements? What do your bowel movements look like (consistency, color)? What does your urine look like (clarity, color)? Do you have any burning, or foul smell to your urine? Do you need laxatives to have a bowel movement? Enemas? Do you experience pain during a bowel movement? | What are the color and odor of the urine? Describe the consistency and color of stools. | Frequency and amount of urination Frequency of bowel movements Amount and kind of laxative, bulk agent, or enema used Lab results: urine and feces |
| c. Exercise | What kinds of physical activity do you engage in? How long has it been since you've done them? What type of work do you do for a living? Are you satisfied with the amount of exercise you get each week? | What is the tone of the client's muscles? Are height and weight proportional? Is atrophy present? | Duration of physical activity Length of time since client has exercised Height and weight |
| d. Hygiene | Describe how you take care of your body. Do you prefer baths, showers, or sink baths? Morning or evening? Do you use deoderant agents or cologne? How often do you brush your teeth? Floss? When did you last visit your dentist? | Are clothes, hair, and nails groomed? What is the condition of scalp and hair? Note odors (body and mouth), makeup, and appearance of teeth. | Frequency of hygiene Frequency of oral care Date of last dentist visit |
| e. Substance use | Do you smoke cigarettes or cigars? What is your understand- | What are the person's nonverbal messages while smoking? Jittery? | Number of cigarettes or cigars smoked during interview |

**Table 4-2** Data Collection of Individual Client Based on Eclectic Assessment Model—cont'd

| Area of data collection | Interactions | Observations | Measurements |
|---|---|---|---|
| | ing of the effects of smoking? Do you inhale the smoke? Do you drink alcoholic beverages? Whom do you drink with? Do you drink alone? Do you smoke marijuana or use any tranquilizers or stimulants (coffee, tea, cola)? What is your understanding of the use of marijuana and drugs? Do you use drugs and alcohol at the same time? | Quick movements? Slow, relaxed movements? Attention span? Ability to understand spoken word? Response time? Note pupil dilation and constriction, hand tremors. | Number of cigarettes or cigars per day Number of drinks per day or week Frequency of use of marijuana and drugs Number of cups of coffee, tea, or cola Amount of marijuana or drugs used at one time |
| f. Sleep and rest | How much sleep and rest do you get each 24 hours? Do you take naps? Do you feel rested with the amount of sleep you get? What helps you sleep (for example, backrubs, music, or warm milk)? How often do you wake up during the night? | What is the client's nonverbal language? Posture Yawning Circles under eyes Concentration on discussion | Number of usual hours of sleep and rest Number of hours sleep and rest needed to feel rested Medication and dose used for sleep |
| g. Sexual activity | Do you feel that your sexual needs are being met? How has your health concern affected your ability or desire to relate sexually? Do your needs coincide with those of your partner? If not, how do you deal with the difference? How are your sexual needs met (for example, intercourse, touching, fondling, or masturbation)? Women: What are your menstrual cycles (periods) like (regularity and discomfort)? How old were you when your first period started? | Note nonverbal communication during discussion: Eye contact Gestures Tone of voice | Frequency of sexual contact<br><br>Date of last menstrual period Usual duration of cycle |

*Continued.*

**Table 4-2**   Data Collection of Individual Client Based on Eclectic Assessment Model—cont'd

| Area of data collection | Interactions | Observations | Measurements |
|---|---|---|---|
| | Do you know how to examine your own breasts?<br><br>Do you have regular Pap smears? | | Frequency of self-examination of breasts<br>Number of pregnancies, abortions, miscarriages |
| 3. Past biophysical health | | | |
| a. Restorative interventions | What major illnesses and surgeries have you had?<br>What treatment did you have for them?<br>Was the recovery uneventful?<br>Did these have an impact on your lifestyle?<br>Are you currently being treated for or affected by these incidents?<br>How have these affected your physical functioning? | Any apparent physical dysfunction or limitations? | Dates of major illnesses, injuries, and surgeries<br>Duration of each hospitalization |
| b. Allergies | Are you allergic to any foods, medications, or other substances (dust or animals)?<br>What is your usual reaction?<br>Have you ever been treated for allergies? | Note appearance of eyes and surrounding tissue, presence of sniffling, need to blow nose.<br>Note condition of skin (redness, scaling) and scratching. | |
| c. Immunizations | Are your immunizations up to date?<br>Did you experience any unusual reactions to the immunizations? | Observe documents of immunizations. | Dates of immunizations |
| d. Growth and development | Was your growth and development as a child the same as for other children your age?<br>Did you feel the same as friends and siblings in developing verbal and motor skills? | Depending on client's age, is the person able to carry on a conversation, verbalize thoughts, and follow directions? | Child development measures (such as Denver Developmental Screening Test)<br>Height and weight |
| e. Foreign travel | Have you traveled out of this country?<br>If so, were you exposed to or did you contract any diseases? | | Dates and duration of travel |
| f. Family health history | Do you have any chronic physical or emotional illness in your family (for example, tuberculosis, diabetes, cancer, hypertension, depression, anxiety, heart disease, kidney disease)? | Observe documents indicating familial diseases. | |

**Table 4-2**  Data Collection of Individual Client Based on Eclectic Assessment Model—cont'd

| Area of data collection | Interactions | Observations | Measurements |
|---|---|---|---|
| B. Psychological health | | | |
| 1. Coping patterns | Who are the people significant (who mean a lot) to you? Who can and do you talk to on a regular basis? How much time do you spend alone? How many people do you relate to each day? Do you go out with and see other people on a regular basis? Do you keep to yourself most of the time? Do you exercise regularly? What type? Do you have anyone to go to in times of need (such as family, friends, clergy, social agency)? What do you do to handle stressful situations in your life (for example, *biophysical:* eat, smoke, become agitated, use nervous gestures, sleep, exercise, drink alcoholic beverages, desire sexual activity; *psychological:* become angry with self, become anxious, intellectualize, withdraw, deny, accept, solve the problem; *sociological:* talk with person involved with stress, talk with noninvolved person, blame others, become angry with others; *spiritual:* talk with clergy, pray, listen to music, read religious books, read mind-soothing poetry or prose)? | Note nonverbal communication: Eye contact Gestures Body language Tone of voice Affect | Number of hours each day spent alone Number of times per day or week client sees family and friends Frequency of times client calls on support persons |
| 2. Interaction patterns | Who are the people in your family? How do you usually express your feelings and thoughts to others (for example, directly and verbally, or indirectly | To whom does the client speak in family? Note nonverbal communication during interaction. | Ages of family members |

*Continued.*

**Table 4-2**   Data Collection of Individual Client Based on Eclectic Assessment Model—cont'd

| Area of data collection | Interactions | Observations | Measurements |
|---|---|---|---|
| | through hints and behavior)?<br>What do you think about voicing your opinion or feelings to family? To friends?<br>Do you find ways to blame others for some things you do?<br>What do you do when others make plans that you aren't particularly interested in?<br>Who initiates activities with family? With friends?<br>How do you feel about the way you interact with others? | Does client answer questions or make comments with direct "I" statements? | |
| 3. Cognitive patterns | How much formal education have you had?<br>Can you read?<br>Did or do you have difficulty with school or learning new things?<br>How do you learn best (watching others or reading)?<br>How are you doing in school or at work? | Note verbal ability:<br>Concrete thought<br>Simple sentences<br>Formal operational thought<br>Complex sentences<br>Vocabulary used<br>Ability to conceptualize | Level of education<br>IQ |
| 4. Self-concept | What is your highest weight?<br>Lowest weight?<br>How do you feel about your weight and appearance?<br>Have you had any physical alterations to your body? Was or is it difficult for you to accept those changes?<br>How have those changes affected your relationships with family? Friends? The way you look at yourself?<br>How do you see yourself in relation to other people (such as family, co-workers, friends)? Better than? Equal to? Less than equal to?<br>What religion and social values were you raised with? Are you comfort- | Note nonverbal communication.<br>What is the nature of the client's clothes? Loose, fitted? Clean? Visible soil?<br>Does the client shield or avoid touching or looking at a certain area of the body?<br>What is the nature of any scars, deformed body parts, or alterations in function?<br>Whom does the client interact with?<br>What is the client's affect?<br>How is client groomed?<br>Hair<br>Clothes<br>Nails<br>Teeth<br>Skin | Height and weight<br>Frequency of eye contact |

**Table 4-2** Data Collection of Individual Client Based on Eclectic Assessment Model—cont'd

| Area of data collection | Interactions | Observations | Measurements |
|---|---|---|---|
| | able with those beliefs and values now? | | |
| | How do you express your thoughts and feelings to others? Are there some situations when you don't? When? | | |
| | What are your goals in the next 5 years? How do you plan to achieve them? (or, Where do you see yourself 5 years from now? How do you plan to get there?) | | |
| | Describe some characteristics of the type of person you'd most like to be. Do you see yourself as that person? Is your description realistic to you? | | |
| 5. Emotional patterns | What type of mood are you usually in (such as calm, depressed, pleasant, happy, excited, or agitated)? | Note facial affect. | |
| | How do you express yourself during mood changes? | | |
| | Do your relations with others change with your moods? How? | | |
| | Are you satisfied with your usual mood? | | |
| | Are you satisfied with your behavior during mood changes? | | |
| 6. Sexuality | Note interactions for B.4. Self-concept | Note observations for B.4. Self-concept | |
| | How do you express yourself as a woman (man)? | What are the person's gender identity and role behaviors? | |
| | Has your health concern changed the way you express yourself as a woman (man)? | Dress | |
| | | Gestures | |
| | | Grooming | |
| | | Nonverbal behavior | |
| | What do you enjoy/not enjoy about being a woman (man)? | Nature of interactions with others | |
| | Do you have any problems regarding what others want you to do as a woman (man) and what you want to do as a woman (man)? | | |

*Continued.*

**Table 4-2**   Data Collection of Individual Client Based on Eclectic Assessment Model—cont'd

| Area of data collection | Interactions | Observations | Measurements |
|---|---|---|---|
| 7. Family coping patterns | What is your occupation? How has being a woman (man) affected your work? How do you show affection toward others? How do you want others to show affection toward you? How does your family handle stress? Be specific for each member of the family. (See B.1. Coping patterns, p. 79) How does your family make decisions? Who has the last word? If someone in the family disagrees with another, what happens? If someone in the family gets sick, who is the caretaker? What is your role or place in the family? | Note nonverbal communication. | |
| C. Sociocultural health | | | |
| 1. Cultural patterns | What social values were you brought up with? Which ones are important to you now? What are and were the traditions in your family? Family gatherings Celebrations Head of home Types of food eaten Religious activities Health care practices Which of these do you participate in? | What type of clothes does the client wear? How is the hair groomed? Stylish? | Frequency of traditional family get-togethers |
| 2. Significant relationships | Who are the significant people in your life? Family? Friends? (Name them.) To whom do you feel closest? Why? How does your family get along as a whole? Is there any major conflict in your family? Whom do you go to when you have a concern or need help? | With whom does the client interact? Note nonverbal communication during client's interactions with others. | Frequency of eye contact, gestures |

**Table 4-2**  Data Collection of Individual Client Based on Eclectic Assessment Model—cont'd

| Area of data collection | Interactions | Observations | Measurements |
|---|---|---|---|
| | How is your family reacting to your health-related concerns? Do they accept them? Are they supportive? | | |
| 3. Recreation patterns | What do you do for fun? How do you feel about leisure time? Do you have hobbies or interests outside of work (such as club memberships, sport activities, children's activities)? Do you have the resources to get involved with your interests? Materials Money Transportation Time What do you know about your community's recreation resources? How long has it been since you participated in any leisure activities? What do you feel or think about that? | Note leisure materials in environment: Books Craft material Woodworking Sport equipment Stereo Collections | Number of hours per day or week spent on leisure activities Time since having leisure activity |
| 4. Environment | What type of dwelling do you live in (multiple or single dwelling)? Are you comfortable where you live? Do you feel you have enough space to yourself? Is your place easy to move around in? Are there sounds, noises, or odors in the environment that are of concern to you? Do you have any pets? If so, what kind? | What is the appearance of dwelling in regard to: Safety Orderliness Cleanliness? Note steps, placement of rooms; shower or tub, and availability; loose rugs. What are the usual sounds, noises, and odors of the environment? | Number of people and rooms in dwelling |
| 5. Economic | Is your income adequate to meet your basic needs for housing and food? How do you plan to pay for health care services? Do you have any concerns about this? | Note nonverbal communication. | Monthly income |

*Continued.*

**Table 4-2**   Data Collection of Individual Client Based on Eclectic Assessment Model—cont'd

| Area of data collection | Interactions | Observations | Measurements |
|---|---|---|---|
| | Do you have health insurance, Medicare, Medicaid coverage? Do you have disability insurance (if appropriate)? | | |
| D. Spiritual health<br>  1. Religious beliefs and practices | What are your religious practices? What is your involvement with church groups and committees? Do you have a religious preference? Do you practice the same religion you grew up with? If not, do you feel any conflict about this? What does your family or significant others think about your differences? | Are any religious artifacts present in the environment? On the client? | Amount of time spent in religious activities per week |
|   2. Values and valuing | What things are important to you in life? Which would you say were most important? How do you incorporate these things into your lifestyle? If not, are you comfortable with this? How do you feel about the social morals you were brought up with? Does this present any conflict for you internally or with your family? How do you see yourself in relation to society? What do you think about helping people you don't know? People you do know? (The same interaction data are relevant to outpatient or inpatient settings.) | What are the indicators of values in the environment? Orderliness Cleanliness Safety Upkeep of furniture, belongings What are the indicators of values in interactions with others? Open dialogue Praise for others Active listening Touch Are there any books or pamphlets regarding things valued by client? Does the client incorporate values into lifestyle? (The same observations can be made in regard to outpatient or inpatient settings.) | (The same measurement data can be made in outpatient or inpatient settings.) |
| II. Review of Systems<br>III. Physical Examination. | | | |

persons in a traditional family. Piaget (1951) provides a model for assessing cognitive development of children and adolescents.

Selye's (1976) stress theory is useful in looking at physiological and psychological coping. Aguilera and Messick (1989) provide a model to work with individuals in crises.

Some models are very limited in scope. The more limited the approach is in scope, the greater the need to combine it with others to provide a multifocal data collection of the client.

## SUMMARY

Nursing models are used as overall guides for data collection. Data collection begins with a data base of preliminary biographical information and discussion of the major concerns and current health status. Additional focused or general information is obtained after selection of a nursing model to guide further assessment. A review of systems and a physical examination are completed to ensure a multifocal and comprehensive assessment. The nature and amount of data obtained depend on the client's health status, type of setting, purpose of interaction, data sources, nurse's skills and knowledge, and resources available. The general guidelines for data collection apply to nursing assessment of the individual client.

## REFERENCES AND READINGS

Aguilera DC and Messick JM: Crisis intervention: theory and methodology, ed 6, St Louis, 1989, The CV Mosby Co.

Bates B: A guide to physical examination, ed 4, Philadelphia, 1987, JB Lippincott Co.

Block GJ and Nolan JW: Health assessment for professional nursing: a developmental approach, ed 2, Norwalk, Conn, 1986, Appleton-Century-Crofts.

Erikson EH: Childhood and society, ed 2, New York, 1963, WW Norton & Co, Inc.

Fitzpatrick JJ and Whall AL, editors: Conceptual models of nursing: analysis and application, Bowie, Md, 1983, Robert J Brady Co.

Gordon M: Nursing diagnosis: process and application, ed 2, 1987, McGraw-Hill Book Co.

Guzzetta CE, Bunton SD, Prinkey LA et al: Clinical assessment tools for use with nursing diagnoses, St Louis, 1989, The CV Mosby Co.

King IM: A theory for nursing: systems, concepts, and process, New York, 1981, John Wiley & Sons, Inc.

Maslow A: Toward a psychology of being, New York, 1968, D Van Nostrand Co.

Nursing Theories Conference Group: Nursing theories: the base for professional nursing practice, ed 2, Englewood Cliffs, NJ, 1985, Prentice-Hall, Inc.

Orem D: Nursing: concepts of practice, ed 3, New York, 1985, McGraw-Hill Book Co.

Piaget J: The psychology of intelligence, ed 2, London, 1951, Routledge & Kegan Paul, Ltd.

Rogers ME: The theoretical basis of nursing, Philadelphia, 1970, FA Davis Co.

Roy Sr C and Reihl JP, editors: Conceptual models for nursing practice, ed 2, New York, 1980, Appleton-Century-Crofts.

Roy Sr C: Introduction to nursing: an adaptation model, ed 2, Englewood Cliffs, NJ, 1984, Prentice-Hall, Inc.

Selye H: Stress without distress, New York, 1974, Lippincott and Crowell, Publishers.

Selye H: The stress of life, New York, 1976, McGraw-Hill Book Co.

# Assessment: Data Collection of the Family Client

JANET W. KENNEY*

## THE FAMILY

There are many definitions of family. Traditionally, the nuclear family, comprised of a married couple and their children by birth or adoption, was the accepted definition. This limited definition of the family, which includes only those members who are legally married and their children, is no longer acceptable, because of the trend toward independence and alternative lifestyles. Today, the nuclear family does not represent the majority of families in the United States. With the changes in family composition and structure, authors use broader criteria to define the family. A "structural" definition of family includes kinship members with differentiated positions in a family system, such as grandparents, aunts, uncles, cousins, and any genetic relatives. A "functional" definition of family is any social group engaged in certain family activities, such as child-rearing, nurturing, socializing, and so forth.

In this book, a family is a group of two or more people living together who are committed to each other. These people may or may not be related by genetics or marriage, but they care about each other. This definition encompasses diverse groups, including single-parent families, extended families, nuclear families, married and unmarried couples, homosexual couples, aging couples, and even communes, convents, and monasteries.

In today's society, the family is the basic biological, psychological, and sociological unit. Sometimes legal implications are also considered impor-

tant in looking at a family. As a *biological* unit, the family produces children, who may inherit genetic traits or have a predisposition to specific health problems such as depression, diabetes, or heart disease. The family as a *psychological* unit interacts with members of the nuclear family and often extended family members, such as grandparents, step-parents, aunts, uncles, and cousins. Family relationships and interactions may profoundly influence each member's values, beliefs, and behaviors.

*Sociological* aspects of the family include the multiple roles and activities or tasks that members carry out both within the family structure and in the community. Ethnic and cultural values, traditions, and practices are often passed on and guide younger family members' behavior patterns. Roles and activities may be viewed within the context of working, learning, socializing, child-rearing, housekeeping, exercising, community functioning, religion, and so forth. The *legal* aspects of the family are found in definitions of the state and local laws, which may impact on the family. For example, decisions regarding who qualifies to pay child support and who is considered a "family member" with visitation privileges in a hospital are determined by legal interpretations.

### Data Collection

The nurse's definition of family guides and influences data collection. Because each nurse grew up and probably lives in some type of family, many nurses have preconceived ideas about how family members "should" interact. Nurses' past and present lived experiences with their own families and others may create personal and emotional

---

*Parts of this chapter were written by Linda L. Delaney, author in the first and second editions.

biases, which can lead to faulty perceptions of the family and inaccurate data collection. For example, during a teenager's prenatal clinic visit, the girl's mother answered each question that the nurse directed at her daughter. The nurse could mistakenly assume that the mother was overly concerned about the daughter or that the daughter was incompetent. However, the daughter may have been too embarrassed to discuss her problems or may have resented her mother's intrusions and felt she was checking up on her.

Nurses must watch that their personal and emotional biases do not influence their perceptions of the family. Also, information for data collection cannot be based on inferences from only one family member. The data need to be validated, sometimes with several family members or other health personnel. Although the family members are the primary source of data, other relevant sources for data collection are:

| | |
|---|---|
| Extended family members | Nursing notes |
| Close friends | Nursing rounds |
| Home and community | Shift reports |
| | Progress notes |
| Medical and social records | Nursing care conferences |
| Health team members | |

Guidelines for assessment were discussed in Chapter 3 and apply to data collection for the family. All three methods of data collection—interaction, observation, and measurement—are used to obtain comprehensive and accurate data. Important points to remember in assessment are listed below:

1. A systematic format is used for data collection.
2. The data are comprehensive and multifocal.
3. A variety of sources is used for data collection.
4. Appropriate methods are used for data collection.
5. The data are verifiable.
6. The data reflect updating of information.
7. The data are recorded and communicated appropriately.

## FAMILY MODELS
### Types of Family Models

Family models were primarily developed within the disciplines of psychology or sociology. Each family model has a unique perspective or way of understanding a family. Family models are categorized as developmental, interactional, structural-functional, or systems models. Some theorists' models represent these types, whereas other theorists have combined two or more basic family models into a comprehensive model. For example, the Calgary family model combines the structural-functional and systems models with the developmental model. Characteristics of the basic four categories of models are shown in Table 5-1.

### Selection of Family Model

Selection of a model usually occurs during the initial contact with the family, as described in Chapter 1. The nurse gathers preliminary data and considers what constitutes health for this family, what prevents this family from achieving health, and what nurses can do to facilitate the family's health. The nurse's viewpoint may be based on family development with its stages and tasks, the family as a dynamic interacting group, the family as a system interacting with subsystems and supra-systems, or the family as a structural-functional unit. The nurse considers possible factors that prevent this family from achieving optimum health. Finally, the nurse considers potential nursing strategies that may achieve optimal family health. The nurse who is familiar with several different models is able to rapidly compare the family's preliminary data with the models and to identify the "best fit." For example, the family with an adolescent diabetic may have difficulty regulating the teenager's activ-

**Table 5-1**  Types of Family Models

| Developmental | Interactional | Systems | Structural-functional |
|---|---|---|---|
| Nuclear family | Unity of interacting personalities | Social system with interacting parts | Social system |
| Sequential family life cycle | Dynamic life process | Structure | Composition |
| Tasks and responsibilities | Multiple changing roles | Permeable boundaries | Values-beliefs |
| Goal orientation | Perception of self and others' interactions | Interaction with environment | Daily tasks |
| | | | Communication |
| | | | Power/control |
| | | | Roles |
| | | | Equilibrium |

ities and food intake. One nurse may choose a developmental model to examine family tasks and responsibilities at this stage. Another nurse may believe that an interactional model with a focus on family member's roles would be the best model for the same situation. There is no correct model for each family situation. The selection of a family model is based on how the nurse perceives and defines family health, factors preventing health, and nursing.

A family model can be used alone, in combination with a nursing model, or as a supplemental model when working with an individual client. Some practitioners are more familiar with and prefer one model; other practitioners, with knowledge of a variety of family models, use an eclectic approach and try to choose a model they feel best fits or is most appropriate to the family situation.

Throughout the life cycle or during its lifetime, each family experiences change and transitions as members grow, move, seek new opportunities, or become ill. Change may be *situational,* such as job loss, advancement, divorce, death, illness, or poverty, or *maturational,* such as marriage, pregnancy, parenthood, or advanced age. Each change, whether positive or negative, may create stress on family members. The change and resulting stress may alter family members' roles and the way they interact with each other. Nurses work with individual family members and with families as a whole. During a family member's illness, especially if the person is hospitalized or is diagnosed with a chronic disease, family members experience change and, usually, stress. The nurse uses family models to identify patterns and trends of family interactions and behaviors and to assist families to find or develop strengths, resources, and healthy interactions.

## FAMILY MODELS APPLIED IN NURSING
### Developmental Models

Although several family developmental models are available in the literature, Duvall's (1977) model is the most well-known. This model is based on the premise that the life cycle of families follows a universal sequence of development. Although the developmental model emphasizes ongoing stages and changes over time, it shares similarities with a systems model. The family is viewed as a social system, characterized by interrelated, interdependent roles and positions, relatively semiclosed boundaries, ongoing adaptive processes, and task performance. Each stage represents major developmental tasks and responsibilities for the family to accomplish, as shown in Table 5-2.

Within each stage, Duvall has identified eight basic tasks. These tasks are performed during each stage, but are unique for each family. The eight basic tasks listed below were described in Chapter 2:
1. Provide physical maintenance
2. Allocate or manage resources
3. Determine division of labor
4. Assure members' socialization
5. Expand and reduce family size
6. Maintain communication/order
7. Establish links with society
8. Maintain motivation and morale

The nurse who is working with a family initially gathers preliminary information about the family members' ages, general patterns of living, and perception of family health concerns. The nurse considers what constitutes this family's health, what prevents their health, and how can nursing facilitate their health. The major developmental tasks and the eight basic tasks are compared with the family's health concerns. If the family's health concerns best fit with the developmental model tasks, the nurse selects and uses that model to collect ad-

**Table 5-2**    Major Developmental Tasks for Family

| Life cycle stage | Major developmental tasks |
|---|---|
| 1. Married couple | Establish a mutually satisfying marriage. |
| 2. Childbearing | Adapt to parenthood; establish a satisfying home. |
| 3. Preschool age | Adapt to child's needs and interests; cope with diminished energy and privacy. |
| 4. School age | Encourage children's educational achievements; fit into community of school-age families. |
| 5. Teenage | Balance teenage responsibility and freedom; establish mutual parental interests. |
| 6. Launching | Release young adults while maintaining supportive home base. |
| 7. Middle age | Rebuild marital relationships; maintain ties with other generations. |
| 8. Aging | Adjust to retirement, loneliness, and bereavement. |

Adapted from Duvall E: Marriage and family development, ed 5, Philadelphia, 1977, JB Lippincott.

ditional data. For example, a middle-aged married woman with grown children is scheduled for a mastectomy. The woman expresses concern about maintaining her relationship with her spouse and seeking employment to support their children in college. The nurse can use Duvall's model to assess the marital relationship in the middle-age stage and focus on the tasks of establishing communication and managing resources.

Assessment of the family using Duvall's model is illustrated in Table 5-3, with the data collection tools of interaction, observation, and measurement. This assessment guide is a representative sample of data, and is not intended to be all-inclusive. Additional data can be beneficial. Duvall's model is applicable to traditional families, but has limited use with cohabiting couples and communal families.

## Interactional Models

Interactional models were first developed by philosophers in the early twentieth century to describe social interaction. These models focused on how individuals define themselves in relation to their situation. Current interactional models view the family as a unity of interacting personalities,

*Text continued on p. 94.*

**Table 5-3**  Data Collection of the Family Client Based on Duvall's Model

| Task | Interactions | Observations | Measurements |
|---|---|---|---|
| **Physical maintenance** | | | |
| Shelter | Where do you live? What type of community is it? Do you have a stove, refrigerator, washer, dryer? Do you rent or own your home/apartment? Who lives with you? What are your major problems in your home? | Type of housing (apartment, house) Condition of rooms, furniture and appliances (cluttered, neat) Light and heat sources, odors, noise Safety features—fire/smoke detectors, locks on doors, windows, screens | Number of rooms, bathrooms |
| Clothing | | Type of clothes on family members (suitability to weather, condition of clothes) Compare adults/children's attire | |
| Food | What does your family eat for breakfast, lunch, dinner, snacks? How often does your family eat out? | Snacks and food visible in kitchen Physical appearance of family members Condition of skin, hair, nails, eyes | Three-day diet recall Height and weight—appropriate |
| Health care | Do you have a family physician? Who? When did you last see the physician? Why? What immunizations have your family members had? Do you have a family dentist? When did family members have their last dental check-up? Have your family had their eyes checked? When? | Condition and color of teeth Presence of eyeglasses | Frequency of physician and dental visits |

*Continued.*

**Table 5-3**   Data Collection of the Family Client Based on Duvall's Model—cont'd

| Task | Interactions | Observations | Measurements |
|---|---|---|---|
| **Resources** | | | |
| Financial | Who is employed in your family? What do they do?<br>What are your major regular expenses?<br>How do you make ends meet?<br>What would you like to buy or need that you cannot afford now? | | Total amount of family income, regular expenses, debts, family savings |
| Time | How do family members spend their time in a typical week, weekend?<br>Who has the most free time, and the least free time? | In the home, what activities are family members doing? | Number of hours adults are away at work |
| Energy | What activities of family members regularly take the most energy?<br>What types of activities do family members do for relaxation? | Appearance of family members (energetic, strong, weak, lethargic, happy, depressed) | |
| Relationships | Which family members are the most helpful?<br>Which members require the most care and time? Describe how.<br>How do family members share authority, respect, and affection? | Who talks to whom in what manner?<br>Who volunteers information, help, affection?<br>Who asks for information, help, affection? | A sociogram of family members relationships |
| **Division of labor** | | | |
| Employment | What types of employment do family members have (accounting, sales, sewing in the home, delivering newspapers)?<br>What hours do family members work outside/inside the home? | | |
| Household responsibilities | Who plans, shops, prepares, and cleans up after meals?<br>Who decides, who does household chores?<br>Who cleans, who does the laundry?<br>Who shops for clothing and household goods?<br>Who decides where the money is spent? | What is the condition of the rooms (neat, cluttered, clean, dusty)?<br>Are home chores kept up with, or is there laundry to be done, dishes to wash, mail to sort? | |

**Table 5-3**   Data Collection of the Family Client Based on Duvall's Model—cont'd

| Task | Interactions | Observations | Measurements |
|------|-------------|--------------|--------------|
| Care of members | Who takes care of the children, elderly, incapacitated? Who looks for illnesses and seeks health care? | | Ages of children and elderly |
| Yard and car | Who takes care of pets? Who maintains the yard, farm? Who handles car maintenance? | Types of pets | Number of pets Size of yard Number of cars |
| **Socialization** | | | |
| Eating | What are mealtimes like for your family? How do the children behave during meals? How do family members feel about other members' eating habits? | In the home, are children's manners and interactions appropriate for their age? Do they use knife, fork, and spoon appropriately? | |
| Interactions | How well do family members get along with each other? To whom is each member closest? Who fights with whom? Verbally or physically? Who comforts whom? | Who sits close together or apart from others? Who talks to whom? Who has eye contact, touch? | Number of times members touch, have eye contact |
| Sexuality | How do family members express their sexuality (behavior, appearance, verbally)? Are family members comfortable with the way others express their sexuality? | Appearance of family members (hair combed, makeup, jewelry, tight or loose clothing, revealing or concealing clothing, attractive vs disarray) | |
| Expressing feelings | How do family members express joy, sorrow, anger, frustration? Are other family members comfortable with the ways each member expresses feelings? | Behavior patterns of family members (touch, posture, stance, facial expressions, closeness, or distance) | |
| **Expansion and reproduction** | Do you plan to have any (more) children? How do you feel about the number of children you have? Are you using birth control? Which method? Are you satisfied? At what age do you feel your children will be on their own? How do you feel about your children | Nonverbal expressions between husband and wife (touch, smile, eye contact, distancing) | Number of children desired Ages of children currently at home Number and age of children living outside family home |

*Continued.*

**Table 5-3**   Data Collection of the Family Client Based on Duvall's Model—cont'd

| Task | Interactions | Observations | Measurements |
|------|-------------|-------------|-------------|
| **Expansion and reproduction**—cont'd | leaving? Where will they go? Will your parents or in-laws be living with you in the near future? Will any special accommodations be necessary (diet, avoid stairs, commode)? How will this affect your family lifestyle? | | |
| **Order and communication** | Who makes decisions about how family members spend their leisure time together and apart (sports, vacations, education)? | Who talks to whom in the family? What tone and attitude are used among members? | |
| Decision-making | How are decisions communicated to other family members? Who establishes the family rules? What are the rules (homework, late hours, bedtime, meals, snacks, friends)? Are rules rigid or flexible? How is discipline handled? By whom? | Who answers questions? Who interrupts? Types of discipline (saying "no," spanking, slapping, verbal put-downs, sending child from room) | Number of interruptions |
| Affection | How do family members show approval and love for each other? What are each member's special needs? Do family members recognize and try to meet other members' needs? What things do members like and dislike about family members? | Ways of touching and expressing affection between family members | |
| **Community-neighbors** | Who are the close friends of family members? How often do members get together with friends? Which schools do your children attend? How do you and they feel about their school? What stores and services | Which friends visit home, hospital? Are there cards, pictures, or flowers from friends? Types of neighborhood, stores, services, transportation | Number of friends Number of hours children spend at school |

**Table 5-3**   Data Collection of the Family Client Based on Duvall's Model—cont'd

| Task | Interactions | Observations | Measurements |
|---|---|---|---|
| | (post office, library, transportation) are convenient for your family? Do family members regularly use neighborhood recreational areas? How do you monitor family members' activities outside the home (drugs, alcohol, groups, movies, hang-outs)? | Facial expressions and gestures | |
| Organizations | Does your family attend church regularly? Are family members active in any clubs or organizations (scouts, athletic, musical, PTA, civic)? How do family members feel about participating in local clubs and organizations? What is the relationship between employed family members and their co-workers? | Religious symbols in home; worn as jewelry Trophies, medals, awards, pictures | Number of hours members spend in clubs/ organizations A sociogram of the family's relationships with community organizations |
| **Motivation and morale** | What are the family goals? Individual member's goals? What plans do you have for reaching those goals? Are goals shared by all members? How does the family handle members' achievements/success (promotions, good grades, awards)? | Members' tone and affect, posture, and gestures when speaking Who speaks up and how often? | |
| | How does the family handle a member's failures? How does the family encourage members to do better? What happens in the family when the going get rough? When there is a crisis? What's special about your family? What special things does your family do together? | Types of punishments (criticism, withholding TV or treats, sent to bedroom) Special projects such as decorations, games, traditions | |

and focus on the internal family dynamics. These models are based on the premise that individuals selectively note and assess their surroundings through a continuous process of interpretation in which they define the situation and determine their actions. Individuals constantly form and revise their actions through interpretation of each other's actions. Interactions are considered roles that family members carry out; however, environmental interaction is not considered important. Life is viewed as a process rather than a state of equilibrium.

Satir (1972) developed a simple, yet broad model to examine family interactions (Table 5-4). This model focuses on how family members' roles are enacted and how role performance is perceived in each family. Four major concepts of family life are addressed: *communication* patterns, *self-worth* of family members, *rules* about how members should feel and act, and the family's *links to society*. Healthy families are seen as having open communication patterns among members, high perceptions of each member's worth, flexible rules that are clearly defined, and successful interactions with established networks in society. Satir's major concepts are more fully described in Chapter 2.

First, the nurse gathers preliminary information about the family, compares this information with the nurse's view of a healthy family, and considers factors preventing their health and strategies to facilitate health. The nurse who decides that the family's health concerns best fit Satir's model, would apply this model throughout the nursing process. For example, a family in which the 38-year-old father has had a heart attack seeks the nurse's assistance. The mother and young children are very upset about the father's prognosis and finances. The nurse believes that if the family members openly discuss these problems (communication), strengthen each member's feelings of self-worth, and identify community resources (links to society) for assistance, their concerns would decrease. Each of these areas requires changes in family members' roles. The nurse first must consider the typical way members relate to each other in their accustomed roles, listen to their viewpoints (yet not take everything at face value), and understand how each member perceives the situation.

Satir's model is sufficiently broad to encompass different types of families, including couples, single-parent families, and small groups. However, the model does not address the family structure and health. Supplemental models, which address these aspects, can be combined with Satir's model.

**Table 5-4**   Satir's Concepts as Related to a Healthy Family

| Major concepts | Healthy families |
| --- | --- |
| Communication | Open, direct, clear, honest; share feelings and needs |
| Self-worth | High self-esteem, integrity; responsibility, compassion, and love |
| Rules | Known to all members, clear; flexible and allow individual freedom |
| Links to society | Trust and have many friends; belong to various groups and clubs |

Table 5-5 illustrates how the nurse collects data using Satir's model with interaction, observation, and measurement tools. This assessment guide suggests possible questions, but it is not all-inclusive.

## Structural-Functional Models

In structural-functional models, the family is viewed as a social system, with the focus on the family composition (structure) and members' interactions (functions) during socialization and communication. Systems theory is usually integrated within this model; family members are viewed as interacting subsystems and community groups represent suprasystems. Friedman's (1986) family model depicts the typical concepts in a structural-functional model, with some additional concepts included, as shown in Table 5-6, and described in Chapter 2.

The *structure* of the family considers the immediate family members—their names, ages, and the relationship of those who reside together. The family composition includes extended members who are actively involved with the immediate family. Data are collected about the immediate family and relevant extended family members. The extent and depth of data collection about the family structure depend on the purpose of the interview. A genogram is constructed to clarify the relationships and relevant data about each family member. The health, genetic influences, and occupation of the immediate and extended family members are considered very important in the genogram (see Fig. 5-1, p. 97).

The Green's nuclear family, as shown in Fig. 5-1, includes Joe and Jane, who have been married 20 years, and their two children, Josie and Jake. On Joe's side of the family, his father, John, died of

**Table 5-5**   Data Collection of the Family Client Based on Satir's Model

| Concept | Interactions | Observations | Measurements |
|---|---|---|---|
| **Communication** | Which family members talk together regularly?<br>Are there any members who seldom talk?<br>What topics do family members discuss together?<br>What topics are only discussed between certain members?<br>Are family communications superficial or in-depth?<br>Which family members express their feelings about others? Which members seldom express their feelings? How are feelings expressed?<br>How does each member feel about the other family members?<br>What happens when family members disagree? Does anyone feel threatened?<br>How do members communicate their needs? | Who speaks to whom? Who gets involved in discussions and who does not contribute to the conversation?<br>Do family members have eye contact when addressing each other? How often?<br>Is discussion open? Spontaneous? Friendly? Closed? Halting? Are meanings hidden?<br>Do family members sit close or touch each other?<br>Do members show empathy toward each other? Do members feel understood? | Number of times each person speaks<br>Number of times members interrupt each other<br>A sociogram showing family members' relationships |
| **Self-worth** | How does each member feel about himself or herself?<br>Do family members trust each other?<br>What is special about this family and each member?<br>Who nurtures the family and who is the disciplinarian?<br>What is the family emotional climate (happy, angry, exhausted, chaotic, indifferent)? | What words are used to describe family members (sweet, mean, bossy, kind)?<br>What tone is conveyed (authoritative, docile, critical, ingratiating)?<br>What attitude is displayed (caring, responsible, apathetic, passive)?<br>What is the body posture of members (rigid or relaxed)? | |
| **Rules** | What family rules are known to all members?<br>What are your family's rules about spending money? Household chores? Discipline? Schoolwork? Television?<br>What activities are members encouraged to participate in or to avoid?<br>Are there rules about privacy or use of words?<br>Who makes the rules in your family?<br>Are family rules firmly adhered to or flexible?<br>How are rules enforced? | How do members behave while discussing rules: body posture, eye contact, tone of voice?<br>Were any rules noticed during interview with family (eg, children sent to do homework, father expecting dinner at a specified time, mother upset when someone left a room cluttered)? | Number of rules |

*Continued.*

**Table 5-5**   Data Collection of the Family Client Based on Satir's Model—cont'd

| Concept | Interactions | Observations | Measurements |
|---|---|---|---|
| **Rules**—cont'd | What happens when a rule is broken? How do members feel about family rules? How do rules get changed? | | |
| **Links to society** | To what community organizations or groups do family members belong? How often do members participate in community educational, recreational or cultural programs/groups? Would you like the family to be involved more or less in community activities? Why? How do family members contribute to the community? What kinds of support does your family receive from the community? | Were there any signs of family participation in community activities, such as trophies, sports equipment, awards, notices, religious symbols? | A sociogram of the family's links to community agencies |

**Table 5-6**   Friedman's Structural-Functional Family Model

| Structural components | Functional components |
|---|---|
| Family composition | Affective |
| Value systems | Physical necessities and care |
| Communication network | |
| Role system | Economics |
| Power structure | Reproduction |
| | Socialization and placement |
| | Family coping |

emphysema at age 65. Joe's mother, Alice, is 60 years old and has heart disease. John and Alice were divorced after 10 years of marriage. Joe's older brother, Jim, died recently at 45 years of age in a car accident; his sister, Jean, who was adopted, is alive and well. Joe is 38 years old and has been an alcoholic for 20 years. His wife, Jane, is 38 years old and has diabetes and recently had a mastectomy for breast cancer. On her side of the family, her mother, Carol, died at age 50 of uterine cancer. Her father, Tom, is 62 years old and has diabetes, hypertension, and obesity problems. Jane's younger sister, Julie, age 37, is obese and separated from her husband, Fred, after 17 years of marriage.

They have three young children who are alive and well. Joe and Jane have two teenagers, Josie, who is 18 years old and pregnant, and Jake, a 15-year-old with allergies. As can be seen from Fig. 5-1, a three-generational genogram can provide clear information about the age, relationships, and health of family members.

Structural data also include information about (1) family values, (2) communication patterns among members, (3) roles of each member, and (4) power structure patterns. Healthy families work toward specific goals, and the structure serves to facilitate the accomplishment of these goals.

The functions of the family are the activities and interactions of members to achieve their goals. Functions describe the family's purpose or how the family meets individual member's needs and those of society. Friedman (1986) identifies six family functions: (1) affective, (2) physical necessities and care, (3) economic, (4) reproductive, (5) socialization, and (6) coping. These functional components are interrelated with each other as well as interactive with the structural components. Change in any one component usually affects other components. (Each component in the structural-functional model is described in Chapter 2.)

In working with a family, the nurse initially gathers preliminary information about the family situation and compares these data with optimum

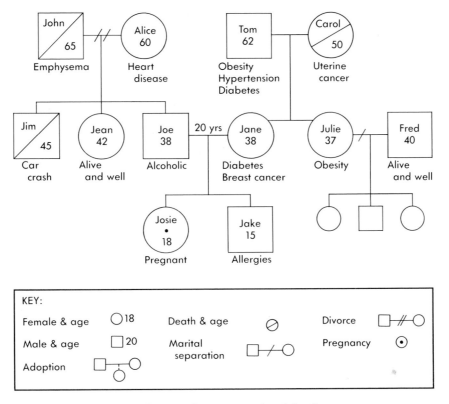

**Fig. 5-1.** The Green's three-generational family genogram.

family health, factors preventing their health and nursing. Then, the nurse decides whether the structural-functional model fits this family situation. For example, a young family with two preschoolers, one of whom is slightly retarded, is having difficulty sharing the increased burdens of caring and planning for the handicapped child. Areas of concern that the nurse identifies are family communication patterns, roles, power, economics, physical care, and coping. The nurse thinks that by increasing the parents communication about handling the problems (including financial) created by the presence of a handicapped child and sharing their roles and power, the family may strengthen their coping abilities. Thus, the nurse selects the structural-functional family model to continue gathering assessment data and uses this model for the family nursing process.

The basic structural-functional model provides a broad framework to assess the family. This model can easily be applied to different types of families and is useful to the nurse who is working with a family for an extended period of time. However, the basic structural-functional model is limited to the present view of the family and focuses on family equilibrium and stability. Growth, change, and disequilibrium in the family are minimized. Therefore, Friedman incorporates relevant aspects from developmental and systems models into her structural-functional model. Biological data about individual family members are also needed for a comprehensive view of the family. Data collection based on Friedman's model is shown in Table 5-7. This guide is a representative sample of questions and does not include all possible data. Additional data can be included as needed. (A family case study applying Friedman's model is presented in Chapter 16.)

**An Eclectic Model**

The Calgary Family Assessment Model (Wright and Leahey, 1984) was developed at the University of Calgary. This broad comprehensive model incorporates a structural-functional approach, with the systems and developmental perspective. There are three major concepts—family structure, development, and functions—each with numerous subconcepts, as shown in Table 5-8. The family is viewed as a social system, composed of members who interact with each other, with extended family members, and with the community. Boundaries are considered semipermeable and may change over time. The focus is on how family members interact to achieve instrumental and expressive functions of the family. Each subconcept in this model is described in Chapter 2.

*Text continued on p. 102.*

**Table 5-7**  Data Collection of the Family Client Based on Friedman's Structural-Functional Model

| Concept | Interactions | Observations | Measurements |
|---|---|---|---|
| **Structural** | | | |
| Family composition | Genogram data | | |
| Value system | What inherent and cultural/ethnic values are important to your family (work/productivity, education, individualism, materialism, cleanliness/orderliness, achievements health, family, religion)? How are these values conveyed to family members and acted upon? Do any value conflicts currently exist among family members? How do major family values affect the family's health and functioning? | Are value-laden objects in the home (numerous books, expensive home furnishings, framed diplomas/awards, sports equipment/trophies, medicine)? | Number of value-laden objects: type |
| Communication | How do family members share their needs and feelings? Is communication open, closed, tolerant, or receptive among family members? Who talks with whom, and in what manner? Which family/personal issues are open/closed to discussion? What are the emotional issues for the family? How often does the family discuss issues together as a group? | Note degree of functional/dysfunctional communication among family members (congruence between verbal and nonverbal communication and between content and intended message). Which family members listen, are attentive, receptive, encourage feedback, validate information, share views? What tone/affect is used by each member? Is there eye contact or touch among members? | A sociogram of family members' relationships |
| Role system | What formal (dyadic) roles does each family member fulfill (husband-wife, father-mother, sister-brother, mother-daughter)? What informal (implicit) roles does each member assume (breadwinner, nurturer, scapegoat, compromiser, negotiator, distractor, dominator)? How does each family member carry out both formal and informal roles? How do family members feel about their own and other members roles? Are there any role conflicts (supermom)? | Who answers what questions? Who cares for children, pets? Who prepares meals, handles bills, purchases household supplies? Who maintains car, yard? Who runs errands, chauffeurs others? | |

**Table 5-7** Data Collection of the Family Client Based on Friedman's Structural-Functional Model—cont'd

| Concept | Interactions | Observations | Measurements |
|---|---|---|---|
| | Are members able to change roles? | | |
| Power structure | What topics/issues does the family discuss and make decisions on (vacations, education, major purchases, community activities, household chores)? | What are the nonverbal behaviors of family members during this topic of discussion (voice tone, eye contact, posture, touch)? | A sociogram depicting power structure |
| | What decision-making processes are used by the family (consensus, bargaining, compromise, coercion)? | | |
| | How does your family make decisions? | | |
| | Who makes what decisions? How important are these decisions to the family? Who usually has the "last word?" | | |
| | What types of power does each family member have (authority, seniority, expert/experience, reward, coercive, affectional)? | | |
| | Are there any member coalitions in your family (mother-father, mother-daughter)? | | |
| **Functional** | | | |
| Affective | What are the needs of each family member? | Are members aware of and responsive to the needs and feelings of each other? | |
| | How does each member express his/her needs? | | |
| | How do members respond to other family members: needs for privacy, recreation, socialization; work pressures, financial burdens; household tasks? | | |
| | Who does each member share special problems with and feelings? | | |
| | Are each member's needs, interests, and unique qualities respected by others? | | |
| | How do family members nurture and support each other? | | |
| | Are your family members close or distant? | | |
| | What makes each member special? | | |

*Continued.*

**Table 5-7**    Data Collection of the Family Client Based on Friedman's Structural-Functional Model—cont'd

| Concept | Interactions | Observations | Measurements |
|---|---|---|---|
| **Functional**—cont'd | | | |
| Physical necessities and health care | Where do you live? What type of community is it? Do you have a stove, refrigerator, washer, dryer? Do you rent or own your home/apartment? Who lives with you? What are your major problems in your home? | Type of housing (apartment, house) Condition of rooms, furniture, and appliances (cluttered, tidy) Light and heat sources; odors, noise Safety features: fire/smoke detectors, locks on doors, windows, screens Type of clothes on family members (suitability for weather, condition of clothes) Compare adults'/children's attire | Number of rooms, bathrooms |
| | What does your family eat for breakfast, lunch, dinner, and snacks? How often does your family eat out? | What snacks and food are visible in kitchen? Physical appearance of family members Condition of skin, hair, nails, eyes | Three-day diet recall Height and weight |
| | Do you have a family physician? Who? When did you last see the physician? Why? What immunizations have your family members had? | | Frequency of physician and dental visits |
| | Do you have a family dentist? When did family members have their last dental check-up? | Condition and color of teeth | |
| | Has your family had eye examinations? When? How does your family maintain their health (check-ups by physician, dentist, nutrition, exercise)? What types of physical activity (work, recreation, exercise) does each member participate in regularly? What drugs (OTC) and prescriptions do family members take regularly? How do you decide a family member is ill? | Presence of eyeglasses Condition of family members' skin, eyes, teeth, weight to height proportion | |
| Economics | Who is employed in the family? What types of occupations/skills do they have? What are your sources of income (occupation, social | | |

**Table 5-7**   Data Collection of the Family Client Based on Friedman's Structural-Functional Model—cont'd

| Concept | Interactions | Observations | Measurements |
|---------|-------------|-------------|-------------|
| | security, stocks and bonds, interest from savings, alimony, child support, welfare, aid for dependent children [ADC])? <br> What are your major regular expenses (housing, food, clothes, school, health care, transportation, insurance)? <br> What types of insurance does your family have (life, health, dental, car, homeowners)? <br> Are you able to adequately meet your family's needs with your income? | | |
| Reproduction | Do you plan to have any (more) children? <br> How do you feel about the number of children you have? <br> Are you using birth control? Which method? Are you satisfied? <br> At what age do you feel your children will be on their own? How do you feel about your children leaving? Where will they go? <br> Will your parents or in-laws be living with you in the near future? Will any special accommodations be necessary (diet, avoiding stairs, commode)? How will this affect your family lifestyle? | Nonverbal expressions between partners (touch, smile, eye contact, distancing) | Number of children desired <br> Ages of children currently at home <br> Number and age of children living outside family home |
| Socialization and placement | What are your family's views of such child-rearing practices as discipline, autonomy, dependence, reward and punishment, age-appropriate behaviors, learning, watching TV, friendship? <br> What do you consider appropriate behavior for your children—during mealtimes, at school/nursery, with peers, with personal cleanliness, use of language? | How do children react to a stranger (nurse)? <br> How are children and older family members regarded by the adult members (joy or burden, helper or helpless, with pride or despair)? | Number of community groups/organizations each member participates in <br> A sociogram showing family connections with community groups |

*Continued.*

**Table 5-7**    Data Collection of the Family Client Based on Friedman's Structural-Functional Model—cont'd

| Concept | Interactions | Observations | Measurements |
|---|---|---|---|
| **Functional**—cont'd | What community groups/ organizations/services are family members involved in regularly? <br><br> What cultural beliefs or social class factors influence your family members activities? | Are there any visible signs/ symbols of community involvement, such as trophies, religious symbols, sports equipment, newsletters? | |
| Family coping | What types of problems has your family experienced recently: death, divorce, job loss/promotion, new member, moves, arrests, health concerns? <br><br> How does your family usually handle problems and increased stress (coping strategies)? <br><br> What resources/strengths does your family have or seek (relatives, friends, information, spiritual, community agencies)? <br><br> What are family members' inner strengths (patience, wisdom, humor, problem-solving, sharing thoughts/ feelings, seeking information)? | | |

As the nurse begins working with a family and gathers preliminary data, the family health concerns are compared with the nurse's view of family health, factors preventing health, and nursing. If the family concerns are complex and diverse, the nurse may choose the Calgary Family Model to obtain a comprehensive assessment of interacting family components. Then the nurse explores those concepts which seem most relevant to the family's concerns. The breadth and depth of data collection for each concept are based on the family's concerns and priorities. Use of too many concepts may provide irrelevant data, whereas an inadequate amount of data may provide a distorted view of the family. The nurse must obtain sufficient data in the relevant areas and strive to integrate these data within the three major concepts for a holistic assessment. Thus, the nurse moves back and forth among the major concepts and subconcepts during data collection to fill in data gaps as additional data

are needed. Data collection for each concept in the Calgary Family Model is illustrated in Table 5-9. This guide represents areas of data that can be obtained; however, the examples are not all-inclusive.

The Calgary Family Model is very useful during assessment, because it can be applied to various types of families, such as single-parent, blended, and communal families. It also includes extended family members. Another advantage of this model is that it integrates sociocultural, ethnic, and community data. However, family members' biological data and the family's goals and values may need to be added to present a complete holistic view of the family.

**SUMMARY**

Each of the four models for family data offers a different perspective of the family and focuses on unique family characteristics. Nurses who perform family assessments must be aware of their own

*Text continued on p. 109.*

**Table 5-8**  Calgary Family Model

| Family structure | Family development | Family functions |
|---|---|---|
| **Internal** | Developmental stage | **Instrumental** |
| Family composition | Developmental tasks | Daily living activities |
| Rank order of members | Attachments | Allocation of tasks |
| Subsystems in family | | |
| Boundaries of family | | |
| **External** | | **Expressive** |
| Culture | | Communication |
| Religion | | Problem-solving |
| Social class status and mobility | | Roles |
| Environment | | Control |
| Extended family | | Beliefs |
| | | Alliances/coalitions |

Adapted from Calgary Family Assessment Model. In Wright LM and Leahey M: Nurses and families: a guide to family assessment and intervention, Philadelphia, 1984, FA Davis Co.

**Table 5-9**  Data Collection of the Family Based on the Calgary Model

| Concepts | Interactions | Observations | Measurements |
|---|---|---|---|
| **Family structure: internal** | | | |
| Family composition and rank order | What are the family members' ages, places of birth, relationships (father, mother, sister, uncles, etc), health status, marital status, occupation? (See genogram, Fig. 5-1.) | | |
| Subsystems | Which family members form subgroups (mother and children, all the children, grandparent and grandchildren)? In these subgroups, who has power/authority, and what is it based on? | Which family members show loyalty to whom? How is this coalition maintained and expressed? | Number of family subgroups |
| Boundary Obtain | What is the source of family income? What is the source of health care information? What social services are being provided? What are entertainment preferences? What schools are attended? | Dress of family members Artifacts or ornaments worn Health status of individual family members Furniture and appliances in home | Family income Number of these health care services sought Number of social services being provided |

**Table 5-9**   Data Collection of the Family Based on the Calgary Model—cont'd

| Concepts | Interactions | Observations | Measurements |
|---|---|---|---|
| **Family structure: internal**—cont'd | What churches are attended?<br>What service does the family want from the nurse? | | |
| Contain | What are the rules about information coming into the system?<br>What (if any) television programs, movies, books, and magazines are censored?<br>Are certain words prohibited?<br>Are certain substances (food, beverages, drugs) banned?<br>What people are not welcome?<br>What services does family *not* want from nurse? | Environmental measures to avoid contact with toxic environmental forces: screens, windows, fence; air filter, air conditioner, furnace<br>Presence or absence of television, radio, reading material | |
| Dispose | Where do unwanted family members go (e.g., unwanted pregnant teen, grandparents, retarded son, or spouse)?<br>What energy is available for suprasystem use, such as family members' activities in community (coaching, Girl Scouts, sports)? | Are old medicines saved and reused?<br>Is garbage collected or lying around the house? | |
| Retain | What goods are retained for future use or heritage (eg, money, silver, jewelry, medicines)?<br>What are family secrets (eg, teenage daughter taking birth control pills, father an alcoholic)?<br>Are family members allowed to leave the system? Who? When?<br>How much energy must each family member devote to system maintenance (supporting the family)?<br>What information does family not want to share with nurse (e.g., about sex or drugs)? | Family collections<br>Pictures and scrapbooks<br>Topics avoided | |

**Table 5-9**  Data Collection of the Family Based on the Calgary Model—cont'd

| Concepts | Interactions | Observations | Measurements |
|---|---|---|---|
| **Family structure: external** | | | |
| Culture/ethnic | What is the family's cultural/ethnic background?<br>What type of cultural/ethnic neighborhood are they living in now?<br>How long have they lived in the U.S.?<br>How does their culture/ethnicity influence their daily lives (diet, socialization, work, relationships, power/authority, household responsibilities)?<br>What languages are spoken in the home?<br>How does their culture/ethnicity influence the health beliefs and health care services? | Presence of symbols or objects representing culture<br>Use of mannerisms and cultural behavior patterns | |
| Religious | What is the family's religion and how actively are members engaged in religious practices?<br>What religious beliefs or values are important to family members? | Presence of religious symbols or artifacts in home/yard | |
| Social class | What are the education level and skills of family members?<br>What are family members' occupations?<br>Which members are currently employed? Where, and what type of work?<br>Does the family receive any supplemental income? If so, from where? | | |
| Environment | Where do you live?<br>In what type of community?<br>Do you have a stove, refrigerator, washer, dryer?<br>Do you rent or own your home/apartment?<br>Who lives with you?<br>What are your major problems in your home? | Type of housing (apartment, house)<br>Condition of rooms, furniture, appliances<br>Light and heat sources, odors, noise<br>Safety features: fire/smoke detectors; locks on doors, windows, screens | Number of rooms, bathrooms |
| Extended family | (See genogram.) | | |

*Continued.*

**Table 5-9** Data Collection of the Family Based on the Calgary Model—cont'd

| Concepts | Interactions | Observations | Measurements |
|---|---|---|---|
| **Family development** | See Chapter 2 Duvall's Family Developmental Model, p. 44. | | |
| Stages | Stages of development:<br>1. Beginning families<br>2. Early childbearing<br>3. Families with preschoolers<br>4. Families with school children<br>5. Families with teenagers<br>6. Launching-center families<br>7. Middle-age families<br>8. Aging families | | |
| Tasks | See Duvall's Data Collection, p. 89.<br>Physical maintenance<br>Resources<br>Division of labor<br>Socialization<br>Expansion and reproduction<br>Order and communication<br>Societal links<br>Motivation and morale | | |
| Attachments | How well do family members get along with each other? To whom is each member closest? Who fights with whom? Verbal or physical? Who comforts whom? | Who sits close together or apart from others? Who talks to whom? Who has eye contact, touch? | Number of times members touch, have eye contact |
| **Family functions: instrumental** | | | |
| Activities of daily living | How do family members spend their time? Weekdays? Weekends? Who works? What hours? Who attends school? What hours? Which members have part-time jobs? Where, doing what, when? Who helps with household chores, pets, child care, yard work? Who runs errands? What recreational/leisure activities do members participate in together? Alone? | What are family members doing during visit (watching TV, eating, homework)? | Number of hours family spend apart and together |

**Table 5-9**  Data Collection of the Family Based on the Calgary Model—cont'd

| Concepts | Interactions | Observations | Measurements |
|---|---|---|---|
| Allocation of tasks | What times are meals taken? Who eats together? When is bedtime for each member? What types of employment do family members have (accounting, sales, sewing in the home, delivering newspapers)? What hours do family members work outside/inside the home? Who plans, shops, prepares, and cleans up after meals? Who decides who does household chores? Who cleans? Who does the laundry? Who shops for clothing and household goods? Who decides where the money is spent? | What is the condition of the rooms Are home chores kept-up, or is there laundry to be done, dishes to wash, mail to sort? | |
| | Who takes care of the children? Elderly? Incapacitated? Pets? Who looks out for illnesses and seeks health care? Who maintains the yard? Farm? Who handles car maintenance? | Types of pets | Ages of children and elderly Number of pets Size of yard Number of cars |
| **Family functions: expressive** | | | |
| Communication | Which family members talk together regularly? Do any members seldom talk? What topics do family members discuss together? What topics are only discussed among certain members? Are family communications superficial or in-depth? Which family members express their feelings about others? Which members seldom express their feelings? | Who speaks to whom? Who gets involved in discussions and who does not contribute to the conversation? Do family members have eye contact when addressing each other—how often? Is discussion open? Spontaneous? Friendly? Closed? Halting? Are meanings hidden? Do family members sit close or touch each other? Do members show empathy toward each other? | Number of times each person speaks Number of times members interrupt each other A sociogram showing family members relationships |

*Continued.*

**Table 5-9**    Data Collection of the Family Based on the Calgary Model—cont'd

| Concepts | Interactions | Observations | Measurements |
|---|---|---|---|
| **Family functions: expressive**—cont'd | How are feelings expressed? How does each member feel about the other family members? What happens when family members disagree? Does anyone feel threatened? How do members communicate their needs? | Do members feel understood? | |
| Problem-solving | Who makes decisions about how family members spend their leisure time together and apart (sports, vacations, education)? | Who talks to whom in the family? What tone and attitude are used between members? | |
| | How are decisions communicated to other family members? Who establishes the family rules? What are the rules (homework, late hours, bedtime, meals, snacks, friends)? Are rules rigid or flexible? | Who answers questions? Who interrupts? | Number of interruptions |
| Roles | What formal (dyadic) roles does each family member fulfill (husband-wife, father-mother, sister-brother, mother-daughter)? What informal (implicit) roles does each member assume (breadwinner, nurturer, scapegoat, compromiser, negotiator, distractor, dominator)? How does each family member carry out both formal and informal roles? How do family members feel about their own and other members' roles? Are there any role conflicts (supermom)? Are members able to change roles? | Who answers what questions? Who cares for children? Pets? Who prepares meals, handles bills, purchases household supplies? Who maintains car? Yard? Who runs errands, chauffeurs others? | |
| Control | How do members influence each other (use of objects or privileges such as money, candy, time together, watching | How do members behave during discussion of rules: body posture, eye contact, tone of voice? | |

**Table 5-9**    Data Collection of the Family Based on the Calgary Model—cont'd

| Concepts | Interactions | Observations | Measurements |
|---|---|---|---|
| | TV; or use of communication and feelings such as hugs, praise, spanking, criticism)?<br>What are the major rules in the family? Who enforces the rules? How are rules enforced? | Were any rules or methods of influence noticed (children praised or scolded, spouse or children reprimanded)? | |
| Beliefs/values | What inherent and cultural/ethnic values are important to your family (work/productivity, education, individualism, materialism, cleanliness/orderliness, achievements, health, family, religion)?<br>How are these values conveyed to family members and acted upon?<br>Are there any value conflicts currently among family members?<br>How do major family values affect the family's health and functioning? | Are there value-laden objects in the home (numerous books, expensive home furnishings, framed diplomas/awards, sports equipment/trophies, medicine)? | Number of value-laden objects-type |
| Alliances/coalitions | Are there any special coalitions/strong ties among your family members (mother-daughter, brother-sister)?<br>What is the nature of these relationships: Who holds the power? What roles do members assume? How strong is the relationship? | Which family members hold similar viewpoints, or stay in close proximity to other members? | |

personal view of the family to avoid gathering false impressions and inaccurate data. The model chosen to guide data collection, and the depth of assessment, depend on the client-family situation, the health care setting or home, and the purpose of the nurse-client interaction. Comprehensive data collection includes biological, psychological, sociocultural, and spiritual data. Frequently, supplemental data or a different type of model are added to a family model for a complete family assessment.

**REFERENCES AND READINGS**

Beavers WR: Psychotherapy and growth: a family systems perspective, New York, 1977, Brunner/Mazel, Inc.

Bross AE: Family therapy: principles of strategic practice, New York, 1983, The Guilford Press.

Clements IW and Buchanan D: Family therapy: a nursing perspective, New York, 1982, John Wiley & Sons, Inc.

Clements IW and Roberts FB, editors: Family health: a theoretical approach to nursing care, New York, 1983, John Wiley & Sons, Inc.

Duvall EM: Marriage and family development, ed 5, Philadelphia, 1977, JB Lippincott Co.

Fife BL: A model for predicting the adaptation of families to medical crises: an analysis of role integration, Image 17(4):108, 1985.

Friedman MM: Family nursing: theories and assessment, ed 2, New York, 1986, Appleton-Century-Crofts.

Getty C and Humphreys W: Understanding the family: stress and change in American family life, New York, 1981, Appleton-Century-Crofts.

Gurman A and Kniskern D, editors: Handbook of family therapy, New York, 1981, Brunner/Mazel, Inc.

Hart SK and Herriott PR: Components of practice. In Hall J and Weaver B, editors: Distributive nursing practice: a systems approach to community health, Philadelphia, 1977, JB Lippincott Co.

Hymovich D and Barnard MU, editors: Family health care, vol. I, New York, 1979, McGraw-Hill Book Co.

Kandzari JH and Howard JR: The well family: a developmental approach to assessment, Boston, 1981, Little, Brown & Co.

Kane CF: Family social support: toward a conceptual model, Adv Nurs Sci 10:18, 1988.

Levitt MB: Families at risk: primary prevention in nursing practice, Boston, 1982, Little, Brown & Co.

Logan BB and Dawkins CE, editors: Family-centered nursing in the community, Menlo Park, Calif, 1986, Addison-Wesley Publishing Co.

Miller JR and Janosik EH: Family-focused care, New York, 1980, McGraw-Hill Book Co.

Miller SR and Winstead-Fry P: Family systems theory in nursing practice, Reston, Va, 1982, Reston Publishing Company.

Olson DH, McCubbin HI et al: Families: what makes them work, Beverly Hills, Calif, 1983, Sage Publications.

Satir V: Peoplemaking, Palo Alto, Calif, 1972, Science and Behavior Books.

Stevenson JS: Issues and crises during middlescence, New York, 1977, Appleton-Century-Crofts.

Whall AL: Family system theory: relationship to nursing conceptual models. In Fitzpatrick J and Whall A, editors: Conceptual models of nursing: analysis and application, 1983, Bowie, Md, Robert J Brady Co.

Wright LM and Leahey M: Nurses and families: a guide to family assessment and intervention, Philadelphia, 1984, FA Davis Co.

# CHAPTER 6

# Assessment: Data Collection of the Community Client

KAREN A. SAUCIER
JUDITH A. BARTON

Community nurses have traditionally included nursing assessments of whole communities. The focus of the nursing assessment is on the community's health status rather than the individual's health status. Historically, community assessment was first seen as a nursing practice role by Florence Nightingale. Nightingale was concerned with assessing the physical and social environment as a possible cause of illness. Nightingale's own community assessments included an analysis of the 1861 census data of England, which served as the foundation of England's sanitary reform acts (Kopf, 1986). She also included community assessment as a nursing role for district nurses. District nurses, as conceived by Nightingale, were to visit families within a certain geographical district for the purpose of improving the health status of that particular community. These nurses were to assess both the physical and social environments of the community in order to determine what health teaching and social reform programs were needed by the community (Montero, 1985). From its earliest history, the nursing profession has viewed community assessment as an important nursing role directed toward improving the health of whole communities.

Today, recommitment toward community assessment is a vital nursing practice role (APHA, 1980; ANA, 1980; AACN, 1986). This recommitment coincides with research findings that demonstrate the important role that physical and social environments play in health and disease (Lalonde, 1974; Cassel, 1976; Rodgers, 1984). Nursing can make an important contribution to community health by considering the current ecological perspective on health and disease. Knowledge of community assessment is now considered essential for the baccalaureate nurse.

The purpose of this chapter is to provide basic frameworks for conducting community assessments. In the following section, multiple definitions of community are discussed as the target or unit for nursing assessment.

## DEFINITIONS OF COMMUNITY AS TARGET OF ASSESSMENT

The first step in designing a community assessment is to define the community to be assessed. This step is necessary because of the many definitions applied to the concept of community. Goeppinger (1982) discusses how nursing tends to use the term *community* to mean a *geopolitical community* (a geographical area with boundaries such as city limits and a political structure for managing the area), as well as a *community of shared functions* requiring interaction (a community whose members share functions such as the growing and distribution of food which in turn requires interactions among members of the community).

Shamansky and Pesznecker (1981) incorporated the geopolitical aspects of community with the shared functional aspects in a nursing model that included three interdependent factors: (1) *people factors* (persons who constitute a community), (2) *space and time factors* (the history and geographical/environmental features of a community), and (3) *for what purpose factors* (the functional processes carried out in the community, such as lines of communication, government policies, and educational services).

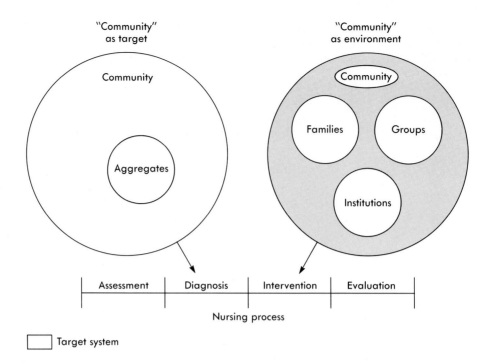

**Fig. 6-1.** Comparison of "community" as target or environment. (From McKay R and Segall M: Methods and models for the aggregate. Copyright 1983 American Journal of Nursing Company. Reprinted from Nursing Outlook 31(6):329, 1983. Used with permission. All rights reserved.)

Public health officials responsible for protecting the health of persons who reside within a given geopolitical area prefer to define community as a *population* or an *aggregate group*. An *aggregate group* is defined as a group of individuals who share common personal or environmental characteristics, but who may or may not interact with one another (Williams and Highriter, 1978). An aggregate group that shares a personal characteristic but different environments is the entire group of unemployed persons in the United States. An example of an aggregate group that shares a common environmental characteristic is all persons who live in a particular neighborhood. By defining community as an aggregate of individuals, the public health official can target subgroups within the greater geopolitical community for clinical or environmental services.

McKay and Segall (1983) incorporated the concept of the aggregate as a community for assessment in a nursing model. The purpose of the model is to compare "community" as the *target* of assessment and diagnosis with "community" as the *environment* for intervention and evaluation. In this model illustrated in Fig. 6-1, the aggregate is viewed as a subsystem of the geopolitical community. In other words, the aggregate should never be considered in isolation. Aggregates are always a part of, are affected by, and affect the greater geo-

political community. This model includes all but the planning components of the nursing process and moves from assessment on the community level to intervention within community organizations and families and government.

When the focus is on assessment and diagnosis, the aggregate within the context of the greater community is considered the target system. When the focus is on intervention and evaluation, the concept of community is defined as the environment for the target system. For example, the nurse may target high school seniors as an aggregate within the context of the greater community. Therefore, a thorough assessment of this group within the context of the greater community is conducted. A primary diagnosis emerging from this assessment is that high school seniors have a serious drug abuse problem. As interventions concerned with this identified problem are planned, carried out, and evaluated, the concept of community is defined as the environment for the target system of high school seniors. The emphasis in the McKay and Segall model is that community assessment involves knowing how the aggregate and greater geopolitical community are interrelated. This knowledge is needed in order to diagnose and intervene on the community level.

Rodgers (1984) agrees with McKay and Segall's definition of community as both a target and an environment. Rodgers further points out that the problems of aggregates overlap with those of the greater geopolitical community. In other words, if the aggregate at risk within a geopolitical community is pregnant teenagers, interventions must be directed toward both the aggregate and the geopolitical community. Perhaps an intervention with the teenagers involves a class on labor and delivery. On the geopolitical community level, an intervention may involve instituting a teen pregnancy prevention program. In conclusion, Rodgers points out that aggregate health assessments require a shorter time frame for analysis and intervention and are less complex than greater community health problems. Greater community health problems require regional and national level analysis and intervention, which in turn require a longer time frame.

This chapter focuses on the aggregate within the context of a geopolitical environment. Nursing and general models serve as guides to the community client assessments. General data collection considerations, techniques, and sources for community data collection are described. Three conceptual models for aggregate assessment within the context of a geopolitical environment are presented. The model that a nurse selects to guide the assessment of the aggregate depends on the type of aggregate, the aggregate characteristics, the model's focus, and the nurse's preference among other factors. One non-nursing model and two nursing models for community assessment are presented. Each model is followed by a chart, with guidelines for data collection based on the model's concepts. These guidelines for data collection focus on the aggregate as the designated community client.

## DATA COLLECTION
### General Data Collection Considerations

The collection of meaningful data about a community depends on the nurse's gaining entry successfully into the community. According to Goeppinger and Schuster (1988:262), "gaining entry or acceptance into the community is perhaps the biggest challenge in assessment." Activities such as participation in community events, demonstration of interest in community leaders, and the use of an assessment guide can be successfully utilized.

The nurse maintains confidentiality after entry into a community has been accomplished. Protecting the identity of community members who provide sensitive or controversial data is a critical issue for the nurse conducting a community assessment (Goeppinger and Schuster, 1988).

**Table 6-1**  Methods and Sources for Data Collection

| Method | Source of data |
| --- | --- |
| Informant interviews | Community or aggregate members |
| Participant observation | Observations in social setting(s) |
| Secondary analysis | Census data, historical accounts, diaries, court records, minutes, previous community studies |
| Constructed surveys | Community or aggregate members |
| Windshield surveys | Observations of community from automobile |

### Techniques and Sources for Data Collection

The primary goal of data collection is to acquire meaningful and useful information about the community and its health. A systematic and informed nursing assessment in partnership with the community is obtained by means of a variety of techniques and resources.

There are five methods of collecting community data: informant interviews, participant observation, secondary analysis of existing data, constructed surveys, and windshield surveys. The community health nurse should attempt to collect data using several different methods because no method is without bias. The process of using multiple complementary methods is termed *triangulation*. These five methods and sources are described below and summarized in Table 6-1.

*Informant interviews* are conducted by directly questioning community residents. The nurse uses appropriate communication techniques in directed conversation with selected members of a community. These interviews can be structured involving specific questions or unstructured, in which the informants guide the interviews. Data gathered through informant interviews are considered subjective and can yield valuable information about the resident's perspective of health values and health care. For example, how do the residents perceive their community health care services? Such data are recorded in the resident's own words and noted as direct quotations in the interaction column of the assessment tool.

The nurse uses *participant observation* by observing what is occurring in selected settings. The nurse observer looks and listens for significant events and occurrences that are taking place and systematically records these observations. Relevant conversations of community residents are noted and recorded in the interaction column of the assessment tool. Places where people gather (such as town meetings or barbershops) can be a source of data collection utilizing participant observation.

*Secondary analysis* used by the nurse is analysis of records, documents, and other previously collected data. The nurse may not have to collect new data when conducting the community assessment. Such data may already exist in the form of census data, historical accounts, diaries, previous studies of the community or aggregate, court records, minutes from community meetings, and research studies of other community workers. These are invaluable sources of information that can reveal the characteristics of the community as well as the attitudes of people in the community and how they cope with their lives on a daily basis.

In *constructed surveys,* community or aggregate members provide answers to specific written or oral questions based on a random sample of the population. This technique is costly and time-consuming and is used only when other resources have been exhausted. For example, if a nurse is interested in abortion attitudes and if very little information is available through other techniques, a survey of community members may provide useful information about this issue.

The nurse can conduct a driving tour of the geopolitical community as a technique for data collection. *Windshield surveys* use observations through the window of an automobile as a way of collecting information about a community's environment. As an initial data collection technique, a windshield survey often reveals common characteristics about the way people live, where they live, and the type of housing they live in. A nurse can observe the presence or absence of street people, where people "hang out", and the social atmosphere of neighborhoods (Goeppinger and Schuster, 1988).

## GENERAL SYSTEMS ASSESSMENT MODEL

The reader is encouraged to review Chapter 2 for a detailed presentation of the basic concepts and tenets of general systems theory. The systems approach can assist the nurse to understand the relationships within a complex system such as a community. Systems theory provides an approach for defining a specific community and for organizing assessment data into a meaningful format for decision-making, priority setting, and program planning (Higgs and Gustafson, 1985). According to Hazzard (1975:384), "one advantage of systems theory is that it puts the total system at the core, and the concern is with the whole and not the parts."

A system has been previously described as a "set of components or unity interacting with each other within a boundary that filters both the kind and the rate of flow of input and output to and from the system" (Von Bertalanffy, 1968). A system has both structure and process, and both must be addressed when conducting the community system assessment.

### Structure

The structure of a system can be defined as a static arrangement of a system's parts at any given time. A significant feature of a system is its hierarchical structure. Boundaries are specified, thus determining what is inside the system and what is outside the system. In terms of community assessment, the *system* is considered to be the target community. The target community could be a geopolitical community, such as a town, or a population aggregate, such as adolescent parents. The *subsystem* is a smaller system included within a designated system. An example of a subsystem is a religious group that exists within the designated community system. The *suprasystem* is the larger system of which the system is a part. It is everything that is *not* included within the identified system, such as a state, a country, or a continent. However, the suprasystem has great relevance to the system and to the assessment process.

The identified community system interacts constantly with the suprasystem while the subsystems exist in dynamic interplay within the system. Relationships among subsystems, system, and the suprasystem must be considered for a full understanding of the dynamics of any given system (Hazzard, 1975). The hierarchy of systems in a typical geopolitical community is illustrated in Fig. 6-2.

### Process

Process refers to the dynamic change among and between the components of the system—how the system works to meet goals. This process of responding to internal and external stimuli assists the system to maintain a sense of balance or equilibrium. See Fig. 6-3 for an illustration of the concepts from systems theory that apply to the dynamic processes between and among components of the total system.

Boundaries maintain the integrity of the system. These may be geographical, such as rivers or building walls, or socioeconomic, such as poverty. Cultural boundaries, such as language, may also exist to define the system's parameters. The boundaries of an aggregate community are common characteristics of the group (such as being an alcoholic or a

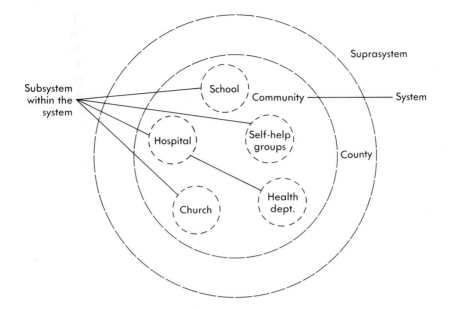

**Fig. 6-2.** Hierarchy of a community system.

**Fig. 6-3.** Diagram of flow of input, throughput, output, and feedback in a community.

pregnant adolescent) or a common environmental factor (such as residence in an urban slum area).

Boundaries control the exchange of matter, energy, and/or information into and out of the system. When this exchange is directed toward the system from the suprasystem, it is called *input.* An example of input for an aggregate with multiple sclerosis is a decrease in disability benefits from Medicare. The exchange from the system to the suprasystem is termed *output.* An example of output from the multiple sclerosis aggregate is the formation of a political advocacy committee. *Throughput* is formed as the inputs are processed and the output is developed. An example of throughput is the aggregate's initial response, such as letters to the editor in a local newspaper.

Because some portion of the output or results of

the throughput is returned to the system, the result is termed *feedback.* Feedback may be positive or negative. Positive feedback maintains disequilibrium within the system, whereas negative feedback tends to return the system to a state of balance. An example of positive feedback would be no response from Medicare or political leaders after being contacted by the aggregate's political advocacy committee regarding the reduced disability. Negative feedback would be the reestablishment of disability benefits from Medicare based on congressional action. Positive feedback therefore maintains the disequilibrium because of a lack of response, whereas negative feedback implies systemic action which promotes constructive changes.

The processes of throughput, output, and feedback have both beneficial and disruptive effects on the system. However, any action has the potential for both growth-producing and growth-inhibiting effects on the community system (Neuman, 1982). Table 6-2 illustrates how the nurse can collect data on an aggregate as the target of community assessment based on the major concepts of general systems framework.

## COMMUNITY-AS-CLIENT ASSESSMENT MODEL

Based on nursing theorist Betty Neuman's (1982) systems model, the Community-as-Client Model was developed by Anderson, McFarlane, and Helton (1986). This model was created to illustrate public health nursing as a synthesis of public health and nursing. The model is presented in Fig. 6-4. Concepts from the model guide both the assessment and the analysis. The reader is encouraged to review Neuman's Systems Model in Chapter 2 to assist in the understanding of the Community-as-Client Model.

The community assessment wheel as depicted in Figs. 6-4 and 6-5 as shown on pp. 118 and 119 guides the assessment phase according to the model. The community core (the aggregate) and the eight subsystems surrounding the core direct the collection of data. Techniques and sources for data collection for the core and the eight subsystems follow.

### Aggregate Core

The *core* represents the people who constitute the designated community-based aggregate. It includes the values, beliefs, and history of the aggregate. The people who make up the core are influenced by and in turn influence the eight subsystems of the greater community within which they reside. According to Anderson, McFarlane,

**Table 6-2**   Data Collection of the Community Client Based on a General Systems Model

| Structure/process | Interactions | Observations | Measurements |
|---|---|---|---|
| **A. Structure** | | | |
| 1. Target system | Do members of the aggregate say that they are stigmatized by others because of a shared characteristic such as being overweight? | Are boundaries for the aggregate natural or artificial? For example, does the commonality for the aggregate involve an artificial boundary (high-rise apartment complex for the elderly) or a natural boundary (shared characteristic of being a pregnant teenager)? Within the aggregate's artificial boundary, are fire standards applied to the high-rise elderly complex? Is the lighting adequate in the hallways? What is observable about the aggregate's shared characteristic(s)? For example, is the observable characteristic an overweight population? | What is measurable about the aggregate? What are the statistics relating to age distribution, sex ratio, marital status, income level, occupation, educational levels, ethnic background, religion, nationality? |
| 2. Subsystem | Is there interaction among members of the aggregate? Is this interaction cooperative or conflictive? | Can you actually observe formal or informal subgroups within the target aggregate? For example, can you attend a support group sponsored by the aggregate for the purpose of taking field notes? | |

**Table 6-2** Data Collection of the Community Client Based on a General Systems Model—cont'd

| Structure/process | Interactions | Observations | Measurements |
|---|---|---|---|
| 3. Suprasystem | What is the relationship between the aggregate and the greater community? Is there cooperation? Conflict? Is there an understanding and caring attitude for the aggregate? What agencies best serve the needs of the aggregate? What agencies could assist the aggregate but currently do not do so? What professionals best serve the needs of the aggregate? | | What statistical data are available on the number of services designed specifically for the aggregate? For example, are there specific health clinics, how many, what is the utilization rate? |
| **B. Process** | | | |
| 1. Input | Is the aggregate open to input from the greater community? Open to assistance and support from the greater community? Is funding available for the aggregate's care? Are protective services available for the aggregate? | Statistically, is there an increase in the number of persons included in the aggregate? For example, are number of persons to be included in the aggregate of homeless persons increasing statistically? | What is the amount of funding available from the greater community for the aggregate? What health and recreational facilities can be found in a particular neighborhood aggregate? |
| 2. Output | How does the aggregate respond to input from the greater community? Does the aggregate have political power, or is the aggregate low in power? What mechanisms are used by the aggregate in response to input from the greater community (e.g., lobbying groups or self-educational groups)? | Can any political action groups be observed? | |
| 3. Throughput and feedback | Is the aggregate in a state of equilibrium or disequilibrium? (In other words, is the aggregate experiencing stability or anxiety and disorganization?) | | Statistically, do records demonstrate an increase or decrease in services available for the aggregate? Are agencies and professionals responding to the aggregate's output with added services, (negative feedback)? Is the aggregate's output being ignored, (positive feedback)? |

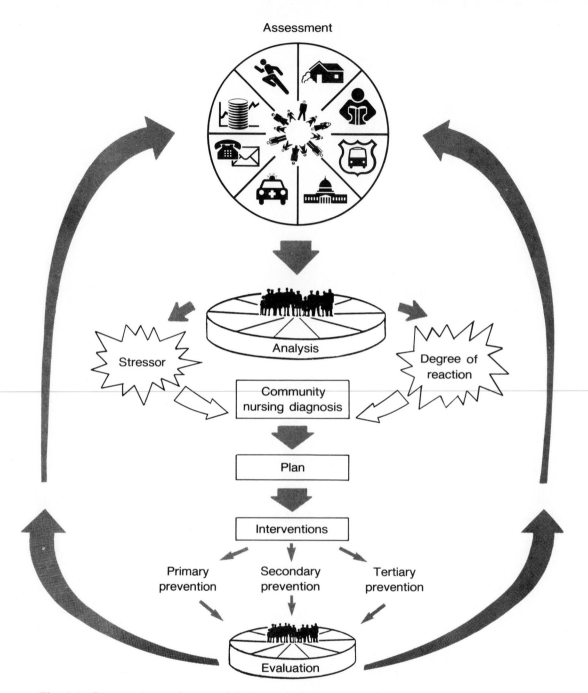

**Fig. 6-4.** Community-as-client model. (From Anderson ET and McFarlane JM: Community as client: application of the nursing process, Philadelphia, 1988, JB Lippincott Co, p 158.)

and Helton (1986:220), "the people and subsystems in dynamic interaction comprise the whole of the community. As a system this whole represents more than simply the sum of its parts."

### Self-concept

In order to assess the core, the community nurse must learn about the people who make up the aggregate core. What makes the identified aggregate different from any other aggregate? Just as an assessment of an individual client in-

cludes self-identity, an assessment of an aggregate community is incomplete without the aggregate's "self-concept." How the aggregate views itself is usually based on history and traditions from the past. How does one find out what kind of self-identity the aggregate has of itself? Ask the membership! Each aggregate community often thinks of itself in terms of such descriptors as "we are friendly," or "we just leave each other well-enough alone." These perceptions can reflect whether the members of an aggregate see themselves as being

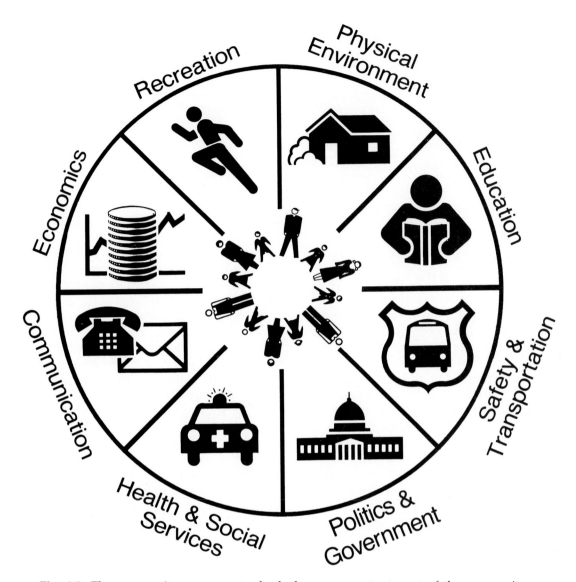

**Fig. 6-5.** The community assessment wheel, the assessment segment of the community-as-client model. (From Anderson ET and McFarlane JM: Community as client: application of the nursing process, Philadelphia, 1988, JB Lippincott Co, p 170.)

connected to each other or not. Listen to the aggregate members as they communicate with each other. Are they proud of being a member of the designated aggregate, or are they ashamed of or apathetic about being a member of the aggregate? As Klein (1965:303) states, "it is reasonable to expect that differing community images would lead to quite varied responses" in terms of health care service utilization. In other words, a poor self-image and feelings of shame or apathy could serve as a resistance to health care service utilization.

### History

Another area in core assessment concerns the changes that an aggregate has experienced over time and its response to those changes. Understanding the history of the aggregate, such

as how and when it was identified as an aggregate, assists the nurse to assess change and community response over time. Was the aggregate stigmatized early in its history, as was the aggregate of AIDS patients? How has the aggregate responded to system changes such as technical advancements in medicine? How has the aggregate of parents of premature babies responded to the "high tech" nursery? Did parents accept turning over their baby to technology, or did they insist on being more involved in the care of their child? An aggregate's ability to mobilize resources in response to problems significantly affects how the aggregate will respond to future interventions. Community nurses can assist an aggregate within the greater community in maintaining its equilibrium. As such, knowledge about the aggregate's past can

**Table 6-3**  Age at Onset of Marijuana Use

| Age at survey | Birth year | High school class | Percent of users | Median age at first use |
|---|---|---|---|---|
| 12 | 1967 | 1985 | 4% | 11 years |
| 14 | 1965 | 1983 | 26% | 13 years |
| 16 | 1963 | 1981 | 43% | 14 years |
| 18 | 1961 | 1979 | 60% | 15 years |
| 20 | 1959 | 1977 | 68% | 16 years |
| 25 | 1954 | 1972 | 63% | 17 years |
| 30 | 1949 | 1967 | 51% | 20 years |
| 35 | 1944 | 1962 | 34% | 25 years |

This hypothetical table is based on research findings by Clayton and Ritter (1985).

give perspective to the present and make realistic health planning possible.

*Statistics*

Indices of the aggregate are somewhat more difficult to obtain than those of the individual client. Indices for the aggregate client are demographics, vital statistics, and health statistics. The assessment includes the morbidity/mortality rates and distributions of sex, age, ethnicity, and race. Other indices are education, occupation/employment patterns, and socioeconomic standing. Morbidity statistics provide a picture of the aggregate in terms of the incidence and prevalence of specific diseases associated with the aggregate.

Indices of the aggregate can be found in the literature associated with the aggregate. Volunteer organizations associated with the aggregate are also a source of indices. For example, the American Heart Association at the local or national level has statistical information on the aggregate of cardiac patients. The nurse determines the aggregate density (number of aggregate members included in the geopolitical space); age, ethnic, race, and gender distribution; socioeconomic characteristics (income, education, employment); and marital status. These demographic data are examined in a historical context. Aggregate communities often experience age-related shifts over time. For example, statistics in Table 6-3 demonstrate a downward shift in the age at which adolescent drug use begins (Clayton and Ritter, 1985). Appropriate planning for an aggregate of adolescent drug abusers would consider the historical shift in beginning age for drug use.

The relationship between aggregate demographic characteristics and the health status of the aggregate has been well established. The links among ethnicity, socioeconomic status, and educational status are of utmost importance if health planning is to be effective. For example, an aggregate of lower socioeconomic persons living near a

toxic dump site has less power to clean up their environment than an aggregate of higher socioeconomic persons. The health statistics (morbidity and mortality) for an aggregate located in one region are compared with a similar aggregate located elsewhere to determine the significance of the health statistics. The health statistics for the target aggregate should also be compared with general population health statistics. These comparisons provide clues as to what health problems exist in a particular aggregate and the effectiveness of existing health services.

*Culture*

The values, beliefs, and religious practices of the aggregate membership comprise another facet of the core. Certain aggregates have a wide range of cultural factors to be considered because culture can influence people's health. The aggregate of drug-abusing adolescents is an example. Drug abuse by adolescents is found in all ethnic, racial, and socioeconomic groups. Some aggregates are more homogeneous in terms of culture. An aggregate of workers, such as migrant farm workers, would be skewed toward the Hispanic culture. It is especially important to determine the aggregate's attitudes toward health in general. Is health care a priority among the members? Is health valued, as evidenced by observations of preventive health practices? An assessment of health values can reveal where health fits into the aggregate's priority structure.

The culture of the aggregate is often difficult to assess during the initial phase. The nurse as a community outsider interacts with members of the aggregate in order to assess the aggregate culture. Norms and values are intangible and become apparent to the nurse only through direct involvement with the group membership. Each aggregate is unique, with different values, belief systems, and practices rooted in tradition. These characteristics evolve and continue to exist because they meet the needs of a particular community (Anderson and McFarlane, 1987).

### Social Networks/Support

Dean (1986:544) contends that "social networks strongly influence people's well-being and should therefore be included in any client assessment." Social networks are identified by examining the degree of social isolation that exists for the aggregate. Aggregates with inadequate social support networks experience more stress and use fewer available resources (McKinley, 1973). Whom do they call when they need health advice or have health problems? Examples of data collection activities associated with social networks include asking members of the aggregate to identify individuals and agencies that give emotional, informational, and material support.

## Interacting Subsystems (see Fig. 6-5 on p. 119)
### Physical Environment

The physical geopolitical community has a significant effect on the health status of aggregate members. An aggregate of elderly persons may reside in a high-rise apartment complex. An aggregate of hypertensive black clients may reside in particular neighborhoods. An aggregate of persons with lung disease may reside in a highly polluted urban environment.

The assessment of the physical environment for the aggregate is similar to the physical examination of the individual client: all five senses are used to collect pertinent data. A physical examination of the environment for the aggregate involves a "hands-on" approach. Perhaps a "feet-on" approach would be more descriptive! Shumway and Wisehart (1969) suggest a walking tour of the environment. They advise that "getting a feel" for a community involves a systematic observation to increase sensitivity to the surrounding ecologic elements. For example, one would want to identify through sight and smell the sources of food for a particular aggregate. Does the aggregate prefer fast foods, or ethnic or regional foods?

If the community can be defined by geographical parameters, boundaries are defined and described as clearly as possible. Parameters are defined in several ways: census tracts; natural boundaries, such as rivers or mountains; roads or streets; proximity to needed resources; and isolation or proximity to other communities.

Environmental threats to health such as air, water, noise pollution, and hazardous wastes are major detriments to the health status of a community. Environmental factors such as road conditions, animal population, housing conditions, and general appearance of the community also are noted in the physical assessment of the community.

A community's climate, just like a person's basal temperature, can have a significant effect on health status. A desert or a mountainous climate can affect the lives of the aggregate in dramatic ways. An aggregate of cardiac patients may experience an increased incidence of angina at a high altitude.

### Health and Social Services

The health care delivery system has been described as delivering "two-class" health care: one kind to those who can pay and another kind to those who cannot pay. This division between public and private health services has implications for the assessment of health services for the aggregate within the geopolitical community. Services also can be grouped into type of service and number of persons served. Services can be further identified as being extra-community (outside the geopolitical community) or intra-community (within the geopolitical community). Table 6-4 describes the major components of the health and social services within a geopolitical community and sources of information for data collection.

In addition to gathering data about the services provided and cost to clients, the nurse also examines the quality and use of the services and the degree of coordination among services. Which health and social services are frequently used by the aggregate? Why are some services not frequently used by the aggregate? Is the aggregate being discriminated against by these resources? Are some resources unknown, unaccessible, or unacceptable services for members of the aggregate?

Some appropriate health care sources may not reflect traditional health care roles. For example, in rural communities, the local pharmacist or the lay midwife may be the primary source of health information and therefore would be included in the assessment.

### Economics

The assessment of the economic system includes the major businesses and industries within the geopolitical community. In addition, census information on the local unemployment rate, percentage of families living below the poverty level, major occupations, and median family income are included in the assessment. The economic system essentially represents the goods and services available to community members as well as the patterns of how these resources are distributed (Anderson and McFarlane, 1987). These same indices are assessed within the target aggregate. How does the aggregate compare with the greater geopolitical com-

**Table 6-4**    Health and Social Services

| Component | Sources of information |
|---|---|
| **Health services** | |
| Extra-community *or* intra-community facilities. Once identified, group into categories (eg, hospitals and clinics, home health care, extended care facilities, public health services, emergency care) | Chamber of Commerce |
| | Planning Board (county, city) |
| | Phone directory |
| For each facility, collect data on | Talk to residents |
| 1. Services (fees, hours, new services planned and those discontinued) | Interview administrator or someone on the staff |
| 2. Resources (personnel, space, budget, record system) | Facility annual report |
| 3. Characteristics of users (geographic distribution, demographic profile, transportation source) | |
| 4. Statistics (number of persons served daily, weekly, monthly) | |
| 5. Adequacy, accessibility, and acceptability of facility according to users and providers | |
| **Social services** | |
| Extra-community *or* intra-community facilities. Once identified, group into categories (eg, counseling and support, clothing, food, shelter, and special needs) | Chamber of Commerce |
| | United Way Directory |
| | Phone directory |
| For each facility collect data on the areas 1-5 listed above | |

From Anderson ET and McFarlane JM: Community as client: application of the nursing process, Philadelphia, 1988, JB Lippincott Co, p. 186.

munity in terms of these indices? How does the economic base of the greater geopolitical community affect the health and social well-being of the aggregate? If a community industry that employs primarily males closes, how is the aggregate of female-headed families affected? Is this aggregate now at risk for a higher rate of unemployment?

### Safety and Transportation

Community safety includes protective services such as police and fire services. How safe do members of the aggregate feel? If the aggregate is a minority group residing in a particular neighborhood, do members feel they are given the same safety services as in other neighborhoods? Is safety education being provided? Does the police department assist the community in developing neighborhood watch programs? Does the fire department uphold the standards of fire prevention and evacuation for elderly high-rise housing?

Sanitation services, including water treatment, and environmental pollution control, are assessed within the subsystem of safety. Are there any special risks involved in living in this particular community?

The assessment of transportation includes the sources of transportation for residents. Is mass transit available, and do these services include special handicapped services? What transportation services are available for traveling outside the community? Are emergency transportation services available to all members inside and outside the geopolitical community? Transportation has a significant influence on the ability of the residents to access health care services and is assessed accordingly.

### Politics and Government

The political subsystem of a community can be assessed through a variety of sources: interviews with formal and informal leaders, reading the local newspaper, and observing political action groups. The aggregate may have developed its own political action group. The political values of a community can make a significant difference in health planning and successful health services. If political values lean toward conservatism, the community may have fewer resources for indigent care. The community may value health care as a consumer good rather than a social right (Reinhart, 1984). If the aggregate is a minority group of low socioeconomic status, access to health and social services are affected.

## Communication

Communication patterns, both formal and informal, are an integral component of the community's subsystems. Communication is a necessary process by which people exchange information and interact with each other and is basic to community living. Language is the keystone to the cultural beliefs and health concerns of both the geopolitical community and the aggregate (Robertson, 1981). Assessment of formal and informal communication patterns can reveal how linked together the total community is and what is being communicated regarding health needs and services.

Informal communication tends to occur wherever people gather: post offices, local cafes and bars, recreation centers, and barbershops. Key informants may be identified in such gatherings or collections of people. These key informants are a source of information regarding community beliefs and needs. Other sources of informal communication patterns are bulletin boards such as those found in local supermarkets.

Formal communication sources include all forms of the media: newspapers, television, radio, telephone services, and the postal system. Is the aggregate ever the focus of these formal communication channels? Is the homeless aggregate being written about in the local newspaper? Are the media accounts sympathetic or nonsympathetic to the conditions of the homeless?

## Education

The general educational status of the geopolitical community is assessed by means of census data. Census data includes the number of residents at-tending school, the average years of education for residents, and the percentage of residents who can read. What are the major educational resources available in the community? Has the community responded to a high rate of illiteracy by providing specialized educational services? The target aggregate may include many illiterate persons who are in need of such services.

## Recreation

The recreational resources of a community often reflect the community's interest in relaxation and fitness. An asessment of the community's "fitness" includes exercise and fitness facilities, such as jogging and bicycling trails. In addition, information on the use of these facilities by the general population and the target aggregate is important. Are specialized fitness centers available for the handicapped, such as warm exercise pools? Assessment of the recreation subsystem provides information on the value of health and fitness for the geopolitical community. Does the aggregate share the fitness value of the larger community?

### Summary of Community-as-Client Assessment Model

Anderson and McFarlane's (1988) Community-as-Client Model includes concepts from general systems theory. The model describes specific subsystems found within a community as to content and how each is related to the goal of health. The nurse may use this model as a guide for collecting data on the aggregate as the target of community assessment, as illustrated in Table 6-5.

**Table 6-5** Data Collection of the Community Client Based on Community-as-Client Model

| Structure/process | Interactions | Observations | Measurements |
|---|---|---|---|
| **A. Core structures** | | | |
| 1. Self-concept | How do aggregate members view themselves? (Are there perceptions of feeling good about being a member of the aggregate, or are the perceptions indicative of shameful feelings?) | | Does statistical data indicate a trend toward increasing morbidity rates of clinical depression for the aggregate group? |
| 2. History | How do aggregate members perceive their history as a group with a common personal or environmental characteristic? | | Statistically, when was the aggregate first considered to be at risk? For example, when did morbidity statistics first indicate that smokers were at risk for lung cancer? |

*Continued.*

**Table 6-5**   Data Collection of the Community Client Based on Community-as-Client Model—cont'd

| Structure/process | Interactions | Observations | Measurements |
|---|---|---|---|
| **A. Core structures—**cont'd | How do aggregate members perceive changes that have occurred in health and social welfare programs affecting the group? Have the changes had a positive or negative effect?<br>How has the aggregate responded to changes in the health and welfare system? For example, have self-help groups formed in response to inadequate health care? | | |
| 3. Statistics | | | What are the current statistics for the aggregate on<br>  a. age distribution<br>  b. sex distribution<br>  c. literacy rate<br>  d. educational level<br>  e. morbidity and mortality rates<br>  f. income levels<br>  g. occupational composition<br>  h. ethnicity<br>  i. nationality<br>Have these statistics changed over time? How do these statistics compare with those of other aggregate groups within the greater community? |
| 4. Culture | What are the values and beliefs of the aggregate?<br>Is there a common culture shared by the aggregate such as a belief system which values holistic medicine above western medicine?<br>Is there a special language and tradition for the aggregate?<br>How are health and illness defined by the aggregate? | Can specialized clothing or equipment be observed for the aggregate? | |
| 5. Social network/ support | Do members of the aggregate report a high level of stress?<br>Are there supportive agencies and professionals for the aggregate?<br>What type of support is given by these agencies?<br>Is a strong natural helping network operating for the aggregate? | | |

**Table 6-5**  Data Collection of the Community Client Based on Community-as-Client Model—cont'd

| Structure/process | Interactions | Observations | Measurements |
|---|---|---|---|
| **B. Interacting subsystems** | | | |
| 1. Physical environment | | | What do you see as you walk or drive through the aggregate's identified geopolitical community? Is the environment in good repair or a state of disrepair? |
| | | Are service facilities such as health and social service agencies in close approximation to the target aggregate? Are there smells and sounds in the aggregate's physical environment? | |
| 2. Health and welfare services | What health and social services are available within the geopolitical community? How do members of the aggregate feel about the acceptability and quality of care given by health and social service agencies? Do members of the aggregate perceive any stigmatization by health and social services staff? How are services between health and social service facilities coordinated for the aggregate? What non-traditional health care does the aggregate utilize? Are there specialized health and social services for the target aggregate? | | What statistical data are available on health and social services designed specifically for the aggregate. How many clinics are available? What is the utilization rate? |
| 3. Economics | How does the economic base affect the health and social wellbeing of the aggregate? | | What is the unemployment rate for the aggregate? How does this rate compare with the unemployment rate for the geopolitical community? What percentage of aggregate members are living under the poverty line? What is the median family income? What is the occupational composition? What is the educational level? |

*Continued.*

**Table 6-5**　Data Collection of the Community Client Based on Community-as-Client Model—cont'd

| Structure/process | Interactions | Observations | Measurements |
|---|---|---|---|
| **B. Interacting subsystems—**cont'd | | | |
| 4. Safety and transportation | How safe do members of the aggregate feel within their environment?<br>Do members of the aggregate feel that they are given the same safety services as other aggregates within the geopolitical community?<br>What safety services are available in the geopolitical community (police, fire protection, sanitation services, environmental controls, emergency services)?<br>Are these same safety services available to the aggregate?<br>What public transportation services are available in the geopolitical community?<br>Are special services available for the handicapped? Do the general and specialized transportation services serve the target aggregate? | | What is the crime rate for the geopolitical community?<br>What is the crime rate for the target aggregate? |
| 5. Politics | Does the aggregate have a formalized governing body? If so, what is the structure of the formalized governing body (officers and chairpersons, a board of directors)?<br>What are the political values of the aggregate? Is the aggregate more liberal or conservative?<br>How do the political values of the aggregate compare with the greater community's political values.<br>How do the political values of the greater community affect the health and social well-being of the aggregate?<br>Do members of the aggregate feel that they are represented politically within the greater community?<br>Is power equally distributed within the aggregate? Is the aggregate divided as to | Are there records of organizational charts, minutes of meetings, or newspaper clippings that record events or interactions between the aggregate and the greater community? For example, are there newspaper accounts of the aggregate's struggle in terms of political strength or lack of strength? | |

**Table 6-5**    Data Collection of the Community Client Based on Community-as-Client Model—cont'd

| Structure/process | Interactions | Observations | Measurements |
|---|---|---|---|
| 6. Communication | who has power? Who represents the aggregate in the greater community? How is information communicated within and to the aggregate? What newsletters or bulletin boards are available to the aggregate? Are community leaders available to the aggregate? What are the meeting areas for the aggregate (club room, school, or other)? Do aggregate members attend community meetings? Do they give information? What is done with this information? | | Is the aggregate being focused upon within the media? Can members of the aggregate be observed on television or heard on radio? How many times per week? |
| 7. Education | Do members of the aggregate feel that they need more education or a different type of education? What educational resources are available to the aggregate? Do any of these resources specialize in the education of the aggregate? | What percentage of the aggregate is currently attending school? What is the average number of years in school for aggregate members? What percentage of the aggregate cannot read? | |
| 8. Recreation | What "fitness" facilities are available in the geopolitical community? Are there biking and walking trails? Is there a system of community-sponsored recreational centers? What special recreational services are handicapped-accessible? Do the recreational facilities meet the aggregate needs? What is the value toward "fitness" for the aggregate? How does this value compare to other aggregates within the geopolitical community? | What observations can be made about recreational opportunities? Are there parks in the community? What type of equipment is found in these parks? Are people seen using park equipment? | |

## COMMUNITY COMPETENCE ASSESSMENT MODELS

The two preceding models primarily focus on the status of a community (the indicators of the health of a community such as morbidity and mortality rates) and the structures found within the community (the various subsystems such as health and recreational resources). Although both models address community process or interactions among groups within a community, process is not the emphasis of these assessment models.

Goeppinger, Lassiter, and Wilcox (1982) developed a nursing process-related model for community assessment designed to address the importance of community processes. They recognized that the process perspective of community health is less popular than perspectives that include community status and community structures. The primary focus of the process-related model is community competence. To assess community competencies, the nurse examines the health capabilities and potential health actions of the community. The basic assumption of the community competency model is that health assessments need to include the community's strengths and abilities to improve their own health status.

The model is based on research conducted by Goeppinger and Baglioni (1986), which was designed to discover indices of community competence. These competencies are not considered mutually exclusive, but interrelated. The conditions of competence are described as follows:

1. *Commitment.* Community members demonstrate an attachment to the community. For example, if the community assessed is an aggregate of elderly persons, do the aggregate members have a support group that meets on a regular basis? How many members of the aggregate participate in the support group? These behaviors demonstrate attachment and commitment to the group.

2. *Self-other awareness.* Do community members recognize that not all members agree on community issues? Are members of the community with minority views on issues listened to by others in the community?

3. *Articulation.* How well does the community articulate their needs to the greater community (vertical communication)? In other words, is an aggregate group of working mothers able to organize and inform the greater community of their needs for better day care?

4. *Effective communication.* How well do community groups communicate with one another (horizontal communication)? For example, in a community divided by two primary aggregate groups of whites and blacks, do these two groups communicate with one another? Is that communication effective in meeting both groups needs?

5. *Conflict containment and accommodation.* How does the community deal with conflict? Does the aggregate use a consensus model, or are those of differing opinions expected to conform to the group?

6. *Participation.* Is there evidence of active community-oriented participation? Do members of the community attend the town council meetings? An example of participation would be members of the aggregate organizing a fund raising event and a majority of aggregate members participating in it.

7. *Management of relations with larger society.* How do members of the community obtain external support for their community? An example of good management of relations with the larger society is found in the chronic kidney failure aggregate community. This aggregate community was able to secure medicare insurance coverage for their medical needs, regardless of age.

8. *Machinery for facilitating participant interaction and decision-making.* What mechanisms exist for facilitating interaction among community members? Does the aggregate community have a network system of phone calls among members to keep all members informed on certain issues? Does the aggregate community have a governing board designed to implement the desires of the aggregate?

Assessing community competencies requires a hands-on experience with members of the community. The nurse cannot rely on others' opinions of the community or on statistical data. The nurse must assess the community by interviewing community members. Members of the community define their own competencies. Table 6-6 proposes assessment questions that the nurse may ask to gather information on community competence. These assessment questions are based on Goeppinger's initial method for measuring each of the eight competencies using the Community Residents Survey (CRS) instrument.

## CONCLUSION

Three models for community assessment as applied to the aggregate within a geopolitical community have been presented. The reader should note that although different models are used, the data are often similar. Each model addresses both structural and process aspects of the community with Goeppinger's community competence model emphasizing process aspects. The model that the nurse chooses for the assessment depends on the community setting, the focus, and preference.

**Table 6-6** Data Collection of the Community Client Based on Community Competence Model

| Conditions of Competence | Interactions | Observations | Measurements |
|---|---|---|---|
| A. Commitment | How do members of the aggregate demonstrate a commitment to the welfare of the group? Are there sponsored activities directed toward meeting aggregate needs. (For example, does the aggregate sponsor a program for exchanging material goods needed by members of the aggregate, such as wheelchairs, baby clothes, etc.) | | What percentage of the total aggregate attend monthly support meetings? |
| B. Self-other awareness | Do members of the aggregate express that they have differing needs from the larger community or are aggregate members unorganized and passive about their needs? Do members of the aggregate recognize that not all members of the aggregate have the same needs? Are there mechanisms for recognizing differences among aggregate members? For example, are all members included in decision-making? Do some members receive more services than others? | | |
| C. Articulation | How does the aggregate make their needs known to the greater community? For example, how does an aggregate of homebound frail elderly organize to obtain homemaking services? Does the aggregate sponsor lobbying activities on behalf of the aggregate? | | |
| D. Effective communication | How do members of the aggregate demonstrate that they understand the common element that ties the group together? For example, does the aggregate sponsor a newsletter or a bulletin board? What type of information is conveyed? | | |
| E. Conflict containment and accommodation | How do members of the aggregate express differing opinions? Does the aggregate sponsor a forum for an exchange of ideas on issues affecting the aggregate? How do members of the aggregate work together to settle their differences? Does the aggregate use a competitive model or a consensus model for settling differences? | | |

*Continued.*

**Table 6-6** Data Collection of the Community Client Based on Community Competence Model—cont'd

| Conditions of Compliance | Interactions | Observations | Measurements |
|---|---|---|---|
| F. Participation | How do members of the aggregate demonstrate participation? Are group activities sponsored? Do members join in group activities? | | |
| G. Management of relations with larger society | How do members of the aggregate demonstrate that they are aware of the supports available in the greater geopolitical community? What resources are available and how are these resources used by members of the aggregate? How do members of the aggregate negotiate with larger society for needed services? Is there a collective effort to gain the needed services, or is each member on his/her own? | | |
| H. Machinery for facilitating participant interaction and decision-making | What mechanisms exist (phone calls, personal contacts, membership on boards/committees) for influencing what goes on within the aggregate? | | |

## REFERENCES AND READINGS

American Association of Colleges of Nursing (AACN), Essentials of college and university education for professional nursing: final report, Washington, DC, 1986.

American Nurses' Association (ANA), Division of Community Health Nursing Practice, Conceptual model for community health nursing, Kansas City, Mo, 1980, The Association.

American Public Health Association (APHA), Public Health Nursing Section, The definition and role of public health nursing in the delivery of health care, A position paper, Washington, DC, 1980.

Anderson ET and McFarlane JM: Community as client: application of the nursing process, Philadelphia, 1987, JB Lippincott Co.

Anderson E, McFarlane J and Helton A: Community as client: a model for practice, Nurs Outlook 3 (5):220, 1986.

Cassel J: The contribution of the social environment to host resistance, Am J Epidemiol 104(2):107, 1976.

Clayton R and Ritter C: The epidemiology of alcohol and drug abuse among adolescents. In Brook DW, Brook JW, Lettieri DJ et al, editors: Advances in alcohol and substance abuse #3/4, New York, 1985, Haworth Press.

Dean PG: Expanding our sights to include social networks, Nurs Health Care 7 (10):544, 1986.

Goeppinger J and Baglioni AJ Jr: Community competence: a positive approach to needs assessment, Am J Community Psychol 13:507, 1986.

Goeppinger J, Lassiter PG, and Wilcox B: Community health is community competence, Nurs Outlook 30 (8):464, 1982.

Goeppinger J and Schuster G: Community as client: using the nursing process to promote health. In Stanhope M and Lancaster J: Community health nursing: process and practice for promoting health, St Louis, 1988, The CV Mosby Co.

Hanchett E: Community health assessment, New York, 1979, John Wiley & Sons, Inc.

Hazzard M: An overview of systems theory, Nurs Clin North Am 6:383, 1975.

Higgs ZR and Gustafson DD: Community as client: assessment and diagnosis, Philadelphia, 1985, FA Davis Co.

Klein DC: Community and mental health: an attempt at a conceptual framework, Community Health J 1:301, 1965.

Kopf EW: Florence Nightingale as statistician. In Spradley BW, editor: Readings in community health nursing, Boston, 1986, Little, Brown & Co.

Lalonde M: A new perspective on the health of Canadians—a working document, Ottawa, 1974, Government of Canada.

McKay R and Segall M: Methods and models for the aggregate, Nurs Outlook 31(6): 1983.

McKinley JB: Social networks, lay consultation, and help-seeking behavior, Soc Forces 53(1):275, 1973.

Montero LA: Florence Nightingale on public health nursing, Am J Public Health 75(2):181, 1985.

Neuman B: The Neuman Systems Model, Norfolk, Conn, 1982, Appleton-Century-Crofts.

Reinhart UW: Rationing the health-care surplus: an American tragedy, Nurs Econ 1(4):210, 1984.

Robertson I: Sociology, ed 2, New York, 1981, Worth Publishers, Inc.

Rodgers S: Community as client—a multivariate model for analysis of community and aggregate health risk, Public Health Nursing 1(4):210, 1984.

Shamansky SL and Pesznecker B: A community is . . ., Nurs Outlook March, 1981.

Shumway SM and Wisehart D: How to know a community, Nurs Outlook 17:63, 1969.

Von Bertalanffy L: General systems theory, New York, 1968, George Braziller, Inc.

Williams CA and Highriter ME: Community health nursing: population focus and evaluation, Public Health Reviews VII (3-4):197, 1978.

# Diagnosis: Analysis and Synthesis of Data

PHYLLIS BAKER RISNER

## GENERAL CONSIDERATIONS

After client data have been collected, it must be interpreted and given meaning. The data alone are simply a number of cues or pieces of information obtained from the five senses. These data, or cues, may include client statements, observable signs and symptoms, laboratory values, census data, and reports from professional colleagues. Interpreting the multiple cues is the nursing diagnosis component of the nursing process.

The processes involved in nursing diagnosis emanate from Florence Nightingale's principles of observation and reflection (Bennett, 1986). Nightingale realized that observation alone was of little value unless nurses used their ability to think about what the observations meant. Reflection incorporates introspection, intuition, and recalling cues and relationships. These principles remain essential in this critical component of the nursing process—the processing of information to reach an accurate conclusion about the client's health status and concerns.

The nursing diagnosis component of the nursing process consists of two parts: *process* and *product* or the nursing diagnosis statement. Although the diagnostic process begins with the nursing assessment, this chapter focuses on the diagnostic *process* or analysis and synthesis of data. The nursing diagnosis statement or *product* is discussed in Chapter 8, which also includes the historical development of the concept.

The analysis and synthesis process is evaluating, interpreting, and giving meaning to the collected data. It is the phase in which conclusions are made regarding the client's health status, such as the client is functional with identified strengths, dysfunctional, or potentially dysfunctional; the client is capable of self-care activities or needs partial to total assistance with self-care requisites; and the client is adapting to environmental stimuli or is ineffectively coping in specific modes of adaptation. If the client is dysfunctional and needs assistance with self-care, or is coping ineffectively, then contributing factors must be specified.

La Monica (1985) and Iyer and associates (1986) refer to the nursing diagnosis component as data processing. Little and Carnevali (1976) describe it as ruling out and ruling in. Aspinall and Tanner (1981) discuss the thinking processes of clinical problem solving. Gordon (1982) identifies nursing diagnosis as process and application. She refers to the use of diagnostic strategies to narrow and test diagnostic possibilities. Carnevali and co-workers (1984) devote an entire book to the diagnostic reasoning process. They describe the probabilistic nature of the act of diagnosis as "the process of inferring the unobservable state of the client from uncertain and observable data presented by the client" (Carnevali et al, 1984:62). Kelly (1985) terms this component the process of clinical judgment. Diagnosing is the terminology used by Carpenito (1987) and Pinnell and deMeneses (1986).

Analysis/synthesis is a decision-making process that ensures individualized nursing care. Most practicing professional nurses perform this mental diagnostic process daily but only document the product (the nursing diagnosis). This text identifies phases in the diagnostic process in an attempt to clarify this critical and complex component of the nursing process. The phases are presented as guidelines to help the novice to be able to understand the elements of the analysis/synthesis process.

This chapter focuses on the cognitive process and discusses the following guidelines for analysis and synthesis:

1. Data are categorized.
2. Data gaps and incongruencies are identified.
3. Cues are clustered into patterns.
4. Appropriate theories, models, concepts, norms, and standards are applied and compared with patterns.
5. Health concerns and strengths are identified.
6. Etiological relationships are proposed.

## Definitions

The *diagnostic process* is a complex decision-making process that requires cognitive and intuitive skills, experience, and a scientific knowledge base. It begins with collecting data or cues (input) through interaction, observation, and measurement; deciding when to probe for additional data and which questions to ask; and when to end the assessment. The data are then processed and interpreted (throughput) by the nurse, based on knowledge, skills, and experience, culminating in the identification of a nursing diagnosis statement (output). The diagnostic process continues with feedback to the client for validation of the concern. Fig. 7-1 depicts the diagnostic process and its relationship to the nursing process.

The diagnostic process is important because the product, the nursing diagnosis statement, is the basis for planning, intervening, and evaluating the client's health concern. The diagnostic process is the professional nurse's responsibility. Mallick (1983) states that the "role of diagnostician should be designated as a primary nursing role."

*Analysis* is the separation of material into constituent parts, the critical examination that defines essential features and their relations. In the nursing diagnostic process, analysis is the categorization of data and the identification of data gaps.

*Synthesis* is the combination of the parts or elements into a single entity. It is "a process of reasoning in which the conclusion is reached directly from given propositions and established or assumed principles" (Stein, 1982). In the nursing diagnostic process, synthesis is the determination of patterns; the application of standards, norms, theo-

ries, and models; the identification of strengths and health concerns; and the delineation of relationships unique to the client.

According to the dictionary, *diagnosis* is "an analysis of the cause and nature of a problem or situation, or a statement of its solution" (Stein, 1982). Diagnose means to distinguish. Nursing is not the only profession to diagnose. Workers in other professions and trades such as auto mechanics, social workers, and physicians make diagnoses. Nurses are responsible for diagnosing *human responses* to health-related issues and concerns, and determining the effects of these concerns on activities of daily living. Human responses can be identified as conditions or situations related to *intrapersonal factors* such as acute or chronic illness, crisis, self, and development; *interpersonal factors* such as communication, role, and support system; and *environmental factors* such as resources, social systems, and ecology.

## COGNITIVE PROCESS

This section identifies the cognitive skills involved in analyzing and synthesizing data. It includes discussions of empirical and personal knowledge base, critical thinking, and decision-making. Kerr's (1987) research specified seven distinct cognitive processes that nurses use in diagnosing client concerns: recode, search, inference, problem identification, hypothesis generation, validation, and prejudgment. Search, inference, and hypotheses generation were the most frequently used. Many of these relate to the data processing components in this text. The recent number of research studies in the area of diagnostic reasoning indicates the importance of the cognitive process in making clinical judgments (Padrick et al, 1987; Porter, 1987; Fitzmaurice, 1987; Myers and Spies, 1987; Garthe, 1987; Westfall et al, 1987; Cianfrani, 1987; and Justice, 1987). The thought process and the structural phases (guidelines) are discussed separately for clarification and use for the novice nurse. In practice, they occur simultaneously, especially with an expert practitioner.

**Fig. 7-1.** The diagnostic process.

## Empirical Knowledge

Analysis and synthesis of client data are influenced by the nurse's scientific knowledge, past nursing experiences, self-awareness, and definition of nursing. With the professionalization of nursing, nursing education is moving from technically focused education to a broader-based university focus. Baccalaureate education provides depth and breadth to the nurse's knowledge base in the sciences and the humanities. The diagnostic process requires a knowledge base that includes anatomy, physiology, pathology, psychology, sociology, anthropology, epidemiology, bacteriology, and nursing science. Knowledge of nursing models, along with skills in critical thinking and decision-making, are also necessary for successful completion of the nursing diagnostic process. Fitzpatrick, acknowledging the need for an empirical knowledge base, states

> The process of diagnosis in nursing involves a knowledge base related to a nursing perspective, an ability to collect data gathered through the observation and assessment processes, the organization of complex and multiple sets of information, and the making of clinical inferences based on the nature and organization of the data. (1987:63)

Empirical knowledge is obtained through the senses and can be verified by others. This logical knowledge is developed through formal education as well as through a conscious learning from clinical experiences.

## Personal Knowledge

Personal knowledge is gained through introspection. The intentional development of self-awareness integrates feelings, values, and experiences, which leads to authenticity of the self. Personal knowledge includes the intuitive elements of nursing. As introspection and integration occur, nurses increasingly trust their use of personal knowledge and intuition. Hammond (1966) identified both intuition and logic as part of clinical inference.

Clinical intuition is grounded in subjectivity according to Young's (1987) exploratory research. She defines clinical intuition as "a process whereby the nurse knows something about a patient that cannot be verbalized, that is verbalized with difficulty or for which the source of knowledge cannot be determined" (1987:52). Others (Gerrity, 1987; Henderson, 1987) focus on the art of nursing with renewed interest in intuition as an essential element in the nursing process and nursing care. Personal knowledge and intuition involve self-receptivity or being open, experience, personal energy, and self-confidence (Young, 1987).

To make accurate clinical judgments, decision-making involves both the empirical and personal knowledge elements. Nurses need a strong, verifiable knowledge base grounded in scientific investigation. In addition, nurses need an awareness of their own personal feelings, values, and experiences, which influence their perceptions of client data.

## Critical Thinking

Critical thinking is sifting through the data and generating ideas about what it means. Processes such as imagining, conceiving, and inferring are used to join ideas. From these processes, an opinion or judgment is formed to interpret the data. Factors influencing critical thinking include short-term and long-term memory (cognitive abilities), experiences of the nurse, the pressure of time, and the risk to hypothesize.

## Decision-making

Decision-making is discriminative thinking and is used to choose a particular course of action. Several models of decision-making may be used for making clinical judgments (Kepner and Tregoe, 1965; Vroom and Yetton, 1973; Easton, 1975; Bailey and Claus, 1975; Bower, 1982; and Bernhard and Walsh, 1990). Aspinall (1979) tested the effectiveness of a decision tree for diagnostic accuracy. Aspinall and Tanner (1981) specify decision points in their model. They describe the thinking strategies used in clinical problem solving as (1) generating multiple alternatives (diagnostic hypotheses or possible explanations of cues) and (2) systematically testing the alternatives against additional information from the client or other sources.

Decision-making is the process of identifying and selecting the best alternatives and includes the elements of deliberation, judgment, and choice. Nurses use decision-making throughout the nursing process. It is especially relevant in analysis and synthesis, because decision-making is used in viewing the data, identifying health concerns and strengths, and determining contributing factors to health concerns.

### Deliberation

Deliberation is a careful consideration of data. It is used in each phase of the diagnostic process. Deliberation uses logic and reasoning to process the data. The nurse's level of expertise and self-confidence also influence how data are considered.

Inductive and deductive logic are thinking strategies in decision-making. Induction involves clustering data into patterns and labeling the patterns. It is reasoning from specific facts to a general conclusion and is the basis for stating hypotheses. An example of induction is taking client cues and seeing if the cues form a pattern. Many nurses use inductive logic in sorting data, examining alternatives and arriving at clinical decisions. For example, a nurse observes that a newly admitted male client is wringing his hands and placing the floor in a bent posture. The nurse needs to explore the meaning of these cues, obtain additional data, and clarify whether the pattern is indicative of pain or anxiety.

Deduction is reasoning from an accepted principle to a particular instance, from the general to the specific. An example of deduction is starting with a conceptual model and then categorizing and processing the data within that particular model. Another example is a nurse intuitively thinking of the concept *pain* while assessing a client exhibiting the behaviors in the example mentioned previously. The nurse then searches for cues or defining characteristics that may verify the client's experience with pain. Both inductive and deductive reasoning are used throughout deliberation.

### Judgment

Judgment is appraising and evaluating the significance, accuracy, adequacy, and appropriateness of the cues and patterns (Kelly, 1985). Judgments are made throughout the diagnostic process, but are essential for categorizing cues and identifying data gaps and incongruencies. They are also used for evaluating alternative hypotheses. Doona (1976) describes four types of judgments used by nurses in clinical practice: *common sense judgment*, which is based on the situation and tradition; *speculative judgment*, which is seeing clients as "a case of ———"without acknowledging individuality; *pragmatic judgment*, which is emphasizing the here and now with little attention to conceptualization; and *ideal judgment*, which includes both situational facts and theoretical understanding. The latter type of judgment is the most useful in diagnostic thinking because it includes evaluating the situational client patterns and applying theoretical knowledge to decide client strengths and concerns.

### Choice

Choice is when the nurse makes decisions in each phase of the diagnostic process by discriminating or choosing among options. Choice is making decisions about what data to collect, how to categorize the data, what data are missing or incongruent, how to cluster the cues, which theories, standards, and norms to apply, what are the inferences and conclusions, and what is the rationale for choosing. Table 7-1 identifies decision choices to be made within each phase of the diagnostic process.

## GUIDELINES FOR ANALYSIS AND SYNTHESIS

This section describes phases in analyzing and synthesizing the data. These phases are not presented as rigid, linear steps to the complex diagnotic process but as guidelines for approaching this component of the nursing process. Analysis incorporates the first two phases as data are categorized and gaps are identified. Phases 3 through 6 represent synthesis while patterns are determined and compared with norms and standards, health concerns and strengths are identified, and etiologic relationships are delineated.

1. *Data are categorized.* The first phase in analyzing data is to organize, group, or sort the cues logically and systematically. Bower and Bevis (1979:110) state that "the method of categorization is not nearly as important as having some systematic way of handling data that everyone understands.'" Decision-making questions in this phase are the following: Is the model being used to categorize the data the most appropriate model for this client? Which cues belong in which category? (See Table 7-1.)

Data may be categorized by nursing or non-nursing models. Individual data may be organized by nursing models such as Roy's (1984) four adaptive modes, Gordon's (1987) functional health patterns, or Carpenito's (1987) bifocal clinical collaborative model. Table 7-2 shows individual data obtained by interaction, observation, and measurement categorized in the bio-psycho-socio-spiritual model. A non-nursing model that is used for individuals is Maslow's hierarchy of needs. Typically, the nurse categorizes data according to the model chosen for the nursing assessment. Other models for families and communities are described later in this chapter.

In some institutions, nursing data collection instruments are being used to categorize data as part of the nursing assessment phase, thereby negating the need for this part of analysis.

2. *Data gaps and incongruencies are identified.* Data gaps and incongruencies indicate areas to further assess and search for cues. The search for data gaps is based on the nurse's knowledge and experience. Decision-making questions to ask in this

**Table 7-1**  Phases in the Diagnostic Process and Decision Questions for Each Phase

| Phase | Decisions |
|---|---|
| Obtain multiple cues:<br>  Nursing assessment<br>    Laboratory reports<br>    Physician notes<br>  Others | What data need to be obtained?<br>Where is it necessary to probe further? |
| Categorize nursing assessment cues | Is the model appropriate to the client situation?<br>Which cues belong in which category? |
| Identify data gaps and incongruencies | What additional data are needed to reach a conclusion,<br>  what data can be obtained later,<br>  what data are inconsistent and need clarification? |
| Cluster data into patterns | Which cues belong in which pattern?<br>Which cues are relevant? |
| Apply and compare theories, concepts, norms, and standards | Which theories, and so on, are appropriate for interpreting patterns?<br>Which patterns fit with the defining characteristics of a nursing diagnosis?<br>How do the patterns compare with the theories, and so on?<br>What are the client's perceptions of "normal?" |
| Infer health concerns and strengths | What are all possible hypotheses, alternatives, and options?<br>What is the probability that each option is present?<br>Which alternatives are not valid;<br>  which hypotheses are valid?<br>Is there enough data to rule out?<br>Is there enough data to confirm?<br>Which patterns are functional; which patterns are strengths?<br>Which patterns are actual, potential, or possible concerns?<br>What is rationale for inferences? |
| Propose etiological relationships | Which cues or patterns may be the contributing factors?<br>Which nursing diagnosis etiology is the "best fit" for data? |

phase are: What additional data are needed to reach a conclusion? What data must be obtained before proceeding with analysis and synthesis? What data can be obtained later and what data are inconsistent, incongruent, and need clarification? Table 7-1 indicates the questions asked in this phase of the diagnostic process. Data gaps are missing data necessary to determine patterns and specific approaches. Table 7-3 identifies data gaps that are missing from the categorized data. Other examples of data gaps that may not be obtained during the initial contact are sexual history, family history and genogram, health history, past coping, and communication patterns.

An incongruency occurs when data are conflicting or inconsistent. An example of an incongruency is a client denying a history of smoking while having an open pack of cigarettes and matches in a pocket and brown stains on two fingers. This incongruency needs to be clarified or validated before defining specific client concerns. Inconsistencies may occur when more than one nurse or nurses with different levels of expertise contribute to the data base, when the person giving the information is not reliable due to anxiety, or physical or mental stress, or when a misunderstanding or incorrect recording occurs (Pinnell and deMeneses, 1986).

**Table 7-2**  Data Categorized According to Bio-psycho-socio-spiritual Model

| | Data* | Model categories† |
|---|---|---|
| I | "I eat one meal a day, usually a hot dog, and drink three or four soft drinks. . . ." | Biophysical, nutrition |
| | "I sit alone all day and watch TV with my cat. . . ." | Biophysical, exercise, and psychological |
| | "I like my life as it is." | Psychological |
| | "I don't want any change. . . ." | |
| | "I live alone. My income is $200 a month. Rent costs me $100 a month and utilities about $50. . . ." | Sociological, economic |
| | "I am 60 years old." | Psychological, developmental |
| O | Skin folds on arms and ankles | Biophysical, nutrition |
| | Walks with cane | Biophysical, exercise |
| | Sits in chair; stares out window; no eye contact | Psychological |
| | Female | Psychological, developmental |
| | Black | Sociological, cultural |
| M | 5 ft 2 in, 300 lb | Biophysical, nutrition |

*I, Interaction, O, observation; M, measurement.
†Limited categories are included in this table. Spiritual data are not included.

**Table 7-3**  Data Gaps Identified

| Data categorization | | Data gaps |
|---|---|---|
| **Biophysical** | | |
| 1. Nutrition | | 3-day diet recall |
| I | "I eat one meal a day, usually a hot dog, and drink three or four soft drinks." | Knowledge of four basic food groups Type and size of soft drink |
| O | Skin folds on arms and ankles | |
| M | 5 ft 2 in, 300 lb | |
| 2. Exercise | | Activities of daily living |
| I | "I sit alone all day and watch TV with my cat." | Range of motion Strength and energy |
| O | Walks with cane | |
| **Psychological** | | |
| I | "I like my life as it is. I don't want any change. . . ." | Self-concept Coping |
| | "I am 60 years old." | Developmental tasks |
| O | Sits in chair; stares out window; no eye contact. Female | Other psychological patterns |
| **Sociological** | | |
| I | "I live alone. My income is $200 a month. Rent costs me $100 a month and utilities about $50." | Significant others Income sources Insurance Transportation |
| O | Black | Values, traditions, norms |
| **Spiritual** | | Beliefs and practices Values and valuing |

Resources are available to assist with this phase. Depending on the category, the nurse may use any of the nursing diagnosis handbooks to review the defining characteristics section given for each nursing diagnosis (Gordon, 1987; Kim, McFarland, and McLane, 1987; Carpenito, 1987a, 1987b; Doenges and Moorhouse, 1988; Gettrust, Ryan, and Engelman, 1985; Townsend, 1988; Roberts, 1987; Houldin, Salstein and Ganley, 1987). Kelly (1985) identifies defining characteristics as signs and symptoms in her sourcebook.

The nurse can compare the cues from each client assessment and analysis category with the defining characteristics of a possible nursing diagnosis and can identify missing cues that would help form patterns. Reviewing the defining characteristics helps the nurse to identify additional questions.

Provision must be made for further assessment to obtain the information identified as data gaps or incongruencies. Some data may be needed prior to progressing to the next phase in data processing. If data may be obtained later, the nurse may continue with data processing.

3. *Cues are clustered into patterns.* Phase 3 is the beginning of synthesis because it is reformulating cues into patterns. Patterns indicate the sequencing of behavior over time. Cues from the nursing assessment and client data from all other sources are examined to determine whether the client's response is an isolated incidence or whether it indicates a pattern. Theile and co-workers (1986:319) state that "within nursing, clinical situations often evolve as a series of pieces, or cues, much as the pieces of a puzzle . . . (and) the fitting together of these cues to form a total picture is termed linking." The cues are clustered or linked together to see what pieces fit together and which is the best or most appropriate fit. *Inductively,* individual cues are evaluated and clustered to form a pattern, or cues may be taken from different assessment categories and clustered to form a pattern. As shown in Table 7-1, questions to ask in this phase are: Which cues are relevant? Which cues are nonrelevant? Which cues belong in which patterns?

Various client response patterns can be examined. The subconcepts that address the client within nursing and other models are used to cluster data into patterns. The North American Nursing Diagnosis Association (1988) has identified nine patterns of human response or interaction: exchanging, communicating, relating, valuing, choosing, moving, perceiving, knowing, and feeling. These nine patterns are part of the Nursing Diagnosis Taxonomy, and appropriate nursing diagnoses are listed under each pattern. A complete list of this taxonomy is

given in Chapter 8. Gordon's (1987) eleven functional health patterns are also frequently used for clustering cues. Gordon's patterns are health perception-health management, nutrition-metabolic, elimination, activity-exercise, sleep-rest, cognitive-perceptual, self-perception–self-concept, role-relationship, sexuality-reproductive, coping-stress tolerance, and value-beliefs. Other examples of patterns are communicating, adapting, health care practices, parenting, populations at risk, and funding of health care. *Deductively,* the nurse examines each pattern and sees what cues fit into each pattern.

Table 7-4 describes how cues from different data collection categories may be clustered to form a pattern. In the example, cues relating to the client's nutritional-metabolic pattern are taken from categories of biophysical, psychological, and sociological data. The activity-exercise pattern has different cues from some of the same categories. Cues that are clustered into a socioeconomic pattern are derived from the physiological, psychological, and developmental patterns. Helpful resources are the defining characteristics listed in the manuals and handbooks of nursing diagnosis (cited in phase 2). The nurse may compare the list of clustered cues, signs, and symptoms with the list of defining characteristics in a specific pattern area. For example, if the client has a cluster of nutritional cues such as one meal a day, a loss of 10 pounds within the past week, and pale conjunctivae, the nurse could review nutritional nursing diagnoses and their defining characteristics for a "fit." In this case, the correct conclusion would be a dysfunctional pattern that is reflective of the defining characteristics in the nursing diagnosis, *nutritional deficit.*

4. *Appropriate theories, models, concepts, norms, and standards are applied and compared with patterns.* Phase 4 is the major phase in the synthesis process, incorporating the data to form a whole. In this phase the nurse applies theories, models, and concepts to explain the clustered data and compares the data with norms and standards. Components or concepts from the model are used in interpreting the data. Models and theories that may be used are nursing systems, human need, perception, and communication. Others that may be used are crisis, family, role, and stress theories. Examples of the application of nursing models include comparing the patterns with Roy's description of adaptive or ineffective behaviors, determining self-care deficits according to Orem, and identifying the stages of the nurse-client relationship, according to Peplau. To apply systems theory, data are interpreted as input, throughput, and output. Decision-making questions in this phase are the following:

**Table 7-4** Cues Clustered into Patterns Using Gordon's Model

| Data Categorization | | Patterns |
|---|---|---|
| **Biophysical** | | |
| 1. Nutrition | | *Nutrition/metabolic pattern* |
| I | "I eat one meal a day, usually a hot dog, and drink three or four soft drinks." | All cues in category<br>"I don't want any change."<br>"I am 60 years old." |
| O | Skin folds on arms and ankles | $50 for food.<br>Black |
| M | 5 ft 2 in, 300 lb | |
| 2. Exercise | | *Activity/exercise pattern* |
| I | "I sit alone all day and watch TV with my cat." | "I eat one meal a day. . . ."<br>"I sit alone all day. . . ."<br>"I am 60 years old."<br>". . . income is $200 a month." |
| **Psychological** | | *Self-perception/self-concept pattern* |
| I | "I like my life as it is. I don't want any change. . . ."<br>"I am 60 years old." | ". . . sit alone . . . watch TV with cat . . ."<br>All cues in category<br>"I live alone." |
| O | Sits in chair; stares out window; no eye contact.<br>Female | |
| **Sociological** | | *Role-relationship pattern* |
| I | "I live alone. My income is $200 a month. Rent costs me $100 a month and utilities about $50." | "I am 60 years old."<br>All cues |
| O | Black | |
| **Spiritual** | | No data available |

Which theories, concepts, norms, and standards are most appropriate for interpreting the patterns? What does the client consider "normal?" Which patterns fit the defining characteristics of a nursing diagnosis? (See Table 7-1.)

Nurses need to know developmental and physiological norms as well as psychological parameters when comparing and interpreting client patterns. Standards used for individuals may include the Metropolitan Life Insurance Company height and weight chart, the four basic food groups, normal ranges of vital signs and laboratory values, and developmental stages (such as Erikson's or the Denver Developmental Screening Test). The data are compared with normal ranges, values, expectations, and data from the client's previous condition.

An important aspect of this phase is the client's perception of "normal," because this may differ from the nurse's assumptions and perceptions. The nurse must learn and take into account the client's

health standards as well as cultural standards. When the client and nurse agree on these standards, mutuality and cooperation are more likely. If they do not agree, further assessment and evaluation may be needed.

Examples of comparing and applying data are given in Table 7-5. In the example, the client's nutritional pattern may be compared with the four basic food groups, adequate daily caloric and fluid intake, and the Metropolitan chart for height and weight. The client's exercise and socialization patterns may be compared with developmental normals while allowing for individuality. Although data gaps exist, the client's income and expenses may be analyzed mathematically and compared with federal poverty guidelines.

*5. Health concerns and strengths are identified.* In phase 5, the nurse identifies client strengths and concerns based on empirical and personal knowledge. This is done by drawing conclusions about client patterns after comparison with theories,

**Table 7-5** Application and Comparison of Theories, Models, Concepts, Norms, and Standards with Patterns

| Patterns | Application and comparison |
|---|---|
| **Biophysical** | |
| 1. Nutrition/metabolic | |
| Skin folds, eats one meal a day, hot dog, 3-4 soft drinks a day, 5 ft 2 in, 300 lb "I don't want any change." "I am 60 years old." $50 for food Black | Caloric intake Basic four food groups Fluid intake Metropolitan Life chart |
| 2. Exercise/activity | |
| "I eat one meal a day." "I sit alone all day . . ." Walks with cane "I am 60 years old." ". . . income is $200 a month" | Maslow physiological Developmental activities |
| **Psychological (self-perception/self-concept)** | |
| ". . . sit alone, watch TV with my cat." Sitting, staring; no eye contact; likes life as is; wants no changes. Female "I live alone." "I am 60 years old." | Developmental theory Maslow self-esteem Psychological theory |
| **Sociological (role-relationship)** | |
| "I am 60 years old." Lives alone, income $200, rent $100, utilities $50 | Role theory Federal guidelines for assistance and poverty |
| **Spiritual** | No data available |

models, concepts, norms, and standards. It is done by inferences, ruling out, and deciding the client's response to a situation or condition. "Inferential reasoning is the process by which the unknown is tentatively inferred or predicted from the known" (Gordon, 1982:168).

Inferences are made about the client's health status, condition, or situation in each of the assessment categories. Various types of client concerns are identified. After interpreting the data, the nurse makes one or more of the following judgments:

- There are no concerns. The client appears to be functioning/coping at an optimum level.
- There are actual concerns. Client data indicate excesses, deficits, or stressors in one or more areas.
- There are potential concerns. The client is at risk.
- There are possible concerns. The nurse has reason to suspect a concern but needs more data or verification of existing data.
- There are client strengths. The client's abilities are identified as assets, strengths, or resources. These strengths are integrated in the plans for nursing care. Examples of strengths and concerns for the individual, family, and community are shown in Table 7-6.

As shown in Table 7-1, decision-making questions to ask in phase 5 are the following: What are all possible hypotheses, alternatives, or options? What is the probability that each alternative is present? Which alternatives are not valid? Which hypotheses are valid? Are there enough data to rule out? Are there enough data to confirm? Which patterns are functional? Which patterns or cues are strengths? Which patterns are dysfunctional, that is, which are actual, potential, or possible concerns? What is the rationale for all the inferences and conclusions? Decision-making models may be applied in this step. Decision-making is a cyclical process of exploring, ranking, and evaluating alternatives, selecting the best alternative, and exploring for new information to confirm or reject the conclusion.

After applying theories, norms, and standards, the nurse hypothesizes about the results, looking at alternative possibilities. This may be referred to as the concept of *branching*, or the generation of several hypotheses that guide the search for additional cues (Gordon, 1982; Aspinall, 1979; Little and Carnevali, 1976). The nurse may identify several options: there may be no concerns evident, or there may be two or three other alternatives. For example, using the client data from the nutritional-metabolic pattern in Table 7-5, alternative options are:

- There are no concerns; the pattern is functional. This option can be ruled out because of the client's height, weight, and nutritional intake.
- The client has alterations in nutrition—more than body requirements because of the cues: 5 ft 2 in, 300 lb, and body folds. This is a tentative confirmation.
- The client has alterations in nutrition—less

**Table 7-6**  Examples of Strengths and Concerns Applied to the Individual, Family, and Community

| Client | Strengths | Concerns |
|---|---|---|
| Individual | Ability for self-care | Decreased self-care |
| | Feelings of independence | Dependence |
| | High morale | Lack of self-esteem |
| | Family support | No family |
| | Many friends | Social isolation |
| | Adequate housing | Inadequate housing |
| | Education | Lack of job skills |
| Family | Past coping experience | Crisis |
| | Open communication | Dysfunctional communication |
| | Adequate financial resources | Inadequate resources |
| | Extended family presence | No support system |
| | Flexible rules | Rigid rules |
| | Defined roles | Confused roles |
| Community | Adequate funding to meet health needs | Inadequate funding |
| | Enthusiastic leadership and interest in health concerns | Disinterest |
| | Health services available | Health services unavailable |
| | Health services accessible | Health services inaccessible |
| | Health services acceptable | Health services unacceptable |

than body requirements because of her 24-hour recall and comparison with the four basic food groups. Because this is a more accurate fit even though the client is definitely overweight, alternative 2 can be ruled out.

In reality, the next phase in data processing would also occur while hypotheses about strengths and concerns are being tested, that is, proposing an etiology or considering contributing factors to the identified concern. However, in this text, the two phases are described separately.

Aspinall and Tanner (1981) list several problems that may result when alternative explanations and options are not considered or tested: overemphasizing the probability of one explanation, omitting the accurate diagnosis in the initial hypothesis, failing to analyze and synthesize all the data because of a narrow focus, and making an incorrect conclusion as a result of speed, stereotypical views, or inexperience. It is also important not to make assumptions and inferences about missing data, but to make conclusions only about known data.

Sometimes there is confusion in differentiating need from concern; *needs* must be gratified for the normal functioning of an individual. Maslow (1970) identified basic needs as physiological, safety, love and belonging, esteem, and self-actualization. A *concern* or problem exists when an individual cannot provide need gratification. According to Bower and Bevis (1979:176), "a problem is an interruption

in the individual's ability to meet a need; it is a difficulty or perplexity that requires resolution." It is preferable to use the term "concern" rather than problem, disability, deficit, or limitation, all of which have negative connotations.

Table 7-7 provides examples of the application of theories, concepts, norms, and standards for making conclusions or inferences about the client's health concerns and strengths. Considering the client's nutritional-metabolic pattern, there is an actual concern because she is deficient in the four basic food groups. There is uncertainty about caloric intake, because it is not known whether the soft drinks are regular or diet; there is uncertainty about fluid intake, because the size of the container that the client uses is unknown; and the client is approximately 75% overweight, depending on the standard used. There is also a concern about her exercise-activity pattern because of her weight, limited mobility, and sedentary life-style. There is a potential concern about socialization, because data indicate that the client has limited social exchange and limited activity and that she lives alone. According to federal guidelines, the client's income is below the poverty level, so this concern needs to be further explored and referred. The client also has only $50 per month to purchase food after paying expenses. There are other possible concerns that need further exploration, such as self-care, elimination, and other biophysical patterns.

**Table 7-7** Inferences of Actual, Potential, or Possible Concerns and Strengths after Application and Comparison of Theories, Concepts, Norms, and Standards

| Applications and Comparisons | Conclusions |
|---|---|
| **Biophysical** | **Biophysical** |
| Nutrition/metabolic | Nutrition/metabolic |
| Four basic food groups | *Actual concern: inadequate intake of basic four |
| Caloric intake | Unknown |
| Fluid intake | Unknown |
| Metropolitan Life chart | *Actual concern: above wt limit for ht |
| Exercise/activity | Exercise/activity |
| Maslow physiological | *Actual concern: |
| Developmental | Decreased mobility |
| | Not doing tasks for level |
| | Sedentary |
| | *Strength: some mobility with cane |
| **Psychological** | **Psychological** |
| Developmental | *Potential isolation concern |
| Maslow | *Possible belonging need |
| Psychological | *Strength: cares for pet |
| **Sociological** | **Sociological** |
| Federal guidelines | *Actual concern: |
| Role | Inadequate income |
| | Below poverty level |
| | *Strength: independent |

*Asterisk indicates concerns for nursing diagnosis.

6. *Etiological relationships are proposed.* In phase 6, the nurse explores and identifies factors influencing or contributing to the list of concerns. The nurse makes inferences and hypotheses about the possible causal relationships of client concerns. These are pivotal judgments in data processing because the statement of etiological relationships gives direction to nursing interventions. As shown in Table 7-1, questions to ask in this phase are: Which cues or patterns may be the contributing factors for the concern, and Which nursing diagnosis etiology is the "best fit" for the identified concerns?

Examples of possible etiologies are shown in Table 7-8. Inasmuch as an actual nutritional concern is indicated in the example by inadequate intake of the four basic food groups and the client's excess

**Table 7-8** Formulation of Etiologic Relationships to Identified Concerns

| Concerns | Possible etiology |
|---|---|
| Actual: nutrition/ metabolic | Lack of motivation |
| | Lack of appetite |
| Inadequate intake | Inadequate income |
| Overweight | Loneliness |
| | Lack of activity |
| Actual: exercise/activity | Lack of motivation |
| Limited mobility | Inadequate income for diversional activities |
| Overweight | |
| Sedentary lifestyle | Lack of transportation |
| | Depression |
| Potential: social isolation | Limited mobility |
| | Lack of transportation |
| | Depression |
| | No support system |
| Actual: inadequate income | Lack of knowledge of resources |
| | Inability to qualify for resources |
| | Beliefs about asking for help |

weight, the nurse must explore probable causes or contributing factors. From the limited data available, the cause could be lack of motivation, lack of appetite, inadequate income, loneliness, or a combination. These factors need to be explored further and validated with the client.

The actual concern about exercise/activity could be related to lack of interest, inadequate income for diversional activities, lack of transportation, depression, or a combination of factors. The client is at high risk for social isolation, which could be influenced by her limited mobility, lack of transportation, depression, and inadequate support system.

The client's inadequate income could be related to her lack of knowledge of resources, her inability to qualify for resources, of her beliefs about asking for help. It is possible that some actual concerns are probable etiologies for other concerns. This situation must be clarified and prioritized with the client. For example, if inadequate income is prioritized as one of the first concerns, exploring the etiology may help solve part of the nutrition and exercise concerns.

It is also possible that one etiologic factor may be related to several concerns. For example, lack of motivation may be a contributing factor for both nutrition and exercise concerns. Guidelines for differentiating the concerns and etiologic relationship(s) are discussed in Chapter 8.

## APPLICATION OF MODELS

The choice of a model for the nursing process is made during the data collection component. The model then provides a structure for categorizing and interpreting the data. It may influence the wording of the diagnostic statement. Examples of models are given for the individual, family, and community in the following section and are also provided in Chapters 2 and 6.

### Individual

Several nursing models may be used for analyzing and synthesizing data about the individual client. Model selection is influenced by factors related to the client, the nurse, and the setting. Client factors to consider are age and health status. Some models such as Orem's may be interpreted as focused on adults who are motivated toward self-care. Others such as Hall's model may be especially appropriate for the rehabilitation client, whereas an interactional model such as Peplau's may better meet the concerns of a mental health client. Several nursing models that are adaptatations of systems theory (such as Roy's, Neuman's, Rogers', and Johnson's) may be used across all clinical areas. Nurses should select models most appropriate to the client's age and health status.

Nurse factors influencing nursing model selection include the nurse's philosophy and knowledge base. Nursing education programs offer a variety of curricular frameworks, some of which use one specific nursing model. Others take an eclectic approach that familiarizes students with several nursing models. Nurses should use models with which they agree and are knowledgeable.

The setting is another factor that may influence nursing model selection. Some agencies (such as acute, long-term, and home care) may have adopted a particular nursing model as a basis for professional practice. Nurses must be knowledgeable of the agency's philosophy and practice base.

When Orem's (1985) model is used, data are categorized according to the universal self-care requisites. The client is then determined to be within one of the three nursing systems: wholly compensatory, partially compensatory, or supportive-educative.

When Roy's (1984) adaptation model is used, data are categorized according to basic physiological needs, self-concept, role function, and interdependence. The patterns are interpreted as adaptive or ineffective. Table 7-9 demonstrates application of the model with the guidelines for analyzing and synthesizing the data. A written summary of the

processed data is then provided; this identifies the model and its components, with application and interpretation of the data.

### Individual Case Study

**Interaction data (from record and client).** Mrs. B is a 75-year-old widow of Appalachian origin who lives alone with her dog in the house she and her husband built in their urban neighborhood 50 years ago. Her husband died 2 months ago. She has four children and five grandchildren, all of whom live out of town. The children write or call her at least once a month. Mrs. B knits items for her grandchildren. She is a retired clerk, and belongs to the Methodist church. Her income includes Social Security, pension, and Medicare. She states, "My name is Sarah. I'm in the hospital for high blood pressure. I haven't taken my medicine for 2 weeks. I just forget to take it. My feet are so swollen that I can't wear my shoes. And another thing, I just can't keep to that low-salt diet."

**Observation and measurement data.** Client is sitting up in hospital bed, smiling. No teeth in mouth. Wears glasses. Walker next to bed. Height 5 ft 3 in, weight 160 lb, temperature 98.6 F, pulse 72 beats per minute and regular, respirations 20 per minute; blood pressure 200/100 (right arm, sitting). Lungs clear but client exhibits shortness of breath. Color pink. Extremities cool to touch. Unable to palpate pedal pulses. Pitting edema 4+ of both ankles and feet. Circumference of right ankle 10 in, left ankle 10½ in.

### Individual Analysis and Synthesis: Roy's Adaptation Model

According to Roy's adaptation model (1984), there are four adaptive modes or ways for the client to cope with environmental changes: physiological, self-concept, role function, and interdependence. This client's data are analyzed according to these four categories.

*Physiological needs* include activity and rest, nutrition, elimination, fluid and electrolyte balance, oxygenation and circulation, endocrine function, skin integrity, the senses, and neurological functions. In the category of *activity and rest*, the first-level assessment data indicate an ineffective response. The regulator behaviors of the cardiovascular system are affecting the client's mobility. The clustered behavioral cues from nutrition, fluid and electrolytes, endocrine function, and self-concept provide the basis for the second-level assessment: identifying the stressors (stimuli). The focal stimuli causing her physical inactivities are the alterations in her circulatory system. Contextual and residual

**Table 7-9**　Analysis and Synthesis of the Individual Client: Roy's Adaptation Model*

| | Analysis | | Synthesis | | |
|---|---|---|---|---|---|
| **1. Data Categorization†** | **2. Data Gaps** | **3. Patterns‡** | **4. Applications/ Comparisons** | **5. Conclusions** | **6. Etiology** |
| **A. Physiological** | | | | | |
| *1. Activity/rest* | | | | | |
|   I　"I can't wear shoes." | Range of motion, sleep, safety | A.　1. All cues<br>    2. 5 ft 3 in, 160 lb<br>    4. Edema (4+)<br>    8. Wears glasses | Physiology, nursing, aging theories | Ineffective: Mobility Potential safety concerns | Circulation |
|   O　Walker beside bed | | B.　Age 75 years | | | Mobility, vision |
| *2. Nutrition* | | | | | |
|   I　"Can't stay on low-salt diet." | Nutritional assessment, knowledge of diet, effect on intake | A.　1. Can't wear shoes<br>    2. All cues<br>    4. Edema (4+)<br>    8. Wears glasses | Nutrition, Metropolitan chart, aging theories | Ineffective: Excessive weight, Noncompliance | |
|   M　5 ft 3 in, 160 lb | | | | | Unknown |
|   O　Edentulous | | B.　Age 75 years<br>D.　Lives alone | | Possible chewing concern | Edentulous |
| *3. Elimination* | Elimination | | | | |
| *4. Fluid and electrolytes* | Intake, salt, elimination | A.　1. Can't wear shoes<br>    4. All cues<br>    6. Has not taken medicine | Physiology, nursing | Ineffective: Excess fluid concern | Lack of medication, diet |
|   M　Edema (4+), right ankle 10 in, left 10½ in | | | | | |
| *5. Oxygenation* | | | | | |
|   O　Color pink, lungs clear | Knowledge of hypertension, past medical history, skin and foot assessment | A.　1. Can't wear shoes<br>    2. Can't stay on diet<br>    4. Edema (4+), R ankle 10 in, L 10½ in<br>    6. All cues | Physiology, pathophysiology, nursing, aging | Ineffective: Oxygenation concern | Alterations in circulation |
|   M　P 72, R 20, BP 200/100 | | | | | |
|   O　Extremities cool to touch; unable to palpate pedal pulses | | B.　States name, location; age 75 years | | | |
| *6. Endocrine function* | | | | | |
|   I　"I haven't taken my medicine in 2 weeks. I just forget to take it." | Knowledge of medication, motivation, daily schedule, sexuality history | A.　1. Can't wear shoes<br>    2. Can't stay on diet<br>    4. All cues<br>    6. All cues | Physiology, pharmacology, nursing, aging | Ineffective: Noncompliant with medication | Forgetfulness, unresolved grief, vision |
|   M　T 98.6. | | | | Adaptive: Temperature | |

*Refer to pp. 143 and 146-147 for clarification of table.
†I, Interaction; O, observation; M, measurement
‡Letters and numbers under 3. Pattern refer to the categories from which the cues were taken.

**Table 7-9** Analysis and Synthesis of the Individual Client: Roy's Adaptation Model—cont'd

| Analysis | | Synthesis | | | |
|---|---|---|---|---|---|
| 1. Data Categorization | 2. Data Gaps | 3. Patterns | 4. Applications/ Comparisons | 5. Conclusions | 6. Etiology |
| 7. *Skin integrity* | Skin and foot assessment | | | | |
| 8. *Senses* O Wears glasses | Hearing, smell, touch, date of last eye exam, acuity | | Physiology, aging | Adaptive: Glasses Potential safety concern | Vision |
| 9. *Neurological function* | Neurological | | | | |
| **B. Self-concept** *Personal self* I "My name is Sarah. I'm in the hospital for high blood pressure." O Age 75 years Appalachian origin Sitting up in bed, smiling | Health maintenance practices, values and beliefs | A. 1. Can't wear shoes 2. Edentulous, 5 ft 3 in, 160 lb 6. Has not taken medicine 8. Wears glasses B. All cues | Psychology, nursing, aging theories, Appalachian culture | Adaptive: Oriented; assess further | |
| **C. Role function** I Retired clerk Knits for grandchildren Husband died 2 months ago Four children, five grandchildren | Developmental tasks Past coping, grieving process | B. Age 75 years C. All cues D. Lives alone with dog, belongs to Methodist church | Role, family, Erikson, aging theories; grief/loss | Adaptive: Several roles Possibly maladaptive: Widowhood | Recent loss of husband |
| **D. Interdependence** I Lives alone with dog Receives Social Security, pension, Medicare Belongs to Methodist church Children write or call once a month | Significant others, pet care, diversional activities, communication, transportation, home maintenance management | B. All cues C. All cues D. All cues | Family, Maslow, aging, nursing theories, economics | Potentially ineffective: Socialization Home maintenance management concern | Lives alone, mobility Mobility |

stimuli are her edematous feet, her inability to wear shoes, and noncompliance with medication and diet. The client's behaviors do not maintain her level of psychological adequacy, so there is an adaptation problem in exercise and rest.* There is also a potential safety concern (an important need according to Maslow, 1970) related to her impaired mobility and possible vision concern. Clients in this age group have a high incidence of home accidents (DHEW, 1979), so an important data gap is an environmental assessment. Other data gaps in this category are range of motion and sleep patterns.

In the category of *nutrition*, the client's height and weight indicate that she is approximately 40 lb overweight according to the Metropolitan chart of 1978. This alteration in nutrition is an ineffective response, so it is maladaptive, although the cause needs further exploration.* The probable stimuli are noncompliance with her low-salt diet, and inactivity. Other possible causes may be decreased vision for food preparation that sometimes occurs with aging, and lack of motivation or appetite as a result of her recent loss and role change. Therefore, a complete nutritional assessment is needed before an etiological relationship can be identified. There is also a concern about the client's ability to eat (chew) because of being edentulous.* Data gaps also exist regarding her knowledge of her diet and the effect of eating without teeth.

There is an important gap regarding *elimination* that must be a priority assessment because of the client's circulatory impairment. *Fluids and electrolytes* are ineffective,* as indicated by the edema (4+), ankle circumferences, and the inability to wear shoes. The influencing factors or stimuli may be the omission of her medication for 2 weeks, or her diet, or both. Data gaps include daily fluid intake, amount of salt in diet, and elimination.

The client's *oxygenation* pattern indicates some strengths, as shown by the clustered cues of pink color, pulse 72, respirations 20, clear lungs, and clarity of thought (orientation to person and place). However, according to Bates (1983), her blood pressure is elevated. This and the pattern of clustered cues from exercise, nutrition, fluids, and endocrine function indicate ineffective *oxygenation and circulation.* Although there are circulatory changes with aging, this client is experiencing alterations that are not within normal limits. The influencing factors and stimuli are her history of hypertension and noncompliance with medication and diet. Data

gaps exist regarding her knowledge of her condition, complete past medical history, and skin and feet assessment (as an indication of the effectiveness of her circulatory system).

In the *endocrine function* category, the client's temperature is adaptive. Her noncompliance with her medication is ineffective* and may be related to sensory overload, unresolved grief, or decreased vision. Data gaps include knowledge of medication, motivation, daily schedule, and sexuality history.

The client's *skin integrity* is a data gap that is a priority need. In the category, *senses*, the client wears glasses, which is adaptive, but her visual acuity is unknown. Other data gaps include the date of her last eye examination and her ability to hear, smell, taste, and touch. There is a potential safety concern related to her vision.*

The final physiological category, *neurological function*, is a data gap, although the client is oriented.

The category of *self-concept* includes personal, physical, and moral self. Interaction and observation data in personal self clustered with the physical self data that appear in other categories indicate that the client is adaptive (she is oriented to person, time, and place and responds appropriately to questions). Further assessment is needed of the client's health maintenance practices (such as breast self-examination, Pap smear, and visits to the dentist, ophthalmologist, and physician) and values and beliefs, or moral self (spiritual and cultural information).

*Role function* consists of role performance, role mastery, and primary, secondary, and tertiary roles. The client's role function is indicated by the primary, secondary, and tertiary roles of retired clerk, widow, mother, grandmother, church member, "pensioner," pet lover, and now patient/client. According to Erikson (1963), the client is coping (adapting) with the ego integrity stage of development because of these roles and the fact that she is not exhibiting signs of despair. Limited data indicate that she appears to be coping with hospitalization. There is a potential role adjustment related to the recent death of her husband, although her adaptation is unknown.* Adjusting to grief and loss is common in this age group, but individual coping varies. Data gaps include developmental tasks, past coping, and grieving.

The *interdependence* category includes affectional adequacy and support systems. The client's support systems are Social Security, pension, Medicare, her church (amount of support is a data gap), her dog, and her family. Although the exact

---

* Asterisk indicates concerns for nursing diagnosis.

amount of income and expenses is unknown, the patterned data indicate that the client has adequate income, but this needs to be explored further. She has been living independently with her dog, which is adaptive. There is now the potential concern of how the client will manage the maintenance of her home and the care of her pet.* There is also the potential concern for social isolation because of her impaired mobility and living alone. According to Maslow (1970), the need for belonging is a necessary basis for developing self-esteem. That her children write or call each month indicates family concern and caring, but data gaps exist as to affectional adequacy and significant others nearby. Other data gaps include caregiver of the dog during the period of the client's hospitalization, diversional activities, communication, transportation, and home maintenance management (for example, how she does her shopping, laundry, cleaning).

The client's strengths are adequate oxygen, temperature regulation, orientation, coping with hospitalization, meeting most developmental needs, and adequate income.

The client's concerns are:

1. Impaired mobility related to alterations in lower limbs, edema, inability to wear shoes
2. Potential for injury related to impaired mobility and possibly decreased vision
3. Nutrition, excessive weight related to noncompliance and other unknown causes
4. Possible nutrition concern related to being edentulous
5. Excess fluid volume related to noncompliance with medication and diet
6. Impaired circulation related to noncompliance with medication and diet
7. Noncompliance of medication related to forgetfulness, unresolved grief, and decreased vision
8. Potential ineffective coping related to possible unresolved grief
9. Potential social isolation related to impaired mobility and living alone
10. Potential impairment in home maintenance management related to impaired mobility, recent loss of husband
11. Incomplete data base (in order of priority): elimination; nutritional and fluid assessment; knowledge of diet, medication, and hypertension; communication; effect of no teeth; visual acuity; range of motion; sleep;

environmental safety; home maintenance management including pet care; motivation; developmental tasks including grieving and past coping; significant others; values and beliefs, health maintenance practices; diversional activities; transportation; daily schedule; sexuality history; past medical history

## Family

Family data are analyzed using models different from those used with individual clients. Four well-established frameworks are systems, structural-functional, interactional, and developmental. Conclusions from family data indicate whether patterns are functional or dysfunctional, adequate or inadequate, altered or potentially altered. Family patterns that are functional are family strengths. Patterns that are not functional need to be clarified and identified as concerns.

If a systems approach is used, the family is evaluated as an open or closed system with rigid, diffuse, or permeable boundaries; functional or dysfunctional self-regulatory mechanisms (throughput); and system overload or deprivation (input or output).

The structural-functional approach is a variation of systems theory. In analysis, the functional and structural components are categorized separately. Structure may be grouped and evaluated according to:

1. Role structure (position, behavior, conflict, strain, sharing, and modification)
2. Value systems (overt or covert rules, priorities, conflicts, and restrictive or flexible)
3. Communication patterns (functional or dysfunctional)
4. Power structure (coalitions and decision-making, classified as dominated, autonomic, or leaderless)

The functional categories are either adequate or inadequate, functional or dysfunctional. These distinctions apply to Friedman's (1981) categories of family function: affection (personality maintenance); socialization and social placement; reproduction; family coping, economy; and provision of physical necessities. An example of this approach is shown later.

The interactional approach focuses on ways family members interrelate. Internal family dynamics are analyzed in this approach as functional, potentially alterable, or altered. Processes or dynamics interpreted are role, status, communication patterns, decision-making, coping patterns, and socialization. This approach is limited and needs to

* Asterisk indicates concerns for nursing diagnosis

be used in conjunction with another model. Satir (1972) uses the interactional process to identify four categories: rules, self-worth, communication, and links to society.

Duvall (1977) and Stevenson (1977) use the developmental approach with family tasks and stages of progression through the life cycle. The collected data are analyzed for clues that identify the stage. Then a descriptive statement is made, noting the developmental needs.

An example of how to use the guidelines of the analysis/synthesis process with a family client is provided (Table 7-10), according to Friedman's (1981) structural-functional model.

**Table 7-10**   Analysis and Synthesis of the Family Client: Structural-Functional Model Applied to Powell Family*

| Analysis | | | Synthesis | | |
|---|---|---|---|---|---|
| 1. Data Categorization | 2. Data Gaps | 3. Patterns | 4. Applications/ Comparisons | 5. Conclusions | 6. Etiology |
| **A. Structure** | | | | | |
| *1. Role* | | | | | |
| a. Age 34 yr, female, co-support, college graduate | Anticipatory plans, feelings | A. 1. All cues 2. Child care B. 2. Graduate, representative, church 5. Work 6. Prenatal care | Psychology, role, family theory, developmental | Multiple roles: Mother, wife, daughter, employee, volunteer, alumna, patient/client, church member | |
| | | | | Potential stress | Multiple roles and role change |
| b. Age 35 yr, male, co-support, college graduate | Anticipatory plans, feelings | A. 1. All cues B. 2. Graduate, Big Brother, church 5. Owns business | Potential stress | Multiple roles: Father, husband, business owner, church member, alumnus | Multiple roles |
| c. Age 3 yr, male | Feelings, preparation | A. 1. All cues 2. Child care | | Son, grandson, brother-to-be | |
| | | | | Potential concern | Role change |
| *2. Values* | | | | | |
| "We share chores." Alone time Together time Attend church Child care by grandparents | Cultural assessment, spiritual assessment | A. 1.a. Graduate B. 5. Works Owns business 6. Buying home Prenatal care | Philosophy, religion, culture | Values: Work, democracy, self-worth, relationship, religion, responsibility, health No apparent conflict: Strength | |
| *3. Communication patterns* | | | | | |
| Couple takes turns speaking and listening, include child. | Patterns with grandparents | A. 1. All cues 2. Share chores | Satir, communication, growth and development | Functional: Strength Child's pattern within normal limits | |

*Refer to pp. 147 and 150-151 for clarification of table.

**Table 7-10**  Analysis and Synthesis of the Family Client: Structural-Functional Model Applied to Powell Family—cont'd

| Analysis | | | Synthesis | | |
|---|---|---|---|---|---|
| **1. Data Categorization** | **2. Data Gaps** | **3. Patterns** | **4. Applications/ Comparisons** | **5. Conclusions** | **6. Etiology** |
| Child speaks in sentences, calls parents Mommy and Daddy. | | | | | |
| 4.  *Power structure* Couple makes decisions jointly. | Past decisions: Outcome and process | A.  2. Share chores 3. Take turns speaking | Satir, decision-making | Share: Strength | |
| **B.  Function** | | | | | |
| 1.  *Affective pattern* Child sitting on mother's lap Couple sitting close, occasionally touching | Need-response, recreation | A.  2. Share chores, together time 3. Take turns speaking, include child 4. Share decisions | Psychology, developmental family, Maslow | Mutual nuturance: Strength | |
| 2.  *Socialization* Husband in Big Brothers Wife representative on neighborhood council | Family history, child-rearing practices, developmental status of child | A.  1. Work, college graduates 2. Child care by grandparents; attend church | Psychology, developmental, communication | Community participation: Strength | |
| 3.  *Reproduction* Pregnancy in seventh month | Sexual history, family planning, maternal reproductive history | A.  1. All cues 2. Together time B.  1. Sitting close | Psychology, family theory | Assess further | |
| 4.  *Family coping* | Past crises, coping mechanisms, resources, anticipatory plans, feelings | A.  1. All cues 2. Share chores, child care, attend church 3. Take turns 4. Joint decisions B.  1. Sitting close 5. Owns business, wife works | Satir, crises, developmental stress | Potential stressor | Birth of sibling |

*Continued.*

**Table 7-10**   Analysis and Synthesis of the Family Client: Structural-Functional Model Applied to Powell Family—cont'd

| Analysis | | | Synthesis | | |
|---|---|---|---|---|---|
| 1. Data Categorization | 2. Data Gaps | 3. Patterns | 4. Applications/ Comparisons | 5. Conclusions | 6. Etiology |
| 5. *Economics* Husband owns small business Wife works in architectural firm | Plans | A. 1. All cues 2. Child care 4. Joint decisions B. 3. Pregnancy 6. Buying home, prenatal care | Economics, family | Potential concern | Loss of income |
| 6. *Provision of physical necessities* Buying three-bedroom home Regular prenatal care | Health maintenance practices Individual health histories | B. 5. All cues 6. All cues | Economics, primary and secondary prevention | Strength | |

## Family Case Study

**Interaction data (from family interview).** Mr. and Mrs. P. are expecting their second child in 2 months; they have a 3-year-old son, Brad. Both parents are college graduates and attend church regularly. They are buying their three-bedroom brick home in a suburban neighborhood. Mr. P. is 35 years old and owns a small business. Mrs. P., age 34, works in an architectual firm and co-supports the family. "We share chores and decision-making. We also have time alone at least once a week in addition to a night out together at least once a month." Mrs. P. is a representative on their neighborhood council. She visits her private physician regularly for prenatal care. Mr. P. is a member of Big Brothers and attends their functions. Child care is provided for Brad by his maternal grandparents. Mrs. P. plans to stay at home for 1 year after the birth.

**Observation.** Brad walks across the room, climbs up on the couch with his parents, and sits on his mother's lap. Couple sitting close together on couch, occasionally touching. Couple takes turns speaking and listening; include Brad in conversation. Brad calls parents Mommy and Daddy. Speaks in complete sentences. Height approximately 3 ft, weight approximately 30 lb.

## Family Analysis and Synthesis: Structural-Functional Model

This nuclear family is analyzed using the structural-functional approach. According to Friedman (1981), family structural dimensions include role, values, communication patterns, and power structure. Family functions are affective patterns, socialization, reproduction, family coping, economy, and provision of physical necessities (food, clothing, shelter, health care).

In the *structural* component, *role* implies ascribed or achieved position in a family. Data from this family indicate that the 34-year-old woman has the roles of wife, pregnant mother, daughter, employee, volunteer, alumna, church member, client, and co-supporter. The 35-year-old man is husband, father, businessman, church member, volunteer, alumnus, and co-supporter. The 3-year-old boy is son, grandchild, and potential brother. With the arrival of the new baby, there are three potential concerns. First, the changes in the woman's role from employed to unemployed as well as her multiple roles may cause increased stress.* Data gaps include anticipatory plans and feelings. Second, there is a potential for sibling rivalry to develop in

*Asterisk indicates concerns for nursing diagnosis.

the 3-year-old.* Data gaps include preparation and feelings of the father and son. Third, there is a potential for stress in the husband due to his multiple roles and added responsibilities.*

The *economic* function involves the provision and allocation of finances, space, and materials. Data reflecting the economic function include husband owning small business and wife working in architectural firm. Other cues with economic implications are purchasing their home, the costs of prenatal care, child care (if any), and joint decision-making. There is a potential concern related to the expected loss of the wife's income.* The data gap includes anticipatory plans.

The last function is the provision of *physical necessities,* including health care. Data indicating this function are that they are purchasing a three-bedroom home, and wife gets regular prenatal care. These are strengths. Data gaps include eating habits, 3-day recall; immunizations; dates of last dental, vision, and breast examinations and Pap smear; use of alcohol and other substances including over-the-counter drugs; exercise, family and individual health history; and knowledge of labor and delivery.

The overall family strengths identified are non-conflicting values, functional communication patterns, shared power, mutual nurturance, links to society, adequate housing, and regular prenatal care.

The family concerns are:
1. Potential stress related to role change
2. Potential for sibling rivalry related to new baby
3. Potential economic concern related to loss of income
4. Maintenance of family health
5. Incomplete data base: anticipatory plans, feelings, past decision outcomes and process, relationship with extended family, family need-response, family recreation, child-rearing practices, developmental level, reproduction history, sexual history, past coping and resources, cultural and spiritual assessments, and health care practices

## Community

Models that may be used for analysis/synthesis of community data are epidemiological, interactional, structural, systems, and nursing models. Gordon's (1982:85) functional health patterns may be adapted to communities. Porter's (1987) categories of community data (personal characteristics of group members, environmental conditions, health care services, and health care needs) can be used for nursing diagnoses about population groups. Conclusions indicate a vulnerable population group, populations at risk, a combination of vulnerable and at risk, need-service mismatch, or need-service match. Another nursing model, the Omaha Classification Scheme (Iyer et al, 1986) also may be used for categorizing community data and identifying patterns. The Omaha sytem groups and processes cues in four major domains: environmental, psychosocial, physiological, and health behaviors.

Neuman's Health-Care Systems Model (1982) is an example of a nursing model that can be used for community as client. The community is assessed and analyzed/synthesized according to basic structure, lines of resistance and defense, and stressors. Conclusions indicate community stressors that are concerns. Regardless of the model used, analysis indicates patterns, resources, and influencing factors that identify strengths, concerns, and high-risk populations. Conclusions and judgments are made about each category of the model. If systems theory is used, data are interpreted according to inputs (what the community obtains, and feedback); throughput (decision-making and communication); output (what the community disposes); boundary maintenance (what the community contains and retains, permeability, and system linkages with the subsystems and suprasystems); and system states of entropy, negentropy, and homeostasis. An example of Klein's (1968) interactional framework is given later.

Community data are interpreted from histograms, frequency graphs, pie charts, statistical maps, tables, and narrative statements. The use of energy flow charts can graphically show interrelationships among systems. Concepts, theories, and standards that may be used for synthesis include communication; group; leadership; motivation; developmental; systems; nursing; public health; epidemiology; primary, secondary, and tertiary prevention; federal poverty guidelines; Environmental Protection Agency and Occupational Health and Safety Agency standards; and cultural, organizational, and political norms. The community may also be evaluated by the criteria identified by the National Commission on Community Health Services (1967) for overall health services of a community:
1. Health services should be comprehensive.
2. Health care should be continuous and coordinated.
3. Health care must be available, accessible, and acceptable.

*Asterisk indicates concerns for nursing diagnosis.

4. Health care requires adequate facilities, personnel, and finances.

An example of how to use the guidelines of the analysis/synthesis process with a community client follows, according to Klein's (1968) interactional framework (Table 7-11).

### Community Case Study

**Interaction data (interview with district council representative).** "Two of us are elected to represent our neighborhood. Not many people vote, though. They just do not seem to care. The two of us attend council meetings monthly. We tell them what we think, too, but they don't always listen."

**Observation data (observations from windshield survey and census report).** Most of the neighborhood consists of single-story frame houses, 30 to 40 years old, with peeling paint. Some have the windows boarded up. Most homes have a television antenna on the roof. The yards are approximately 20 × 30 feet; many are enclosed with chainlink fences. Railroad tracks abut the east and south sides of the neighborhood, a freeway is on the west side, and a large fertilizer factory is on the north side. There are no sidewalks or curbs. The streets have at least one pothole in every other

block. No health facilities are observed. However, there is a parochial school next to a Catholic church, with a sign on a side door of the church indicating a senior citizen center location. A paper boy is delivering the evening paper. There are several elderly women in the neighborhood grocery store. They are dressed in cotton dresses and sneakers, chatting with one another. There is also a neighborhood newsletter attached to the bulletin board in the grocery store.

#### Measurement data: demographic data

| Age (yr) | 0-4 | 5-14 | 15-44 | 45-44 | 45-64 | 65+ |
|---|---|---|---|---|---|---|
| Census tract | 20 | 60 | 100 | 200 | 640 | |
| Males | 11 | 40 | 20 | 75 | 140 | |
| Females | 9 | 20 | 80 | 125 | 500* | |
| Income | | | | | | |
| <$5,000 | 800* | | | | | |
| $5,000-15,000 | 90 | | | | | |
| $15,000-24,000 | None | | | | | |
| $25,000-49,000 | None | | | | | |

*Asterisk indicates concern for nursing diagnosis.

Table 7-11 explains how this data may be analyzed and synthesized according to the guidelines.

**Table 7-11**   Analysis and Synthesis of the Community Client: Klein's Interactional Framework Applied to One Census Tract*

| Analysis | | Synthesis | | | |
|---|---|---|---|---|---|
| 1. Data Categorization | 2. Data Gaps | 3. Patterns | 4. Applications/ Comparisons | 5. Conclusions | 6. Etiology |
| **A. Community as social system** | | | | | |
| 1. *Communication* | | | | | |
| Paper boy with PM paper, TV antennas, bulletin board in grocery, newsletter, women talking in grocery | Other places where people meet (bars, drug store, restaurant); effectiveness of communication | A. 1. All cues 2. Elected representatives 3. Senior citizen center, church, school | Communication, group | Formal and informal methods: Strength | |
| 2. *Decision-making* | | | | | |
| Two elected representatives; few vote | Other leaders; effectiveness of leadership; reason for few voting | B. 1. Demographic | Leadership, group, motivation, developmental, systems | Further assessment | |

*Refer to pp. 151-152 and 154-155 for clarification of table.

**Table 7-11**  Analysis and Synthesis of the Community Client: Klein's Interactional Framework Applied to One Census Tract—cont'd

| Analysis | | Synthesis | | | |
|---|---|---|---|---|---|
| 1. Data Categorization | 2. Data Gaps | 3. Patterns | 4. Applications/ Comparisons | 5. Conclusions | 6. Etiology |
| 3. *System linkage* Parochial school next to Catholic church, senior citizen center in church | Transportation, nonchurch relationships, attendance | A. 1. Newspaper, newsletter, TV 2. Two representatives 4. Freeway | Systems | Some linkage; further assess functioning | |
| 4. *Boundary maintenance* Physical Railroad on two sides, freeway, industry | Route and frequency of emergency runs | B. 1. Demographic | Systems, accessibility | Potential for community isolation | |
| Psychological | Decibel level, noise abatement, zoning, political and social norms | B. 1. Demographic | Systems | Potential for noise pollution | Industry, railroad, freeway |
| **B. Population and environment** 1. *Demographic data* (*see* case study) | Mortality, morbidity, recreational resources, nutrition, services for elderly | A. 3. All cues 4. All cues B. 2. All cues 3. All cues | Epidemiology, developmental, primary and secondary prevention, systems, federal poverty guidelines | Concern: Mostly elderly near or below poverty level | |
| 2. *Physical environment* Frame houses, single story, peeling paint, boarded windows, yards with fences, fertilizer plant, no health facilities, no sidewalks or curbs, potholes | Size of census tract, emission and zoning enforcement, assistance for housing improvement, police and fire | A. 3. All cues 4. All cues B. 1. All cues | Systems, epidemiology, health risks | Concern: Lack of health resources Safety | Lack of sidewalks, peeling paint, boarded windows |
| | | | | Potential concern | Air pollution, industry, freeway |

*Continued.*

**Table 7-11**   Analysis and Synthesis of the Community Client: Klein's Interactional Framework Applied to One Census Tract—cont'd

| Analysis | | Synthesis | | | |
|---|---|---|---|---|---|
| 1. Data Categorization | 2. Data Gaps | 3. Patterns | 4. Applications/ Comparisons | 5. Conclusions | 6. Etiology |
| 3. *Psychological environment* | Values and beliefs; community history, culture, religion; orientation to past, future; plans | B. 1. All cues 2. All cues | Culture, sociology, psychology | Assess further | |

### Community Analysis/Synthesis: Klein's Interactional Framework

Klein's (1968) theoretical perspective of a community includes the community as a social system, population, and environment. The community as a social system includes the categories of communication, decision-making, system linkage, and boundary maintenance. Population and environment components include demographic data and the physical and psychological environments. Community data from one census tract are applied to this framework.

In the first category, community as a social system, *communication* refers to formal and informal methods. Clustered data indicate both methods operating in this neighborhood. Newspapers, television, neighborhood newsletters, and talking at the grocery store are examples. The elected representatives communicate with the council. The senior citizen center, school, and church are part of the communication network also. Data gaps include other places where people meet, such as drugstores, bars, and restaurants. From the limited data, methods of communication appear to be adequate, but the effectiveness is unknown.

*Decision-making* in this census tract is related to the two neighborhood representatives elected to the council. Further assessment is needed regarding identification of informal leaders, effectiveness of the leadership, and reasons for voter apathy. The voter apathy may be related to the demographic data (age and income of population), inadequate motivation, or a feeling of powerlessness.

*System linkage* refers to interdependence among groups within the census tract and between the census tract and the larger community. The Catholic church that houses a senior citizen center is an example of system linkage, as is the newsletter in the grocery store. Newspapers and television programs coming into the neighborhood are a form of linkage, as are the elected representatives being linked to the larger government. The freeway may facilitate system linkage. Data gaps include transportation, nonchurch relationships, participation, and support to the community (inputs of finances and services).

*Boundary maintenance* is indicated in this census tract by the physical boundaries of the railroad track on two sides, an industry on one, and a freeway on the fourth. There is a question as to how these physical boundaries are maintained, affecting accessibility into and out of the neighborhood. Because of the physical boundaries, there is a potential concern of isolation, particularly in regard to emergency vehicles coming into the neighborhood.* Data gaps include routes and frequency of emergency vehicle use. In the psychological realm, there is also a potential noise concern related to the two railroads and the freeway.* Data gaps include decibel level and noise abatement, zoning rules, and political and social norms. Although the physical boundaries may be delimiting, the neighborhood appears to be an open (as opposed to a closed) community. There are exchanges of information (newspapers in, council representatives speaking out) and goods (from industry and to the grocery store).

The second theoretical perspective of a community is population. The *demographic* characteristics indicate that most (63%) of the population in this

*Asterisk indicates concerns for nursing diagnosis.

census tract are widowed or single women, 65 years of age or older, with less than $5,000 annual income. According to the federal poverty guidelines, this is at the poverty level. This population group is at risk for chronic disease, but data indicate there are no health facilities in the tract.* The only services identified thus far that would benefit this age group are the senior citizen center, the church, and the grocery. There is a data gap concerning utilization and acceptability of these existing services. There are also more boys than girls 5 to 14 years of age. The only facilities or services for this age group are the school and the church. There is a potential concern regarding recreational/diversional activities for this group.* There are more women than men aged 15 to 45 years. This statistic and the fact that the majority of the population are women 65 years and older suggest the need for women's health services. Important data gaps that must be assessed are mortality and morbidity, for their epidemiological importance; recreational resources; nutrition; and other services for the elderly and women.

Data describing the *physical environment* clustered with demographic data indicate the following actual or potential concerns:

1. Potential air pollution related to the fertilizer plant, the railroads, and the highway.* This concern is especially important because of the elderly population, who are at higher risk for complications.
2. Safety concerns related to lack of sidewalks, peeling paint, and boarded-up buildings.* Sidewalks are important to all ages for safety, but more so for the elderly, who do not move as quickly nor see as well as younger people. Sidewalks are also an encouragement to walk and exercise, which is good primary health maintenance. The peeling paint has the potential to contribute to lead poisoning, particularly in the younger age group, as well as contributing to psychological depression. Boarded-up homes are a safety hazard that can lead to vandalism and arson. Crime affects the entire neighborhood in many ways, but the elderly feel especially vulnerable.
3. Lack of health services.* This is a real concern; however, availability and accessibility to the nearest facility need to be assessed. Data gaps include size of census tract in square miles, emission and zoning enforcement, services and assistance for housing improve-

ments, and police and fire protection. The *psychological environment* includes values and beliefs, which are a data gap. Other helpful information in this category would be a community history, cultural assessment, religion other than Catholic and numbers who are active, orientation to past and future, and community plans.

The only apparent community strength is communication, although there are many data gaps. The community concerns are:

1. Potential for community isolation related to boundaries
2. Potential for noise pollution related to industry, railroads, and freeway
3. Lack of health and women's health services
4. Safety concerns related to lack of sidewalks, peeling paint, and boarded-up buildings
5. Potential lack of recreational/diversional activities
6. Potential air pollution related to industry and freeway
7. Incomplete data base: places where people meet; effectiveness of communication; leaders and their effectiveness; reason for few voting; transportation; nonchurch relationships; attendance; routes and frequency of emergency runs; decibel level enforcement; zoning, political and social norms; mortality and morbidity; recreational resources; nutrition and other services for the elderly and women; size of census tract; aid for housing improvement; police and fire protection; values and beliefs; community history; culture, religion; orientation to past and future; plans.

## SUMMARY

In this chapter the nursing diagnosis *process* of analysis and synthesis was discussed. The cognitive processes of critical thinking and decision-making were included and integrated with the phases in the process. Guidelines were given for interpreting the data and making inferences. Examples were included for the individual, the family, and the community in the application section.

### REFERENCES AND READINGS

Aspinall MJ: The use of a decision tree to improve accuracy of diagnosis, Nurs Res 28:182, May-June 1979.
Aspinall MJ and Tanner CA: Decision-making for patient care, New York, 1981, Appleton-Century-Crofts.
Bailey JT and Claus KE: Decision making in nursing: tools for change, St. Louis, 1975, The CV Mosby Co.
Bates B: A guide to physical examination, ed 3, Philadelphia, 1983, JB Lippincott Co.

*Asterisk indicates concerns for nursing diagnosis.

Bennett M: Nursing diagnosis: in the beginning, Aust J Adv Nurs 4(1):41, 1986.

Bernhard L and Walsh M: Leadership: the key to the professionalization of nursing, St Louis, 1990, The CV Mosby Co.

Black J: Nursing diagnosis in plastic surgical nursing, Plastic Surg Nurs 7(1):4, 1987.

Black M: Critical thinking, Englewood Cliffs, NJ, 1952, Prentice-Hall, Inc.

Bower FL: The process of planning nursing care, St Louis, 1982, The CV Mosby Co.

Bower FL and Bevis EO: Fundamentals of nursing practice: concepts, roles, and functions, St Louis, 1979, The CV Mosby Co.

Braden CJ and Herban NL: Community health: a systems approach, New York, 1976, Appleton-Century-Crofts.

Campbell C: Nursing diagnosis and intervention in nursing practice, New York, 1984, John Wiley & Sons, Inc.

Carnevali DL, Mitchell PH, Woods NF, and Tanner CA: Diagnostic reasoning in nursing, Philadelphia, 1984, JB Lippincott Co.

Carper BA: Fundamental patterns of knowing in nursing, Adv Nurs Sci 1(1):13, 1978.

Carpenito LJ: Nursing diagnosis: application to clinical practice, ed 2, Philadelphia, 1987a, JB Lippincott Co.

Carpenito LJ: Handbook of nursing diagnosis, ed 2, Philadelphia, 1987b, JB Lippincott Co.

Chang BL, Roth K, Caswell D et al: CANDI: a knowledge-based system for nursing diagnosis, Comput Nurs 6(1):13, 1988.

Cianfrani, KL: The relatedness of cues with diagnostic labels following use of a patient care planning program. In McLane AM: Classification of nursing diagnoses, Proceedings of the Seventh Conference, North American Nursing Diagnosis Association, St Louis, 1987, The CV Mosby Co.

Doenges ME and Moorhouse MF: Nurse's pocket guide: nursing diagnoses with interventions, ed 2, Philadelphia, 1988, FA Davis Co.

Doona ME: The judgment process in nursing, Image 8:27, 1976.

Durand M and Prince R: Nursing diagnosis: process and decisions. In Marriner A: The nursing process: a scientific approach to nursing care, ed 2, St Louis, 1979, The CV Mosby Co.

Duvall EM: Marriage and family development, ed 5, Philadelphia, 1977, JB Lippincott Co.

Easton A: Decision making: a short course for professionals, New York, 1975, John Wiley & Sons, Inc.

Erikson EH: Childhood and society, New York, 1963, WW Norton & Co, Inc.

Field PA: The impact of nursing theory on the clinical decision making process, J Adv Nurs 12(5):563, 1987.

Fitzmaurice JB: Nurses' use of cues in the clinical judgment of activity intolerance. In McLane AM: Classification of nursing diagnoses. Proceedings of the Seventh Conference, North American Nursing Diagnosis Association, St Louis, 1987, The CV Mosby Co.

Fitzpatrick JJ: Etiology: conceptual concerns. In McLane AM: Classification of nursing diagnoses: proceedings of the Seventh Conference, North American Nursing Diagnosis Association, St Louis, 1987, the CV Mosby Co.

Fitzpatrick J and Whall A: Conceptual models of nursing analysis and application, Bowie, MD, 1983, Robert J Brady Co.

Ford JAG, Trygstad-Durland LN, and Nelms BC: Applied decision making for nurses, St Louis, 1979, The CV Mosby Co.

Friedman MM: Family nursing: theories and assessment, New York, 1981, Appleton-Century-Crofts.

Garthe K: Analysis of distinctions between nursing diagnoses-related judgments and disease-related nursing judgments. In McLane AM: Classification of nursing diagnoses. Proceedings

of the Seventh Conference, North American Nursing Diagnosis Association, St Louis, 1987, The CV Mosby Co.

George J, editor: Nursing theories: a base for professional nursing, Englewood Cliffs, NJ, 1984, Prentice-Hall, Inc.

Gerrity PL: Perception in nursing: the value of intuition, Holistic Nurs Pract 1(3):63, 1987.

Gettrust KV, Ryan SC, and Engleman DS: Applied nursing diagnosis: guides for comprehensive care planning, New York, 1985, John Wiley & Sons, Inc.

Gordon M: Predictive strategies in diagnostic tasks, Nurs Res 29(1):39, 1980.

Gordon M: Nursing diagnosis: process and application, New York, 1982, McGraw-Hill Book Co.

Gordon M: Manual for nursing diagnosis, New York, 1984, McGraw-Hill Book Co.

Gordon M: Nursing diagnosis. In Werley E and Fitzpatrick J, editor: Annual review of nursing research, 3:127, 1985, Springer.

Gordon M: Manual of nursing diagnosis 1986-1987, New York, 1987, McGraw-Hill Book Co.

Hammond KR: Clinical inference in nursing: II, a psychologist's viewpoint, Nurs Res 15:27, 1966.

Hammond KR, Kelly KJ, Schneider RJ, et al: Clinical inference in nursing: analyzing cognitive tasks representative of nursing problems, Nurs Res 15:134, 1966.

Hammond KR, Kelly KJ, and Schneider RJ: Clinical inference in nursing: revising judgments, Nurs Res 16:38, 1967.

Henderson V: Nursing process-a critique, Holistic Nurs Prac 1(3):7, 1987.

Hogan RC: Problems in use of nursing diagnosis, Ohio Nurse Rev 62(1):12, 1987.

Houldin AD, Salstein SW, and Ganley KM: Nursing diagnoses for wellness: supporting strengths, Philadelphia, 1987, JB Lippincott Co.

Iyer PW, Taptich BJ, and Bernocchi-Losey D: Nursing process and nursing diagnosis, Philadelphia, 1986, WB Saunders Co.

Justice SLG: Identification of the assessment cues used by cardiac nurses to diagnose chest pain. In McLane AM: Classification of nursing diagnoses. Proceedings of the Seventh Conference, North American Nursing Diagnosis Association, St Louis, 1987, The CV Mosby Co.

Kelly MA: Nursing diagnosis source book: guidelines for clinical application, Norwalk, Conn, 1985, Appleton-Century-Crofts.

Kepner CH and Tregoe BB: The rational manager, New York, 1965, McGraw-Hill Book Co.

Kerr ME: Cognitive processes nurses use in diagnosing patient's problems. In McLane AM: Classification of nursing diagnoses. Proceedings of the Seventh Conference, North American Nursing Diagnosis Association, St Louis, 1987, The CV Mosby Co.

Kim MJ, McFarland GK, and McLane AM: Pocket guide to nursing diagnosis, St Louis, 1984a, The CV Mosby Co.

Kim MJ, McFarland GK, and McLane AM: Classification of nursing diagnoses. Proceedings of the Fifth National Conference, St Louis, 1984b, The CV Mosby Co.

Kim MJ, McFarland GK, and McLane AM: Pocket guide to nursing diagnoses, ed 2, St Louis, 1987, The CV Mosby Co.

King IM: A theory of nursing: systems, concepts, process, New York, 1981, John Wiley & Sons, Inc.

Klein D: Community dynamics and mental health, New York, 1968, John Wiley & Sons, Inc.

LaMonica EL: The humanistic nursing process, Monterey, Calif, 1985, Wadsworth Health Sciences Division.

Lancaster W and Beale P: Decision making in nursing practice. In Lancaster J and Lancaster W: The nurse as a change agent: concepts for advanced nursing practice, St Louis, 1982, The CV Mosby Co.

Lenz ER, Wolfe Ml, Shelley SI et al: Clinical specialty preparation and nurses' interpretation of client situations, West J Nurs Res 8(4):431, 1986.

Little DE and Carnevali DL: Nursing care planning, ed 2, Philadelphia, 1976, JB Lippincott Co.

Lunney M: Nursing diagnoses: refining the system, Am J Nurs 82:456, 1982.

Mallick MJ: Nursing diagnosis and the novice student, Nurs Health Care 8:455, October 1983.

Maslow AH: Motivation and personality, ed 2, New York, 1970, Harper & Row, Publishers, Inc.

Matthews CA and Gaul AL: Nursing diagnosis from the perspective of concept attainment and critical thinking, Adv Nurs Sci 2:17, 1979.

Mitchell PH and Loustau C: Concepts basic to nursing, ed 3, New York, 1981, McGraw-Hill Book Co.

Myers JL and Spies MA: Nursing diagnostic skills: a content analysis of spontaneously generated nursing diagnoses. In McLane AM: Classification of nursing diagnoses. Proceedings of the Seventh Conference, North American Nursing Diagnosis Association, St Louis, 1987, The CV Mosby Co.

National Commission on Community Health Services: Health is a community affair, Cambridge, Mass, 1967, Harvard University Press.

Neuman B: The Neuman systems model: application to nursing education and practice, Norwalk, 1982, Appleton-Century-Crofts.

Newman MA: Nursing diagnosis: looking at the whole, Am J Nurs 84:1496, December 1984.

Newman MA: Nursing's emerging paradigm: the diagnosis of pattern. In McLane AM: Classification of nursing diagnoses. Proceedings of the Seventh Conference, North American Nursing Diagnosis Association, St Louis, 1987, the CV Mosby Co.

Nolan A: Utilizing nursing diagnosis in nursing education, Aust J Adv Nurs 4:51, December 1986-February 1987.

North American Nursing Diagnosis Association: Nursing diagnosis newsletter, 15:1, Summer 1988.

Orem DE: Nursing: concepts of practice, ed 3, New York, 1985, McGraw-Hill Book Co.

Padrick KP, Tanner CA, Putzier D et al: Hypothesis evaluation: a component of diagnostic reasoning. In McLane AM: Classification of nursing diagnoses. Proceedings of the Seventh Conference, North American Nursing Association, St Louis, 1987, The CV Mosby Co.

Parse RR: Man-living-health: a theory of nursing, New York, 1981, John Wiley & Sons, Inc.

Pinnell NN and deMeneses M: The nursing process: theory, application, and related processes, Norwalk, Conn, 1986, Appleton-Century-Crofts.

Porter EJ: The nursing diagnosis of population groups. In McLane AM: Classification of nursing diagnoses. Proceedings of the Seventh Conference, North American Nursing Diagnosis Association, St Louis, 1987, The CV Mosby Co.

Price MR: Nursing diagnosis: making a concept come alive, Am J Nurs 80:668, 1980.

Randall B, Tedrow MP, and Van Landingham J: Adaptation nursing: the Roy conceptual model applied, St Louis, 1982, The CV Mosby Co.

Roberts SL: Nursing diagnosis and the critically ill patient, Norwalk, Conn, 1987, Appleton & Lange.

Rogers ME: An introduction to the theoretical basis of nursing, Philadelphia, 1970, FA Davis Co.

Roy Sr C: Theory construction in nursing: an adaptation model, Englewood Cliffs, NJ, 1981, Prentice-Hall, Inc.

Roy Sr C: Introduction to nursing: an adaptation model, Englewood Cliffs, NJ, 1984, Prentice-Hall, Inc.

Satir V: Peoplemaking, Palo Alto, Calif, 1972, Science and Behavior Books.

Schaefer J: The interrelatedness of decision making and the nursing process, Am J Nurs 74:1852, 1974.

Shortridge LM and Lee EJ: Introduction to nursing practice, New York, 1980, McGraw-Hill Book Co.

Stein J, editor: The Random House college dictionary, rev ed, New York, 1982, Random House, Inc.

Stevenson JS: Issues and crises during middlescence, New York, 1977, Appleton-Century-Crofts.

Tanner CA: Teaching clinical judgment. In Werley, E and Fitzpatrick J: Annual review of nursing research, 5:153, 1987, Springer.

Tanner CA, Padrick KP, Westfall UE, et al: Diagnostic reasoning strategies of nurses and nursing students, Nurs Res 36(6):358, 1987.

Theiele JE, Baldwin JH, Hyde RS, et al: An investigation of decision theory: what are the effects of teaching cue recognition? J Nurs Ed 25(8):319, 1986.

Thomas S: Nursing diagnosis: what is it? Aust J Adv Nurs 4(3):41, 1987.

Tinkham CW, Voorhies EF, and McCarthy NC: Community health nursing: evolution and process in the family and community, New York, 1984, Appleton-Century-Crofts.

Titler MG: Implementation of nursing diagnoses in nursing education, Nurs Clin North Am 22(4):987, 1987.

Townsend MC: Nursing diagnoses in psychiatric nursing: a pocket guide for care plan construction, Philadelphia, 1988, FA Davis Co.

Turkoski BB: Nursing diagnosis in print, 1950-1985, Nurs Outlook 36(3):142, 1988.

US Department of Health, Education and Welfare: Healthy people: the surgeon general's report on health promotion and disease prevention, Washington, DC, 1979, DHEW.

Vroom VH and Yetton PW: Leadership and decision-making, Pittsburgh, 1973, University of Pittsburgh Press.

Watson J: Nursing: human science and health care, Norwalk, Conn, 1985, Appleton-Century-Crofts.

Westfall UE, Tanner CA, Putzier D, et al: Activating clinical inferences: a component of diagnostic reasoning in nursing, Res Nurs Health 9(4):269, 1986.

Westfall UE, Tanner CA, Putzier D, et al: Errors committed by nurses and nursing students in the diagnostic reasoning process. In McLane AM: Classification of nursing diagnoses. Proceedings of the Seventh Conference, North American Nursing Diagnosis Association, St Louis, 1987, The CV Mosby Co.

Wiedmann J and North H: Implementing the Omaha classification system in a public health agency, Nurs Clin North Am 22(4):971, 1987.

Williams SR: Essentials of nutrition and diet therapy, ed. 6, St Louis, 1990, Times Mirror/Mosby College Publishing.

Young CE: Intuition and nursing process, Holistic Nurs Pract 1(3):52, 1987.

Yura H and Walsh MB: The nursing process, ed 5, New York, 1988, Appleton & Lange.

PHYLLIS BAKER RISNER

# CHAPTER 8

# Nursing Diagnosis: Diagnostic Statements

## GENERAL CONSIDERATIONS

The *product* of the diagnostic *process* is the nursing diagnosis statement or label. The nursing diagnosis is based on the assumptions that: (1) it is an essential component of the nursing process for the purpose of planning client care; (2) it flows from the analysis and synthesis and is not identified in isolation; and (3) it is the responsibility of the professional nurse. The nursing diagnosis is also an independent function and a statement of nursing judgment.

This chapter discusses what nursing diagnoses are and when they started, reviews misconceptions about them, explores why they are important, and illustrates how to write them. Examples of nursing diagnoses from the perspective of the individual, family, and community as client are related to selected models. Guidelines for determining nursing diagnostic statements are explained in detail throughout the chapter and are cited here:

1. The nursing diagnosis is a statement of an actual or potential health concern.
2. The nursing diagnosis is written as a descriptive and etiological statement.
3. The nursing diagnosis is concise and clear.
4. The nursing diagnosis is client centered, specific, and accurate.
5. The nursing diagnosis provides direction for nursing interventions.
6. The nursing diagnosis is the basis for independent and collaborative nursing actions/interventions.
7. The list of nursing diagnoses reflects the client's current health status.
8. The list of nursing diagnostic statements is validated.

## DEFINITION: WHAT ARE NURSING DIAGNOSES?

There are many definitions of nursing diagnosis in the theoretical and clinical literature. Definitions are stated as process or product. The process definitions focus on decision-making and hypothesis testing. The product definitions refer to nursing diagnosis as the outcome or the result of the decision-making process, as a set of labels or a list. Following are a few definitions of nursing diagnosis:

Gebbie (1975), who documented The First National Conference on the Classification of Nursing Diagnosis, provides a product definition:

. . . the judgment or conclusion which occurs as a result of nursing assessment.

The American Nurses' Association (1980) cites a process definition and definition of nursing:

Nursing is the diagnosis and treatment of human responses to actual or potential health problems.

Shoemaker (1984:109) offers both a process and product definition:

. . . a clinical judgment about an individual, family, or community which is derived through a deliberate systematic process of data collection and analysis. It provides the basis for prescriptions for definitive therapy for which the nurse is accountable. It is expressed concisely and it includes the etiology of the condition when known.

Gordon (1987:3) relates a product definition:

. . . terms used to summarize assessment data . . . (and) describe clients' actual or potential health problems . . . clinical judgments made by professional nurses.

Kelly (1985:17) states a process and product definition:

The determination and statement of a clinical judgment in which a clients' response to a change in health status is described in terms of the effect on routines or activities of daily living and life-style in an individual, group, or community.

Carpenito (1987b:5) gives a product definition:

. . . a statement that describes the human response (health state or actual/potential altered interaction pattern) of an individual or group which the nurse can legally identify and for which the nurse can order the definitive interventions to maintain the health state or to reduce, eliminate, or prevent alterations.

In this text, the nursing diagnosis statement is defined as the product of the diagnostic process, which is defined separately in Chapter 7. A nursing diagnosis is a clear, concise, and definitive statement of the client's health status and concerns that can be affected by nursing intervention. It is the product of the nursing diagnostic process and is derived from inferences of assessed validated data. Naming the conclusions as well as validating them is the final phase in the diagnostic process.

## HISTORICAL PERSPECTIVE: WHEN NURSING DIAGNOSES BEGAN

Nurses have made judgments about client concerns since the beginning of the profession. In the past 30 years, nursing has progressed through several stages of professional growth and development. An essential component of the growth was the search for professional identity including defining the domain of nursing. The term *nursing diagnosis* was first used in the 1950s. McManus (1950) was one of the first to recognize the identifying and diagnosing of nursing problems as a function of the professional nurse. Fry (1953) further clarified the concept by adding the word "nursing" to diagnosis. The term *nursing diagnosis* continued to evolve during the 1960s with increased use of the nursing process. Abdellah's list of 21 nursing problems was one of the first attempts to classify nursing concerns (Kelly, 1985).

During the 1970s, nurses became increasingly interested in the concept of nursing diagnosis. In 1973, the American Nurses' Association included nursing diagnosis as an integral part of the nursing process in the publication of the *Generic Standards of Nursing Practice*. A national task force of nurse professionals from practice, education, and research have been working on a typology or taxonomy of nursing diagnosis since 1973. The First National Conference Group for Classification of Nursing Diagnosis was organized by Gebbie and Lavin at St.

Louis University (Gebbie, 1976). Later renamed the North American Nursing Diagnosis Association (NANDA), the group meets on a regular basis to facilitate acceptance of a common list of nursing diagnoses, to examine and evaluate the current list of accepted nursing diagnoses, and to explore theoretical bases for the taxonomy. The current NANDA-approved list of nursing diagnostic categories for clinical use and testing appears on p. 163. The current list includes new diagnostic categories approved in 1988 and also revised categories. Most of the handbooks, manuals, and pocket guides include the definition, defining characteristics, and etiology for each nursing diagnosis (Doenges and Moorhouse, 1988; Carpenito, 1987a; Gordon, 1987; Kim et al, 1987; Duespohl, 1986; Gettrust et al, 1985).

Currently, the term *nursing diagnosis* is described in the American Nurses' Association Social Policy Statement (1980) and is mandated in the revised nurse practice acts in several states. The concept also appears in the revised national board examination for registered nurses. Nursing diagnosis research and literature have increased significantly in the past five years. Most schools of nursing integrate nursing diagnosis into their curricula. According to the Joint Commission for the Accreditation of Healthcare Organizations, nursing diagnoses are recommended as an effective means of documentation. Many nurse specialty organizations and groups now use the NANDA taxonomy or have adapted it for their particular specialty. There are at least two specialty handbooks: one for psychiatric nursing (Townsend, 1988) and one for critical care (Roberts, 1987). Other examples of journal articles about nursing diagnoses in specialty areas are:

Critical care nursing: Clark, 1987; Carpenito, 1987c; Breu, Dracup, and Walden, 1987

Long-term care: Rantz and Miller, 1987a, 1987b

Nursing education: Titler, 1987; Guzzetta, 1987; Nolan, 1987; Lunney, 1986; Lee and Strong, 1985

Perioperative nursing: Stanfield, 1987; Malen, 1986

Peritoneal dialysis: ANA, 1987

Plastic surgery nursing: Black, 1987; Hutcheson, 1987

Psychiatric nursing: Berry, 1987; Brown et al, 1987

Short-term unit—emergency, obstetric, operating room and postanesthesia recovery: Maibusch, 1987.

Although great advances have been made in the development and implementation of nursing diagnosis, the concept still needs to be clarified and refined. As the concept of nursing diagnosis develops, there is continued professional debate about (1) whether or not it is a taxonomy (Porter, 1987b; Rasch, 1987; Dialogue, 1987), (2) categories and labels within the taxonomy (Jenny, 1987), (3) the theoretical foundation of the categories (Fawcett, 1986; Harrington, 1988; Frissell, 1988), and (4) whether the dysfunctional focus of nursing diagnosis is appropriate for the nursing domain (Schlotfeldt, 1987).

Most research studies have been descriptive, but Gordon (1985) indicates the need for both qualitative and quantitative designs. Other scholars identify the need for systematic testing of the NANDA taxonomy and for more validation studies (McLane, 1987b; Fehring, 1987).

## MISCONCEPTIONS: WHAT NURSING DIAGNOSES ARE NOT

In defining what nursing diagnoses are and understanding their development, it is also helpful to clarify possible areas of confusion. There are at least eight potential areas for clarification. The list of misconceptions begins with one of the most common problems in accepting the term *nursing diagnosis*—the misunderstanding brought about by its confusion with the term *medical diagnosis.*

1. *The nursing diagnosis is not the medical diagnosis.* The medical diagnosis identifies and labels a precise pathological condition. It is made to prescribe treatment, to cure a disease, or to reduce an injury. The medical diagnosis describes a disease or syndrome that is classified as one of medical diagnoses listed in the International Classification of Diseases. The nursing diagnosis describes the effects of the symptoms and the pathological condition on the client's activities and lifestyle. It is the statement of the client's behavioral response to the condition or situation. For example, a client with a medical diagnosis of hyperthyroidism could have one or more of the following nursing diagnoses:

Alteration in nutrition (less than body requirements), related to inadequate intake
Activity intolerance, related to generalized weakness
Altered comfort, related to heat intolerance
Potential for injury, related to unsteady mobility
The nursing diagnosis is *not* hyperthyroidism.

The medical diagnosis is an important component of the individual client's total condition and must be considered in the provision of comprehensive nursing care. However, there is no consensus among the nursing profession about *how* to incorporate the medical diagnosis into the client's plan of care. Nurses acknowledge two domains in providing client care: (1) the *nursing domain*, which is independent and related to judgments regarding the client's health status and its effect on daily living (nursing diagnosis) and (2) the *biomedical domain*, in which nurses have collaborative responsibilities (implementing physicians' orders) and independent responsibilities (using knowledge, experience, skills, and clinical judgment) to monitor and assess the client's pathological condition or medical diagnosis (Gordon, 1982b; Carpenito, 1983; Carnevali, 1984).

Options for incorporating the medical diagnosis into the client's plan of care are controversial. One option is to state the medical diagnosis as an etiological factor in the nursing diagnostic statement. The rationale is that although the medical diagnosis is the physician's domain, specific independent nursing actions (monitoring, assessing, and analyzing the data) need to be done, as well as implementation of the physician's orders.

Another option is to translate the medical diagnosis into terminology that spells out the client system affected (such as musculoskeletal impairment of upper right extremity, rather than fractured right arm). Neither option is acceptable by the North American Nursing Diagnosis Association Classification system. However, because the NANDA system is still evolving, some nurses use the above options while they continue to explore others.

A third option for addressing the biomedical domain is to consider the client as being at risk to respond to the medical diagnosis and to include this potential in the nursing diagnosis list. For example, a client with a medical diagnosis of diabetes could have several nursing diagnoses as a result of the diabetes, such as altered skin integrity related to lack of knowledge, altered nutrition related to eating habits, and anxiety related to becoming insulin-dependent. Another nursing diagnosis could be potential responses related to diabetes. Because specific nursing activities are related to the medical diagnosis, the nursing diagnosis of potential alteration in response to diabetes would assure that the independent monitoring activities of assessing for hypo- and hyperglycemia, skin condition, and the client's reaction to the medical treatment are included in the nursing plan of care.

2. *The nursing diagnosis is not the diagnostic test.* The nursing diagnosis reflects the specific effect(s) of a diagnostic test on the client. Examples of diagnostic tests to which clients may have specific responses are any diagnostic x-ray study, such as gallbladder, upper or lower gastrointestinal series, or mammography; a CT scan or magnetic reso-

nance imaging (MRI); a biopsy; and a glucose toler- ance test. The nursing diagnosis states the client's reaction to the test as shown in the following:

| Incorrect | Correct |
|---|---|
| Cardiac catheterization | Anxiety related to lack of knowledge of procedure |

3. *The nursing diagnosis is not the medical or surgical treatment.* The nursing diagnosis reflects the client's response to the treatment. Examples of treatments to which clients may have specific responses are cast immobilization, chemotherapy, hemodialysis, angioplasty, appendectomy, and tonsillectomy. Possible client responses are fear, anxiety (anticipatory), body image disturbance, depression (reactive), and hopelessness. The nursing diagnosis states the client's individual response to the treatment as shown in the following:

| Incorrect | Correct |
|---|---|
| Radiation therapy | Ineffective coping related to radiation therapy |

4. *The nursing diagnosis is not the equipment.* The nursing diagnosis reflects the client's reaction to the particular equipment. Examples of equipment to which clients may have specific responses are pacemaker, Hickman catheter, insulin pump, urinary catheter, and mechanical ventilator. Possible client responses to the equipment may be one or more of the following, depending on the type of equipment: impaired verbal communication, potential for infection, potential impairment of skin integrity, powerlessness, anxiety, potential for injury, self-care deficit, and potential for impaired home maintenance management. The nursing diagnosis states the client's reaction to the equipment as shown in the following:

| Incorrect | Correct |
|---|---|
| Nasogastric tube | Impaired skin integrity of nares related to nasogastric tube |

5. *The nursing diagnosis is not a single conceptual label.* Labels such as "obesity," "immobilization," and "constipation" are too general and do not define the specific concern or show necessary relationships that are needed to develop meaningful individualized nursing orders. Examples of more definitive nursing diagnoses are shown in the following:

| Incorrect | Correct |
|---|---|
| Obesity | Altered nutrition: more than body requirements related to eating habits |
| Immobilization | Impaired physical mobility related to weakness |

6. *The nursing diagnosis is not a statement of the nurse's problem with the client.* Occasionally nurses and clients develop interpersonal or communication conflicts that result in the nurse's labeling the client as "difficult," "demanding," or "impossible." The problem is really the nurse's and may actually interfere with the client's adjustment to the health concern. The staff's problem in coping with the client needs to be differentiated from the client's situation and coping pattern. The nursing diagnosis is the statement of the client's response to hospitalization or a situation including the etiology, if known. The following indicate incorrect and correct nursing diagnoses:

| Incorrect | Correct |
|---|---|
| Uncooperative | Ineffective coping related to unexpected hospitalization |
| Constantly complains | Anxiety related to role change |
| Uses inappropriate language with staff | Fear related to powerlessness |

7. *The nursing diagnosis is not a nursing goal.* Nursing goals are statements of what the nurse should do for the client. "Provision of adequate fluids" is a nursing goal statement. Nursing diagnoses are stated as labels for the client's health status. A nursing diagnosis concerned with fluids could be "potential fluid volume deficit."

8. *The nursing diagnosis is not a single symptom.* The nursing diagnosis consists of two or more defining characteristics and, in some instances, must include particular critical elements. It is not a single symptom such as elevated blood pressure, increased pulse rate, edema, thirst, or weakness. Nurses may use a manual or handbook to identify the need for assessment of additional defining characteristics.

Nurses need to be aware of misconceptions in order to avoid them and to understand how to use nursing diagnoses appropriately. It is also imperative for nurses to validate the client's response or reaction to the medical diagnosis, the diagnostic test, the medical or surgical treatment, and the equipment.

## PURPOSE: WHY USE NURSING DIAGNOSES?

There are several reasons for writing nursing diagnoses—the main reason being that they are a defining characteristic of nursing practice (ANA, 1980). Nursing diagnoses are the basis for the definitive nursing actions for which nurses are accountable (Shoemaker, 1984). The following is a summary of many of the important reasons for using and writing nursing diagnoses. Nursing diagnoses:

- Contribute to the identity of nursing as a profession
- Provide a mechanism for professional accountability
- Facilitate nurses' autonomy in judgments about client care
- Contribute to the knowledge base of nursing as a science
- Can be used as "key conceptual criteria around which the standards are developed" (Swehla, 1988:18; Dixon and Walker, 1986)
- Are used for communication of professional judgment; they provide a common frame of reference for nurse peers (Creason, 1987; Gordon, 1987)
- Contribute to continuity of care (Hanna and Wyman, 1987)
- Demonstrate effectiveness and quality of care (Gordon, 1987; Treu and Brague, 1987; McCourt, 1987; Maas, 1986); quality assurance programs based on nursing diagnoses provide valuable information to nurses and to the health care system
- Promote collaboration among members of the health care team (Herberth and Gosnell, 1987)
- Provide a mechanism for costing out nursing services (Maas, 1986; Gordon, 1987)
- Provide the basis for generating computerized nursing care plans (Smaldone, Greenberg, and Perez, 1988; Chang et al, 1988; Mehmert, 1987; Brennan and Romano, 1987; Bloom, Leitner, and Solano, 1987; Coler and Vincent, 1987)
- Provide the basis for intershift reporting (Kilpack and Dobson-Brassard, 1987; Bolger and Asghari,1987)
- Provide the basis for a national Nursing Minimum Data Set (Werley, 1987)

Maas (1986:39) focuses on the advantages of nursing diagnoses from a nursing administration viewpoint and identifies the following additional reasons for using nursing diagnoses. Nursing diagnoses are the "keystone for effective nursing administration," because they:

- Are the basis for a research-based practice
- Enable nurses to aquire power and authority for influence
- Are the basis for staff development as well as quality assurance programs (also Brown et al, 1987)
- Can be used to define staffing specifications and to determine case-mix classification (also Sanford, 1987)
- Promote communication among nurses by

clarifying shared goals that focus collective actions

The most frequently identified purposes for nursing diagnoses in Turkoski's (1988) review of nursing diagnosis literature from 1950 through 1985 were to improve delivery of care, to facilitate intraprofessional communication, to validate nursing functions, to measure nursing work loads, and to increase autonomy. All these reasons explain why nurses should use nursing diagnoses.

There are also reasons why nurses may be hesitant to write nursing diagnoses. They fear the risk of making a judgment that others can read. Some fear ridicule or criticism; others fear making an error or not being "perfect." These fears are usually ill founded, because most peers are willing to participate and contribute assistance if asked. Nurses have been making diagnoses for years by identifying client concerns, but now professionals are being held accountable for their critical thinking and inferences. Only through practice does writing nursing diagnoses become easier. Although most diagnoses reflect a probability rather than a certainty, it is better to state a strong possibility than not to decide anything. Indecision may indicate a lack of knowledge, self-confidence, or courage.

Nursing diagnoses contribute to the identification of independent nursing judgments within a science-based profession. Nurses must become proficient in writing accurate nursing diagnoses that are appropriate to client concerns and that meet the guidelines in the following section.

## GUIDELINES: HOW TO WRITE A NURSING DIAGNOSIS

An excellent reference and the first place to start when writing a nursing diagnosis is the list of approved nursing diagnoses from the North American Nursing Diagnosis Association (see box on the next page). The NANDA list includes 98 nursing diagnostic labels organized in nine categories or patterns: exchanging, communicating, valuing, choosing, moving, perceiving, knowing, and feeling (NANDA, 1988). Because the taxonomy continues to evolve, nurses may find it necessary to write a nursing diagnosis that is not on the list or to make refinements in the existing list. NANDA encourages communication with their association and with other professional nurses regarding the development of new diagnoses as well as regarding research or comments about the current taxonomy.

The product of the diagnostic process (analysis and synthesis of data) is the translation of the client's health concerns and etiologic relationships

# NANDA Approved Nursing Diagnostic Categories

## Pattern 1: exchanging

Altered Nutrition: More than body requirements
Altered Nutrition: Less than body requirements
Altered Nutrition: Potential for more than body requirements
Potential for Infection
Potential Altered Body Temperature
Hypothermia
Hyperthermia
Ineffective Thermoregulation
Dysreflexia
Constipation
Perceived Constipation
Colonic Constipation
Diarrhea
Bowel Incontinence
Altered Patterns of Urinary Elimination
Stress Incontinence
Reflex Incontinence
Urge Incontinence
Functional Incontinence
Total Incontinence
Urinary Retention
Altered (Specify Type) Tissue Perfusion (renal, cerebral, cardiopulmonary, gastrointestinal, peripheral)
Fluid Volume Excess
Fluid Volume Deficit (1)
Fluid Volume Deficit (2)
Potential Fluid Volume Deficit
Decreased Cardiac Output
Impaired Gas Exchange
Ineffective Airway Clearance
Ineffective Breathing Pattern
Potential for Injury
Potential for Suffocation
Potential for Poisoning
Potential for Trauma
Potential for Aspiration
Potential for Disuse Syndrome
Impaired Tissue Integrity
Altered Oral Mucous Membrane
Impaired Skin Integrity
Potential Impaired Skin Integrity

## Pattern 2: communicating

Impaired Verbal Communication

## Pattern 3: relating

Impaired Social Interaction
Social Isolation
Altered Role Performance
Altered Parenting
Potential Altered Parenting
Sexual Dysfunction
Altered Family Processes
Parental Role Conflict
Altered Sexuality Patterns

## Pattern 4: valuing

Spiritual Distress (distress of the human spirit)

## Pattern 5: choosing

Ineffective Individual Coping
Impaired Adjustment
Defensive Coping
Ineffective Denial
Ineffective Family Coping: Disabling
Ineffective Family Coping: Compromised
Family Coping: Potential for Growth
Noncompliance (Specify)
Decisional Conflict (Specify)
Health Seeking Behaviors (Specify)

## Pattern 6: moving

Impaired Physical Mobility
Activity Intolerance
Fatigue
Potential Activity Intolerance
Sleep Pattern Disturbance
Diversional Activity Deficit
Impaired Home Maintenance Management
Altered Health Maintenance
Feeding Self Care Deficit
Impaired Swallowing
Ineffective Breastfeeding
Bathing/Hygiene Self Care Deficit
Dressing/Grooming Self Care Deficit
Toileting Self Care Deficit
Altered Growth and Development

## Pattern 7: perceiving

Body Image Disturbance
Self Esteem Disturbance
Chronic Low Self Esteem
Situational Low Self Esteem
Personal Identity Disturbance
Sensory/Perceptual Alterations (Specify) (visual, auditory, kinesthetic, gustatory, tactile, olfactory)
Unilateral Neglect
Hopelessness
Powerlessness

## Pattern 8: knowing

Knowledge Deficit (Specify)
Altered Thought Processes

## Pattern 9: feeling

Pain
Chronic Pain
Dysfunctional Grieving
Anticipatory Grieving
Potential for Violence: Self-directed or directed at others
Post-Trauma Response
Rape-Trauma Syndrome
Rape-Trauma Syndrome: Compound Reaction
Rape-Trauma Syndrome: Silent Reaction
Anxiety
Fear

**Table 8-1**   Relationship of Descriptive Part of Nursing Diagnosis Statement to Defining Characteristics in NANDA Taxonomy*

| Descriptive label | Defining characteristics |
|---|---|
| **Individual** | |
| Altered patterns of urinary elimination | Dysuria, frequency, hesitancy, nocturia, retention, urgency, and/or incontinence |
| Powerlessness (severe) | Verbalization of having no control (eg, situation, outcome, or self-care), depression over physical deterioration occurring despite compliance with regimes, and/or apathy |
| **Family** | |
| Altered sexuality pattern | Reported difficulties, changes, or limitations in sexual behaviors or activities |
| Disturbance in role performance | Denial of role, conflict in roles, change in self-perception of roles, changes in others' perceptions of roles, change in physical capacity to resume roles, lack of knowledge of role, and/or change in usual patterns or responsibilities |

*From Gordon M: Manual of nursing diagnosis 1986-1987, New York, 1987, McGraw-Hill, Inc.

into nursing diagnosis statements. The structure or format of the diagnostic statement is the way in which the data are translated into words that precisely state the client's situation and health concerns. According to the NANDA taxonomy, each nursing diagnosis label/statement infers a specific definition with defining characteristics and etiological parameters (Table 8-1).

The guidelines that follow are provided to assist nurses in writing or validating a statement of the client's health concerns and strengths. These guidelines are *not* sequential steps, but are presented according to types of client concerns, format, and validation. Guidelines are discussed in terms of types of client concerns, which include actual recognized, actual unrecognized, potential, possible, and no concerns (strengths). In addition, format guidelines are provided in relation to writing statements of clarity, specificity, direction for nursing intervention, and independent actions. The final guidelines relate to compiling and validating the list of health concerns.

1. *The nursing diagnosis is a statement of an actual or potential health concern.* Five types of client concerns may be identified. As discussed in Chapter 7, conclusions may indicate actual concerns (recognized and unrecognized), potential concerns, possible concerns, or no concerns (strengths). The term *concern* is more appropriate than *problem, weakness,* and *limitation* (which have negative connotations) and *need.* As stated previously, we all have needs, and when needs are not being met there is concern. Rather than stating the individual's nursing diagnosis as "need for sex" or "need for fluid," these could be stated as "sexual dysfunction related to medication effects" or "debilitated state and fluid volume deficit related to feeding self-care deficit."

An incorrect family nursing diagnosis is "need to improve communication." A correct diagnosis is "altered family processes related to ineffective communication or family schedules." An incorrect community nursing diagnosis is "need for citizen participation," which could be stated as "apathy or powerlessness related to lack of citizen participation."

The following discussion identifies specific nursing diagnoses for each type of client concern:

a. *The nursing diagnosis is a statement of an **actual** client concern **(recognized)**.*

These concerns are existing responses with which the client agrees. They occur as a result of a medical diagnosis, a situation, or a condition. The concerns are stated in terms of the client's response to these factors and may be expressed as a stressor (Little and Carnevali, 1976), a deficit (Orem, 1985), or ineffective behavior (Roy, 1984), depending on the conceptual model used for the assessment or data processing. It is also possible to identify the concerns according to the wording of the specific nursing model in the analysis/synthesis, then to label them according to the NANDA-approved nursing diagnosis list. Many nurses are now using the NANDA list to state individual client concerns. The following are examples of individual and family actual nursing diagnoses from the approved list:

| Individual | Family |
|---|---|
| Activity intolerance | Altered role performance |
| Altered health maintenance | Altered parenting |
| Body image disturbance | Altered family processes |
| Dysfunctional grieving | Parental role conflict |
| Ineffective breathing pattern | Altered sexuality patterns |
| Spiritual distress | Ineffective family coping |

Although some NANDA categories and labels may be adapted for community nursing diagnoses, they were written for the individual and the family. Community nursing diagnoses of actual concerns must meet the same guidelines as those used for the individual and the family; that is, the descriptive part of the statement must describe the client's response to a situation or condition and the etiology reflects the contributing factors. The Omaha Classification Scheme (Iyer et al, 1986:273) lists the following environmental nursing diagnoses which could apply to the community as client: income deficit, sanitation deficit, safety hazards, and abuse (child/adult). Porter (1987a:311) also identifies possible community nursing diagnoses related to population groups. Examples are "vulnerable population group at-risk (school children), in need of caries prevention"; "vulnerable population group (elderly), in need of cardiovascular screening"; "need-service match, related to existing cardiovascular screening service."

b. *The nursing diagnosis is a statement of an **actual** client concern **(unrecognized)**.* Actual (unrecognized) concerns are existing conditions identified by the nurse but not acknowledged by the client. The client may deny the concern or may acknowledge the concern but refuse to do anything about it. Respecting the client's autonomy, the nurse lists the concern on the health status list but notes that it is unresolved or inactive. An example of an actual concern that the client may acknowledge, but does not want to change is "alteration in nutrition: more than body requirements," "noncompliance," "altered health maintenance," or "altered growth and development." Actually, the concern may be any of the nursing diagnosis labels for the individual or family. The community may also deny or not wish to change an identified unhealthy response.

c. *The nursing diagnosis is a statement of a **potential** client concern.* Potential concerns are those that are high risk or probable. Potential nursing diagnosis statements are usually two-part statements with the risk factors replacing the etiology. An example of an individual potential concern is "potential for injury related to mobility impairment or sensory-perceptual deterioration." Because a potential concern can be the client's response to the medical diagnosis, the nursing diagnosis statement is a "potential alteration related to the medical diagnosis" (e.g., hypertension, diabetes, or arthritis). The nursing actions include assessing and monitoring this collaborative biomedical concern. The same descriptive label, "potential for injury," used for the individual can also be used for the family, but the risk factors may be different, such as related to lack of safety precautions or lack of safety education.

Another family nursing diagnosis could be "potential altered parenting related to ineffective role model" or "unrealistic expectations of self and partner." A potential community nursing diagnosis could be "potential for injury related to inadequate funding for sidewalk repair" or ". . . related to high crime neighborhood."

d. *The nursing diagnosis is a statement of a **possible** client concern.* A possible concern is one that has not been verified or validated. The nurse suspects or has a strong hunch that a concern may be present, but additional data are needed to rule out or confirm its viability. This is similar to a hypothesis that needs to be accepted or not accepted; it is the nurse's impression from previous experience and an "inner knowing." The client's condition may be indicative of one of the nursing diagnosis definitions but with inadequate data on the defining characteristics. It may be stated as "possible depression" or "impression of confusion, source undetermined/unknown etiology."

e. *The nursing diagnosis is a statement of client **strengths**.* If the client, with or without a medical diagnosis, is coping and functioning adequately, with no perceived concerns, then the nursing diagnosis is a conclusion that may be stated in a positive manner (as opposed to a concern or problem statement). One of the issues related to developing nursing diagnoses is that the original focus was on negative terms about health problems.

Popkess-Vawter and Pinnell (1987:1211) suggest that strength-oriented nursing diagnoses can be made from the approved list of nursing diagnoses by stating them positively, such as "adequate health maintenance," "functional grieving," "regular elimination," "controlled pain," or "effective parenting." The NANDA list contains a couple of positive labels such as "family coping: potential for growth" and "health seeking behaviors." If nurses choose to use the accepted list for positive nursing diagnoses, it is necessary to use judgment in narrowing the list and focusing on those two or three that are most relevant to the client's developmental level and condition. Duespohl (1986) and Houldin and co-workers (1987) identify positive or well nursing diagnoses in their manuals. An example for an individual client (Houldin et al, 1987) is "adequate accident prevention practices related to awareness of unhealthy and unsafe practices." A family strength is "productive family processes related to role flexibility and consensual decision-making." Stolte (1986:27) supports positive nursing diagnoses and suggested the following examples: "adaptive coping with chronic illness related to adequate family supportive mechanisms"; ". . . integrity related to satisfaction of having raised a family well, having planned for retirement, and being content with decisions made during life." Other examples of using nursing diagnoses for health promotion are "effective health management related to use of personal and community resources and age-appropriate developmental tasks" (Lee and Frenn, 1987:984). Independent nursing actions for the client with no concerns or strengths include support, praise, reinforcement, encouragement, and provision of health information or health alternatives.

If client strengths are not stated as nursing diagnoses, they may be identified and listed at the conclusion of the analysis/synthesis or on a separate list. Strengths that could be noted for the individual are effective coping, numerous situational supports, adequate finances, and knowledge or acceptance of condition. Examples of family strengths are effective parenting, role acceptance, cohesiveness, and open communication. Community strengths could be enthusiastic leadership, adequate health resources, available health facilities for all age groups, and participatory decision-making.

Client concerns may be stated as actual (recognized or unrecognized), potential, possible, and strengths. The format for each type of statement is indicated in the following:

| Types | Parts of Statements* |
|---|---|
| Actual diagnoses (dx) | = Dx label + etiology (+ signs/symptoms) |
| Potential dx | = Modifier + dx label + risk factors |
| Possible dx | = Modifier + dx label (+ source unknown) |
| Strength dx | = Modifier + dx label (+ positive factors) |

*Parentheses indicate optional information.

2. *The nursing diagnosis is written as a descriptive and etiological statement.*

a. *The first part of the statement is descriptive.* It identifies the client response to an "actual or potential disturbance in life processes, patterns, functions or development" (Gordon, 1976). The descriptive part is the specific label for the response and may be any of the 98 NANDA nursing diagnoses labels. The descriptive statement can be initially verified by consulting a handbook or manual that contains a list of defining characteristics and comparing the list with the client's data base. Table 8-1 shows the relationship of the descriptive statement to the defining characteristics (Gordon, 1987).

Examples of descriptive statements for the indi-

vidual are "altered patterns of urinary elimination," "impaired physical mobility," "sleep pattern disturbance," or "hopelessness." Examples for the family are "altered parenting," "sexual dysfunction," "altered family processes" or "parental role conflict." Descriptive community nursing diagnostic statements are "ineffective coping," "fear," "altered or dysfunctional communication," "impaired social interaction," "spiritual distress," or "decisional conflict." (Community nursing diagnoses are *not* part of the NANDA taxonomy and should be written according to the client's response to a situation and stated in terms of the model used for assessment/analysis/synthesis. However, the NANDA list may be used as a resource because many of the patterns are applicable.)

b. *The second part of the statement is the etiology.* The etiology states the contributing or influencing factor(s) of the health concern. This part of the statement indicates the nurse's perception of the probable causative factor(s) and must allow for flexibility and exploration. It is possible that one client concern may be influenced by several factors such as:

Environmental: odors, lighting, noises
Sociological: language, finances, support system
Spiritual: rituals, practices, beliefs
Physiological: fluid deficit/excess, hypothermia
Psychological: fear, anxiety, low self-esteem

An example of a concern for an individual client with multiple etiologies is "sleep pattern disturbance related to fear of impending surgery, noisy environment, and pain." Etiologies or related factors are identified in most nursing diagnosis manuals, which may be consulted when writing the nursing diagnosis statement.

Examples of correctly written nursing diagnostic statements with both descriptive and etiological parts for the individual are "self-feeding deficit related to pain," "impaired skin integrity related to physical immobilization," and "alteration in nutrition: more than body requirements related to dysfunctional eating patterns." Examples written for the family are "altered parenting related to lack of attachment behaviors" and "altered family processes related to hospitalization of income provider." Examples of the two-part statement for the community are "social isolation related to cultural beliefs," "spiritual distress related to community disaster (tornado)," "fear related to increased drug activities," and "high infant mortality rate related to inadequate funding for prenatal services and lack of knowledge among pregnant teenagers."

c. *The nursing diagnosis statement can be written in three parts: descriptive, etiological, and clustered cues.* The three-part PES format was identified by Gordon (1976) as health problem (P), etiology (E), and the defining cluster of signs and symptoms (S). This format may be helpful to students learning to write nursing diagnosis because the S is the rationale for naming the concern. Including the cluster of signs and symptoms as part of the statement encourages accountability and verifies the diagnostic process. An example of PES is "anxiety related to hospitalization as evidenced by restlessness, insomnia, facial tension, and statement of increased helplessness." One of the criticisms of the three-part statement is that it is not concise; however, it meets many of the other important guidelines such as being client centered and specific.

d. *The descriptive and etiological parts of the nursing diagnosis statement are joined by the words "related to."* The words "related to" indicate a relationship between the health concern and a contributing or influencing factor. These words are not as legally or causally defining as "due to."

3. *The nursing diagnosis is concise and clear.*

Until a complete taxonomy is available, it will be necessary for nurses to think and communicate concisely without loss of accuracy. Clarity and conciseness facilitate communication among peers and health team members. A concise, clearly stated diagnosis will be read and understood as opposed to a lengthy paragraph that takes time to read and unravel. For example, there is no need to write "client" or "patient," because such terms are implicit. Examples of nursing diagnoses in addition to the NANDA list are given by Campbell (1984), Lunney (1982), Shortridge and Lee (1980), Gordon (1987), Duespohl (1986), and Carpenito (1987a).

When lists of nursing diagnoses are not available or when none of the existing labels fits the clinical situation, nurses may create their own nursing diagnostic statement. However, the statement should reflect a particular cluster of cues that is indicative of the label. The label is usually derived from the model used during assessment and analysis/synthesis of data. The following terms may be helpful in writing an unlisted nursing diagnosis. The client's response to the condition, state, or situation may be expressed as:

| | |
|---|---|
| Alteration in | Interruption of |
| Potential for | Depletion of |
| Impairment of | Disturbance in |
| Lack of | Unresolved |
| Inadequate | Difficulty in |
| Deficit in | Noncompliance with |
| Diminished | Nonparticipation in |
| Insufficient | Inappropriate |
| Inability to | Maintaining |
| Failure to | Reduced |

Adjectives can be used with the the label to allow nurses to prioritize certain conditions. The following adjectives may be helpful in clarifying the statement:

| | |
|---|---|
| Acute | Maximum |
| Chronic | Mild |
| Full | Minimum |
| Intermittent | Occasional |
| Severe | Sporadic |
| Complete | Moderate |
| Partial | |

An example of a vague nursing diagnosis is "client has open area on foot and complains of pain." This could be restated as the following nursing diagnoses: "impairment of skin integrity of right heel related to immobility" and "pain related to impairment of skin integrity of right heel." The second nursing diagnosis could be further clarified by adding an adjective, acute or chronic, to describe the pain.

4. *The nursing diagnosis is client centered, specific, and accurate.* Client-centered diagnoses are stated in terms of the client's response to intrapersonal, interpersonal, and environmental stressors. The nursing diagnosis focuses on the client rather than the stressor. An incorrect statement would be "cluttered home related to impaired home maintenance management." A client-centered nursing diagnosis would be "impaired home maintenance management related to insufficient family organization or planning as evidenced by disorderly surroundings and accumulation of dirt and food."

The statement must be precise identification of the client's actual or potential health concern, rather than a general concept or categorization. This precision is necessary for accurate communication and appropriate nursing interventions to be planned and implemented. If an incorrect conclusion is stated, the goals, interventions, and evaluations will be inappropriate and ineffective.

5. *The nursing diagnosis provides direction for nursing intervention.* The descriptive and etiological parts of the nursing diagnosis are the basis for planning nursing intervention. The descriptive part of the statement that reflects the client response provides the foundation for the client goals of health promotion, restoration, and maintenance of the response/condition/situation. Specific client outcomes with associated nursing strategies are derived from the etiological part of the statement. Nursing strategies vary according to the etiological factor(s). In other words, the improvement of the client response is directly influenced by the effectiveness of the individualized nursing interventions. Nursing actions also include monitoring the

actual or potential response for improvement, and so forth. An example of a nursing diagnosis for an individual in which the etiology directs the nursing strategies is "ineffective airway clearance," which could be related to an infection, an obstruction, decreased energy and fatigue, trauma, or perceptual/cognitive impairment. The client outcomes and nursing interventions are directed by the correct and accurate etiological statement.

In the previous example, although some of the monitoring interventions would be similar, most of the nursing strategies would be different for each etiology. The overall goal regardless of the etiology, is an improvement in the airway clearance. How the goal is met is influenced by the correct intervention for the specific etiology. An example of a nursing diagnosis for an individual with a preventive goal is "potential for injury related to home safety hazards." The nursing strategies would be methods of helping the client decrease or eliminate the safety hazards, individualized according to the client's condition, situation, and developmental level. The client goal is to decrease the potential for injury or to prevent injuries.

A family nursing diagnosis with differing interventions according to the etiology is "altered parenting." If the etiology is "lack of available role model," the interventions would focus on finding a positive role model and/or referring to a support group. If the etiology is "lack of knowledge," the nursing interventions would be directed toward teaching-learning activities. Or, finally, if the etiology is "perceived threat to own survival," the nursing intervention would focus on the client's physical and emotional safety.

6. *The nursing diagnosis is the basis for independent and collaborative nursing actions/interventions.* The nursing diagnosis must be within the legal and educational parameters of nursing. Independent nursing interventions are activities of health promotion and education, disease prevention, nursing treatment (restoration or maintenance), and referral. The nurse identifies all areas of health concerns, including those for which others' expertise is needed. The independent nursing action for those concerns must be to refer to the appropriate resource. For example, if a nursing diagnosis is "anxiety related to inadequate finances," the nursing action is referral of the client to the social worker, welfare department, or Social Security office. Because anxiety can affect the client's ability to respond to nursing interventions for other nursing diagnoses, it must also be considered.

Collaborative nursing diagnoses and interventions are related to the biomedical domain of nursing. The physician is responsible and accountable for diagnosing, prescribing, and treating the client's pathological condition. Nurses are responsible and accountable for assessing and reporting the client's response to the medical diagnoses and the treatment regimen. The nurse's knowledge and expertise regarding signs and symptoms of progress or potential complications of the client's pathological condition contribute to the biomedical aspect of the client's care. Equally important, however, is the nurse's holistic approach to the client's concerns and the identification of concerns appropriate for nursing interventions to promote, maintain, or restore health. Carpenito (1987b) incorporates collaborative concerns in her model.

7. *The list of nursing diagnoses statements reflects the client's current health status.* The nursing diagnoses are compiled into a list that is sometimes referred to as the *problem list*, but it is *not* the list of nursing or medical problems. The list reflects the concluding statements or nursing diagnoses that were derived after analysis and synthesis of the client data. The list should include all actual, potential, and possible health concerns. Provision should also be made to note the status of each concern: active, inactive (unrecognized, unacceptable to client, not a priority at this time), or resolved. The list provides a capsule view of the client's health status. The following is an example of a list of client concerns or the nursing diagnoses list:

| Nursing diagnosis | Active | Inactive | Resolved |
|---|---|---|---|
| Activity intolerance r/t* immobility | 2/3/90 | | |
| Social isolation r/t socio-cultural dissonance | | 2/3/90 | |
| Potential altered parenting r/t financial stress | | | 2/5/90 |
| Possible noncompliance: medication | 2/3/90 | | |
| Potential for effective coping r/t discharge | 2/3/90 | | |
| Incomplete data base r/t ongoing assessment | 2/3/90 | | |
| Collaborative concerns | | | |
| Potential complication: contracture | 2/3/90 | | |

*r/t, related to.

In addition to the nursing diagnosis statements of client concerns, at least two additional statements may be added, which contribute to comprehensive client care and meet the criteria for client concerns. Because all planning for client care begins with the accurate list of concerns, it is important to consider these two areas. The first relates to *discharge planning.* Plans for discharge and termination of the nurse-client relationship should begin at the time of the client's admission to the agency. One way to incorporate plans for discharge is to place a statement on the list of client concerns. There are no standard statements but the following are statements that may be used, which are all related to discharge planning:

Potential for growth
Potential for effective coping
Potential for positive adjustment
Potential for health seeking behavior
Potential for anxiety

The etiology of discharge planning/termination provides the opportunity for immediate planning of appropriate nursing interventions. Including a statement about termination helps the nurse incorporate the discharge plans into other interventions and not wait until the last minute before client dismissal. The plans may also reflect outcomes and strategies about the nurse-client relationship, interpersonal communication, or the stages of a working relationship.

The second additional statement refers to the client's *incomplete data base.* Because assessment is ongoing and it is impossible to obtain all relevant data during the initial client contact at admission, it is important to provide a strategy for obtaining the client information identified as data gaps after the analysis/synthesis process. There is no standard statement; however, adding a statement to the list allows for plans to obtain the data. The statement may be written as "incomplete data base related to ongoing assessment," or simply as "incomplete data base" followed by a list of data gaps. The statement meets the criteria of a client concern, because it is the client's data base and plans include the client goal of participating by providing the information, with the nursing intervention to assess and obtain the data.

The list of nursing diagnoses is reflective of the client's changing condition and responses. The initial list is not a fixed entity; it is flexible with the expectation of being updated. Nursing diagnoses made after initial data collection are usually tentative and require further assessment and validation.

As long as the client has a health concern, there will be continued adaptation and change in response to it. The nurse needs to assess these changes and adapt the nursing diagnoses and interventions to them. For example, after additional assessment, the nursing diagnosis may be changed from "anxiety related to impending surgery" to "fear related to body image disturbance." Professional nurses continually use the diagnostic process to update and individualize client care.

8. *The list of nursing diagnostic statements is validated.* There are two elements in validating nursing diagnoses. The first relates to the cluster or pattern of signs and symptoms that defines the diagnosis. This validation involves reviewing the data that led to the judgment, and verifying their sufficiency and accuracy. The nurse also evaluates the rationale on which the diagnosis is based to reinforce the reasonable degree of probability.

The second validation is one of the most important aspects of nursing diagnosis and may be the one most frequently omitted. This second phase of validation is collaborating with the client in the confirmation of the nursing diagnosis. Collaboration is an essential component of successful change for three reasons. First, working together is the basis of a trusting relationship, which is more likely to provide accurate and valid data. Second, the trusting relationship provides the client with an anchor and support for risking and for changing behaviors. Third, the collaborative relationship indicates mutual influence. According to Orlando (1961), if there is no mutual validation, the nurse is engaging in a nontherapeutic activity.

In presenting the perceptions and interpretations to the client, one approach is to state: "After looking at the information you gave me, it seems to me that there are a few areas we may be able to help you with. You told me that _____ was bothering you. I was wondering if you also saw _____ as something we could work on. Here are some other areas I would like you to tell me about. _____ What do you think about this one?"

The client's acceptance of the diagnostic statements usually indicates mutuality. If the client does not perceive the nursing diagnosis as accurately indicating a health concern, there is no mutuality and even the most comprehensive and sensitive nursing plans will be meaningless. Nursing care cannot exist in a vacuum, striving for written perfection without client participation. When the client does not acknowledge a health concern, the nurse may record the diagnosis as inactive, indicating it is still a concern but unacknowledged by the client.

Client involvement from the beginning establishes a participatory relationship and encourages the self-care concept. The only exceptions to this second phase of validation would be an emergency or an unconscious client.

After the list of diagnoses is validated, priorities must be determined. After the client and nurse are in agreement with the list of health concerns, they must rank the diagnoses according to client need for nursing intervention. Setting priorities provides a logical approach to a multiplicity of concerns and is discussed in the following chapter.

## POTENTIAL ERRORS IN WRITING NURSING DIAGNOSES

The handbooks and manuals of nursing diagnosis are very helpful in writing nursing diagnoses; however, a few common errors still need to be avoided. Potential errors that can be used to critique the written list of nursing diagnoses are presented below.

### Reversing the Clauses

In the diagnostic statement, the client response is the first part of the statement and the etiology is the second part. Reversing the parts will cause difficulty in communicating and planning, because the etiology is the basis for nursing intervention to modify or alleviate the response. Sometimes it may be confusing, but the nurse must use clinical judgment to clarify the response and the contributing factor(s). Examples of reverse clauses for the individual, family, and community are as follows (r/t means related to):

| Incorrect | Correct |
|---|---|
| Physical immobilization r/t impaired skin integrity | Impaired skin integrity r/t physical immobilization |
| Support system deficit r/t altered parenting | Altered parenting r/t support system deficit |
| Community crisis r/t dysfunctional grieving | Dysfunctional grieving r/t community crisis |

### Restating the Response in the Etiology

The two parts of the diagnostic statement should not say the same thing. In the statement, "ineffective thermoregulation related to individual's temperature fluctuations," the etiological part is actually the definition of the response or descriptive part; both parts have the same meaning. The client response of ineffective thermoregulation is the concern, but the etiology could be trauma, immaturity, or aging, among others. Examples for the individual, family, and community are given here.

| Incorrect | Correct |
|---|---|
| Functional incontinence r/t involuntary urination | Functional incontinence r/t altered environment |
| Altered family processes r/t inability to carry out family functions | Altered family processes r/t birth of first child |
| Impaired communication r/t reduced interaction | Impaired communication r/t divisive issue |

### Including More Than One Concern in Descriptive Clause

Sometimes more than one actual or potential concern may be related to the same etiology. However, because the outcomes are different for each concern, it is necessary to write each concern separately. For example, rather than writing "diversional activity deficit and impaired home maintenance management related to physical immobility," these should be stated as two separate concerns because the outcomes are different for each concern. The correct statements would be "diversional activity deficit related to physical immobility" and "impaired home maintenance management related to physical immobility."

### Including Value Judgments in the Statement

The diagnostic statement is derived from clinical judgments made from verifiable data. The statements also must remain free of bias and not reflect the nurse's value judgments. There is a difference between clinical and value judgment. Value judgments include words like poor, good, bad, and unhealthy. An incorrect nursing diagnosis statement is "altered role performance related to poor developmental progress." A correct one is "altered role performance related to delayed development."

### Stating the Same Response Several Times When There Is More Than One Etiology for One Response

Client's health concerns are usually complex and may be related to more than one etiological factor. In other words, several factors may contribute to one response. For example, a client with diabetes may have several factors that lead to a response of "altered health maintenance." Related contributing factors may be lack of knowledge, lack of financial resources, and spiritual distress. Rather than writing "altered health maintenance" three different times (once for each etiology), because the outcome is the same (for the client to improve health maintenance), it is necessary to make only one nursing diagnosis statement listing all the contributing factors. Separate plans may then be made within the concern for each of the contributing factors, since the interventions are different for each. Attaching each of the etiologies contributes to the overall client outcomes.

### Making a Legally Inadvisable Statement

One way to avoid making a legally inadvisable statement is to use the phrase "related to" rather than "due to" or "as a result of" when joining the

**Table 8-2**  Nursing Diagnoses for the Individual Based on the Eclectic Model

| Model category | Modifier | Response | Etiology | Defining characteristics |
|---|---|---|---|---|
| **Biophysical** | Severe | Impaired skin integrity rt foot | Altered circulation | Open wound 3 cm diameter, rt foot, no drainage |
| | Potential | Altered oral mucous membrane | Ineffective oral hygiene | Coated tongue, halitosis, carious teeth |
| | Possible | Altered thought process | Unknown | Impaired recall |
| **Psychological** | Anticipatory | Grieving | Expected loss of terminally ill spouse | Sadness, crying, change in eating habits |
| | Mild | Anxiety | Perceived threat to self-concept | Expressed concern, facial tension, mildly restless |
| | Severe | Powerlessness | Lifestyle of helplessness | Verbalized no control over life, apathy, sedentary |
| **Sociocultural** | Chronic | Impaired home maintenance management | Lack of knowledge of resources and insufficient finances | States many debts over 1 year, lack of equipment, presence of vermin |
| | | Social isolation | Unacceptable social behaviors and developmental delay | Dull affect, uncommunicative, spits on floor |
| | | Altered sexuality pattern | Fear of pregnancy | Expressed concern about changes |
| **Spiritual** | | Spiritual distress | Intense suffering | Expressed anger toward God, gallows humor, withdrawn |
| | | Hopelessness | Abandonment by family | Passivity, decreased verbalization, decreased affect, increased sleep |

response to the etiology. Another way is not to make potentially libelous statements in the etiology such as "rape-trauma syndrome related to lack of husband's support," "ineffective individual coping related to interference by mother-in-law," or "fluid volume excess related to medication error." Nurses are accountable and responsible for the diagnostic statements, so the legal implications of the statements must be considered.

## APPLICATION OF MODELS TO NURSING DIAGNOSIS
### Individuals

Diagnostic statements are influenced by the assessment instrument used, the model applied in assessment and analysis/synthesis, and the diagnostic classification system. Nursing models that may be used for the individual include Gordon (1987a), Carpenito (1987a), Roy (1984), Orem (1985), King (1981), and others. Models outside the nursing profession may include Maslow (1970) or crisis theory. If Maslow is used, categories would include physiological, safety, belonging, self-esteem, and self-actualization. Crisis categories would include perceptions, situational supports,

and coping mechanisms. Examples are given for the eclectic approach (Table 8-2), Gordon (Table 8-3), and Carpenito (Table 8-4).

The eclectic approach includes biopsychosocial and spiritual concepts and patterns. The biophysiological patterns include nursing diagnoses in the NANDA categories of *exchanging* (such as altered nutrition, potential for infection, fluid volume deficit) and several in the *moving* category, such as impaired physical mobility, sleep pattern disturbance, altered growth and development, and the self-care deficits. The psychological patterns may include the NANDA categories *choosing* (ineffective individual coping, noncompliance), *perceiving, knowing,* and *feeling*. The sociocultural patterns include all the nursing diagnoses in the NANDA category *relating* and a few from the category *choosing* (ineffective family coping, family coping, and decisional conflict). The spiritual patterns include the nursing diagnoses in the NANDA category *valuing*. Table 8-2 explains the use of the eclectic model for the individual.

In Tables 8-2 through 8-6 in this chapter, the first column identifies the model category. The second column is used for the adjective or modifier that clarifies the client response, and the third column specifies the client response to the situation, state, or condition. The second and third columns together form the descriptive part of the nursing diagnosis statement. The fourth column is the etiology or in a potential nursing diagnosis, the risk factors. The etiology includes the contributing factors—environmental, physiological, psychological, and sociological, or, according to Carpenito (1987b), pathophysiological, treatment related, situational, and maturational. The last table column is the rationale for identifying the client response. It includes the defining characteristics, clustered cues, or signs and symptoms.

Gordon's (1987a) model includes 11 functional health patterns: health perception-health management, nutritional-metabolic, elimination, activity-exercise, sleep-rest, cognitive-perceptual, self-perception–self-concept, role-relationship, sexuality-reproductive, coping-stress tolerance, and value-belief. Examples are given for three of the patterns in Table 8-3.

Carpenito (1987a) includes nursing diagnoses and collaborative problems in her bifocal clinical nursing model. Her manual (1987b) includes 65 approved NANDA nursing diagnosis categories and seven additional categories: impaired communication, health maintenance, potential for infection transmission, alterations in parental role, potential alteration in respiratory function, potential for self-harm, and maturational enuresis. Examples of Carpenito's bifocal clinical nursing model (1987a,b) are shown in Table 8-4 for the client with a medical diagnosis of anemia.

## Family

Whether nursing diagnoses of the family are stated functionally, structurally, or developmentally depends on the model used. These diagnoses may be from one model exclusively or from the approved list of nursing diagnoses. As with nursing diagnoses of individuals, those related to the family may deal with actual or potential concerns or with promoting and maintaining optimum family health.

Table 8-5 offers examples of family nursing diagnoses for several types of models. Major concepts of Beavers' (1977) structural family systems theory that may be used as diagnostic categories are family power structure, degree of family individualism, acceptance of separation and loss, perception of reality, and affect. Functional areas for assessing families are family conflict or harmony, bonding, decision-making and task allocation, roles and rules,

and communication. Satir (1972) is a theorist in this category. Her four assessment areas are communication, rules, self-worth, and social linkages. Duvall (1977) and Stevenson (1977) are developmental theorists who list tasks and stages that can be used as diagnostic categories.

Hart and Herriott's (1977) systems theory categories are processes of adaptation to the environment, integration of the parts, and decisions regarding the first two processes. Other models may also be applied to this format for writing nursing diagnoses. Examples also may be found in the approved list of nursing diagnoses.

The purpose in writing family nursing diagnoses is to help the family achieve or maintain optimum health as it is defined within the model(s) chosen for nursing practice with families.

## Community

Community nursing diagnoses may be stated according to structure or process. Structural diagnoses include those related to demographic characteristics, aggregates (groups with similar characteristics), or systems. Systems include sociocultural, political, recreational, housing, transportation, educational, religious, environmental, economic, and health care systems. Process diagnoses include communication, decision-making, participation, and leadership. Examples are given for structure and process diagnoses in Table 8-6.

Nurses can identify health concerns and affect change in many areas with intervention pertaining to health maintenance, health promotion, health education, consultation, and disease prevention. Many community health nurses are also using the concepts of partnership, participation, and community development. It is the nurse's responsibility to work with the community in identifying the concerns and resources.

Gordon's (1987a) functional health patterns can be adapted for the community as well as the NANDA nine response categories. The category *exchanging* could relate to the community's inputs and outputs, including resources, products, services, and waste, among others. *Communicating* could include formal and informal networks and methods of communication such as printed or electronic media. *Relating* may refer to cultural, societal, and neighborhood patterns including recreational and social service availability and accessibility. *Valuing* includes the community's values such as the work ethic, nondiscrimination, health, environmental safety, and so on. Examples of nursing diagnoses for some of the other NANDA categories are given in Table 8-7.

**Table 8-3** Nursing Diagnoses for the Individual Based on Three of Gordon's Functional Health Patterns

| Model pattern | Modifier | Response | Etiology | Defining characteristics |
|---|---|---|---|---|
| **Health perception-health management** | Total | Health management alteration | Activity intolerance, level IV | Inability to manage own treatment, dyspnea, and fatigue at rest |
| | Potential | Noncompliance: medication | Denial of illness and absence of plans to obtain medication | Presence of risk factors in etiology |
| | | Health maintenance alteration | Lack of material resources | Reported and observed lack of equipment and finances |
| **Activity-exercise** | Total | Self-care deficit, level IV | Uncompensated musculoskeletal impairment | Inability to participate in own care |
| | | Ineffective breathing pattern | Pain | Dyspnea, shortness of breath, cough, nasal flaring |
| | Potential | Joint contracture | Abnormal posture | Presence of risk factors in etiology |
| **Role relationship** | Unresolved | Independent-dependent conflict | Physical activity restriction | Expressed anger, expressed desire for independence |
| | | Translocation syndrome | Move to nursing home | Passive, expressed insecurity and lack of trust |
| | | Altered growth and development: social skills | Multiple caretakers | Unable to meet developmental level skills, dysfunctional interaction |

**Table 8-4** Nursing Diagnoses and Collaborative Problems for the Individual with a Medical Diagnosis of Anemia Based on Carpenito's Model

| Model category | Modifier | Response | Etiology | Defining characteristics |
|---|---|---|---|---|
| Nursing diagnosis | | Activity intolerance | Impaired oxygen transport secondary to diminished red blood cell count | Dyspnea, shortness of breath, increased blood pressure, weakness, fatigue |
| | Potential | Infection | Decreased resistance secondary to tissue hypoxia | Altered production of leukocytes, altered immune response |
| Collaborative problems | Potential complication: transfusion reaction | | | |
| | Potential complication: cardiac failure | | | |
| | Potential complication: iron overload (repeated transfusions) | | | |

**Table 8-5**  Nursing Diagnoses for Families Based on Selected Models

| | Model | Modifier | Response | Etiology |
|---|---|---|---|---|
| A. | Beavers | | Alteration in family *power structure*\* | Illness of breadwinner or inadequate problem solving |
| | | Minimum | Acceptance of family *individualism* | Anger or beliefs |
| | | | Inadequate acceptance of *loss* | Youngest child leaving home, or divorce |
| B. | Satir | | Inflexible *rules* | Misunderstanding or authoritarian values |
| | | | Decreased *self-worth* | Inability to share feelings, altered body image, or confusion from medication |
| | | | Inadequate recreation | Closed *societal links* |
| C. | Functional | Decreased | *Bonding* | Prematurity of infant, cesarean section, or absence of role model |
| | | Potential for | Impaired *parenting* | Inconsistent discipline or lack of knowledge |
| | | | Reversal of *roles* | Chronic illness or absence of extended family |
| | | Temporary | Alteration in family *transaction* | Recent divorce, death of spouse, decreased communication, or discovery of homosexuality |
| D. | Developmental | | Inability to accomplish stage-specific *developmental tasks* | Dysfunctional communication or lack of knowledge |
| E. | Systems | | Deprivation of system *input* | Institutionalization |
| | | | Impaired *decision-making* | Confusion from medication or crisis |
| | | | Decreased safety in *environment* | Physical abuse or alcoholic mate |
| | | | Maintaining *equilibrium* | Adequate coping or open communications |
| F. | NANDA approved (1988) | Compromised | Ineffective family *coping* | Incorrect information, or temporary role change |
| | | Disabling | Ineffective family *coping* | Highly ambivalent family relationship, or unexpressed hostility in one member |
| | | | Potential for growth: family *coping* | Adaptation and progress toward self-actualization |
| | | | Altered family *process* | Situational or developmental transition or crisis |
| | | Actual or potential | Altered *parenting* | Lack of available role model, physical abuse, or lack of support from significant other, lack of knowledge |

\*Italicized words indicate major concepts within models, as mentioned in text on p. 172.

**Table 8-6**  Nursing Diagnoses for Community Health Concerns Based on Structure and Process

| Model | Response | Etiology |
|---|---|---|
| **A. Structure** | | |
| 1. Demographic characteristics | Increased respiratory diseases | Air pollution, overcrowded conditions, or inadequate ventilation |
| | Increased dog bites | Packs of roaming dogs, inadequate code enforcement, or inadequate personnel and facilities |
| | Increased infant mortality rate | Cause unknown, inadequate nutrition, or increased teenage pregnancies |
| 2. Aggregates | Inadequate prenatal facilities | Lack of funds or planning |
| | Increased lead poisoning in toddlers | Substandard housing or lack of prevention or knowledge |
| | Increased dental caries in school-age children | Poor hygiene or lack of knowledge |
| | Increased child abuse | Cause unknown |
| | Inadequate programs for substance abuse | Lack of funds or priority |
| | Lack of genetic counseling | Lack of personnel or knowledge of need |
| | Lack of gerontological services | Lack of planning or funds |
| 3. Systems | Substandard housing | Economic recession, lack of funds for improvement, or high unemployment |
| | Inadequate transportation | Lack of state or federal funds or interest |
| | Decreased maintenance of sewers | Lack of information, personnel or leadership |
| **B. Process** | Decreased communication | Political associations, sectionalism, or anger |
| | Lack of neighborhood participation | Apathy, lack of information, or cultural beliefs |

**Table 8-7**  Nursing Diagnoses for Community Health Concerns Based on Adaptation of NANDA Categories of Choosing, Knowing, and Moving

| Model category | Response | Etiology |
|---|---|---|
| Choosing | Ineffective community coping | Lack of leadership, lack of finances |
| | Noncompliance: communicable diseases reporting | Lack of knowledge, insufficient staffing |
| Knowing | Inadequate school health program | Lack of knowledge, lack of finances, apathy |
| Moving | Social isolation | Lack of public transportation, cultural beliefs |

## SUMMARY

Nursing diagnostic statements are the basis for planning and nursing intervention. It is important that they are clear, concise, definitive statements of the client's actual or potential health status and concerns. The nursing diagnoses must be amenable to nursing action and be validated with the client. The nursing diagnoses are written as descriptive and etiological statements. They may be derived from the approved list of nursing diagnoses or from the professional nurse's experience and use of selected models for practice.

## REFERENCES AND READING

Abdellah F et al: Patient-centered approaches to nursing, New York, 1961, Macmillan, Inc.

American Nurses' Association: Standards: nursing practice, Kansas City, 1973, The Association.

American Nurses' Association: Nursing: a social policy statement, ANA Publication Code: NP-63, 35M, December, 1980.

Aspinall MJ: Nursing diagnosis: the weak link, Nurs Outlook 24:433, 1976.

Baretich DM and Anderson LB: Should we diagnose strengths? No: stick to the problem, Am J Nurs 87:1211, 1987.

Beavers WR: Psychotherapy and growth: a family systems perspective, New York, 1977, Brunner/Mazel, Inc.

Berry KN: Let's create nursing diagnoses psych nurses can use, Am J Nurs 87(9):707, 1987.

Bircher AU: On the development and classification of diagnosis. In Duespohl TA, editor: Nursing in transition, Germantown, Md, 1983, Aspen Systems Corp.

Black J: Nursing diagnosis in plastic surgical nursing, Plast Surg Nurs 7(1):4, 1987.

Block D: Some crucial terms in nursing: what do they mean? Nurs Outlook 22:689, 1974.

Bloom KC, Leitner JE, and Solano JL: Development of an expert system prototype to generate nursing care plans based on nursing diagnoses, Comput Nurs 5(4):140, 1987.

Bolger AM and Asghari F: Sift reports: using nursing diagnosis, Nurs Manage 18(10):17, 1987.

Brennan DT: Outcome criteria and nursing diagnosis in ESRD patient care planning, ANNA J 14(2):131, 1987.

Brennan PF and Romano CA: Computers and nursing diagnoses: issues in implementation, Nurs Clin North Am 22(4):935, 1987.

Breu C, Dracup K, and Walden J: Integration of nursing diagnoses in the critical care nursing literature, Heart Lung 16(6):605, 1987.

Brown KG, Dunn K, Ervin D et al: Nursing diagnosis and process evaluation: implications for continuing education, J Cont Ed Nurs 18(5):172, 1987.

Brown P, Funsch R, Seremet N et al: Linking psychiatric nursing care to patient classification codes, Nurs Health Care 8(3):157, 1987.

Bulechek GN and McCloskey JC: Nursing interventions: what they are and how to choose them, Holistic Nurs Pract 1(3):36, 1987.

Campbell C: Nursing diagnosis and intervention in nursing practice, New York, 1984, John Wiley & Sons, Inc.

Carlson JH, Craft CA, and McGuire AD: Nursing diagnosis, Philadelphia, 1982, WB Saunders.

Carnevali DL et al: Diagnostic reasoning in nursing, Philadelphia, 1984, JB Lippincott Co.

Carpenito LJ: Nursing diagnosis: application to clinical practice, Philadelphia, 1983, JB Lippincott Co.

Carpenito LJ: Handbook of nursing diagnosis, ed 2, Philadelphia, 1987a, JB Lippincott Co.

Carpenito LJ: Nursing diagnosis: application to clinical practice ed 2, Philadelphia, 1987b, JB Lippincott Co.

Carpenito LJ: Nursing diagnosis in critical care: impact on practice and outcomes, Heart Lung 16(6):595, 1987c.

Chang BL, Roth K, Caswell D et al: CANDI: a knowledge-based system for nursing diagnosis, Comput Nurs 6(1):13, 1988.

Clark S: Nursing diagnosis: ineffectual coping. (I, A theoretical framework and II, Planning care), Heart Lung 16(6):670, 1987.

Coler MS and Vincent KG: Coded nursing diagnoses on axes: a prioritized, computer ready diagnostic system for psychiatric/mental health nurses, Arch Psych Nurs 1(2):125, 1987.

Craig DI and Sharp DN: Nursing care plan for a pregnant spinal cord injured patient, Rehab Nurs 83:26, March-April 1983.

Creason NS: How do we define our diagnoses? Am J Nurs 87(2):230, 1987.

Dialogue: Image: J Nurs Scholarship, 87(19):216, 1987.

Dittmann EE and Gould MT: Refinement of nursing diagnosis skills: the effect of clinical nurse specialist teaching and consultation, J Cont Ed Nurs 18(5):157, 1987.

Dixon J and Walker BC: Nursing diagnosis: defining the goal of care, Aust Nurs J 16(5):43, 1986.

Doenges ME and Moorhouse MF: Nurse's pocket guide: nursing diagnoses with interventions, ed 2, Philadelphia, 1988, FA Davis Co.

Dossey B and Guzzetta C: Nursing diagnosis, Nursing 81:34, June 1981.

Duespohl TA: Nursing diagnosis manual for the well and ill client, Philadelphia, 1986, WB Saunders Co.

Duvall EM: Marriage and family development, ed 5, Philadelphia, 1977, JB Lippincott Co.

Erikson EH: Childhood and society, ed 2, New York, 1963, WW Norton & Co., Inc.

Fadden TC and Seiser G: Nursing diagnosis: a matter of form, Am J Nurs 84:470, April 1984.

Fawcett J: Guest editorial: conceptual models of nursing, nursing diagnosis, and nursing theory development, West J Nurs Res 8(4):397, 1986.

Fehring RJ: Methods to validate nursing diagnoses, Heart Lung 16(6):625, 1987.

Fredette SL and Gloriant FS: Nursing diagnosis in cancer chemotherapy, Am J Nurs 81:2031, November 1981.

Frissell S: So many models, so much confusion, Nurs Admin Q 12(2):13, 1988.

Fry VS: The creature approach to nursing, Am J Nurs 53:301, 1953.

Gebbie KM: Development of a taxonomy of nursing diagnosis. In Walter JB et al: Dynamics of problem-oriented approaches: patient care and documentation, Philadelphia, 1976, JB Lippincott Co.

Gebbie K and Lavin MA: Classifying nursing diagnosis, Am J Nurs 74:250, 1974.

Gebbie KM and Lavin MA, editors: Classification of nursing diagnosis, St. Louis, 1975, The CV Mosby Co.

George J, editor: Nursing theories: the base for professional nursing practice, Englewood Cliffs, NJ, 1984, Prentice-Hall, Inc.

Gettrust KV, Ryan SC, and Englemen DS: Applied nursing diagnoses: guides for comprehensive care planning, New York, 1985, John Wiley & Sons, Inc.

Gordon M: Nursing and the diagnostic process, Am J Nurs 76:1298, 1976.

Gordon M: Manual of nursing diagnosis, New York, 1982a, McGraw-Hill Book Co.

Gordon M: Nursing diagnosis: process and application, New York, 1982b, McGraw-Hill Book Co.

Gordon M: Nursing diagnosis. In Werley H and Fitzpatrick J, editors: Ann Rev Nurs Res 3:127, 1985.

Gordon M: Manual of nursing diagnosis 1986-1987, New York, 1987a, McGraw-Hill, Inc.

Gordon M: Implementation of nursing diagnoses: an overview, Nurs Clin North Am 22(4):875, 1987b.

Gordon M and Sweeney MA: Methodological problems and issues in identifying and standardizing nursing diagnoses, Adv Nurs Sci 2:1, 1979.

Guzzetta CE and Dossey BM: Nursing diagnosis: framework, process, and problems, Heart Lung 12:281, May 1983.

Guzzetta CE: Nursing diagnoses in nursing education: effect on the profession, Heart Lung 16(6):629, 1987.

Hall JE and Weaver BR: A systems approach to community health: distributive nursing practice, Philadelphia, 1985, JB Lippincott Co.

Hamilton P: Community nursing diagnosis, Adv Nurs Sci 6:21, April 1983.

Hanna DV and Wyman NB: Assessment + diagnosis = care planning: a tool for coordination, Nurs Manage 18(11):106, 1987.

Harrington LW: The diagnosis dilemma: one preferred remedy, Nurs Health Care 9(2):93, 1988.

Hart SK and Herriott PR: Components of practice. In Hall J and Weaver B, editors: A systems approach to community health: distributive nursing practice, Philadelphia, 1977, JB Lippincott Co.

Henderson B: Nursing diagnosis: theory and practice, Adv Nurs Sci 1:75, 1978.

Herberth L and Gosnell DJ: Nursing diagnosis for oncology nursing practice, Cancer Nurs 10(1):41, 1987.

Houldin AD, Salstein SW, and Ganley KM: Nursing diagnoses for wellness: supporting strengths, Philadelphia, 1987, JB Lippincott Co.

Hutcheson HA: Breast reconstruction using abdominal tissue: a nursing diagnosis approach, Plast Surg Nurs 7(1):11, 1987.

Hymovich DP and Barnard MU: Family health care, New York, 1979, McGraw-Hill Book Co.

Iyer PW, Taptich BJ, and Bernocchi-Losey D: Nursing process and nursing diagnosis, Philadelphia, 1986, WB Saunders Co.

Jenny JL: Knowledge deficit: not a nursing diagnosis, Image: J Nurs Scholarship 19(4):184, 1987.

Kelly K: Clinical inference in nursing, Nurs Res 15:23, 1966.

Kelly MA: Nursing diagnosis source book; guidelines for clinical application, Norwalk, Conn, 1985, Appleton-Century-Crofts.

Kilpack V and Dobson-Brassard S: Intershift report: oral communication using the nursing process, J Neurosci Nurs 19(5):266, 1987.

Kim MJ, McFardland GK, and McLane AM: Classification of nursing diagnosis: Proceedings of the Fifth National Conference, St Louis, 1984a, The CV Mosby Co.

Kim MJ, McFarland GK, and McLane AM: Pocket guide to nursing diagnosis, St Louis, 1984b, The CV Mosby Co.

Kim MJ, McFarland GK, and McLane AM: Pocket guide to nursing diagnoses, ed 2, St Louis, 1987, The CV Mosby Co.

King IM: A theory of nursing: systems, concepts, process, New York, 1981, John Wiley & Sons, Inc.

Knight JH: Applying nursing process in the community, Nurs Outlook 22:711, 1974.

Kruse DH: Promoting nursing diagnoses: keeping your care plans short and simple, Ohio Nurse Rev 67(7):13, 1987.

LaMonica EL: The humanistic nursing process, Monterey, Calif, 1985, Wadsworth Health Sciences Division.

Lee HA and Strong KA: Using nursing diagnosis to describe the clinical competence of baccalaureate and associate degree graduating students: a comparative study, Image: J Nurs Scholarship 18(3):82, 1985.

Lee HA and Frenn MD: The use of nursing diagnoses for health promotion in community practice, Nurs Clin North Am 22(4):981, 1987.

Lengel N: Handbook of nursing diagnosis, Bowie, Md, 1982, Robert J Brady Co.

Leslie FM: Nursing diagnosis: use in long term care, Am J Nurs 81:1012, May 1981.

Little D and Carnevali D: The diagnostic statement: the problem defined. In Walter JB et al: Dynamics of problem-oriented approaches: patient care and documentation, Philadelphia, 1976, JB Lippincott Co.

Lunney M: Nursing diagnosis: refining the system, Am J Nurs 82:456, March 1982.

Lunney M: A framework to analyze a taxonomy of nursing diagnoses. In Kim MJ et al: Classification of nursing diagnoses. Proceedings of the Fifth National Conference, St Louis, 1984, The CV Mosby Co.

Lunney M: Implementing an educational program on nursing diagnosis, J NYSNA 17(4):28, 1986.

Maas ML: Nursing diagnoses in a professional model of nursing: keystone for effective nursing administration, J Nurs Admin 16(12):39, 1986.

MacVicar MG and Archbold P: A framework for family assessment in chronic illness, Nurs Forum 15:180, 1976.

Maibusch RM: Implementing nursing diagnoses, Nurs Clin North Am 22(4):955, 1987.

Malen AL: Perioperative nursing diagnoses: what, why, and how, AORN J 44(5):829, 1986.

Maslow AH: Motivation and personality, New York, 1970, Harper & Row, Publishers, Inc.

McCourt AE: Implementation of nursing diagnoses through integration with quality assurance, Nurs Clin North Am 22(4):899, 1987.

McLane AM, editor: Classification of nursing diagnoses. Proceedings of the Seventh Conference of the North American Nursing Diagnosis Association, St Louis, 1987a, The CV Mosby Co.

McLane AM: Measurement and validation of diagnostic concepts: a decade of progress, Heart Lung 16(6):616, 1987b.

McManus RL: Assumptions of the functions of nursing. In Regional planning for nursing and nursing education, New York, 1950, Bureau of Publications Teachers' College, Columbia University.

Mehmert PA: A nursing information system: the outcome of implementing nursing diagnoses, Nurs Clin North Am 22(4):943, 1987.

Mitchell PH and Loustau C: Concepts basic to nursing, ed 3, New York, 1981, McGraw-Hill Book Co.

Mundinger MO and Jauron GD: Developing a nursing diagnosis, Nurs Outlook 23:94, 1975.

Nolan A: Utilizing nursing diagnosis in nursing education, Aust J Adv Nurs 4(2):51, 1987.

Nursing Diagnosis Newsletter: NANDA approved nursing diagnostic categories, 15(1), Summer 1988.

Orem DE: Nursing: concepts of practice, ed 3, New York, 1985, McGraw-Hill, Inc.

Orlando IJ: The dynamic nurse-patient relationship, New York, 1961, GP Putnam's Sons.

Pinnell NM and deMenses M: The nursing process: theory, application, and related processes, Norwalk, Conn, 1986, Appleton-Century-Crofts.

Popkess-Vawter S: Strength-oriented diagnosis. In Kim, MJ, McFarland, G, and McLane, AM: Classification of nursing diagnosis, St Louis, 1984, The CV Mosby Co.

Popkess-Vawter S and Pinnell N: Should we diagnose strengths? yes: accentuate the positive, Am J Nurs 87(9):1211, 1987.

Porter EJ: The nursing diagnosis of population groups. In McLane AM: Classification of nursing diagnoses. Proceedings of the Seventh Conference, North American Nursing Diagnosis Association, St Louis, 1987a, The CV Mosby Co.

Porter EJ: Critical analysis of NANDA nursing diagnosis taxonomy I, Image: J Nurs Scholarship 18(4):136, 1987b.

Price MR: Nursing diagnosis: making a concept come alive, Am J Nurs 80:668, 1980.

Rantz MJ and Miller TV: Change theory: a framework for implementing nursing diagnosis in a long-term care setting, Nurs Clin North Am 22(4):887, 1987a.

Rantz M and Miller TV: Diagnostics: how diagnoses are changing in long-term care, Am J Nurs 87(3):360, 1987b.

Rasch RFR: The nature of taxonomy, Image: J Nurs Scholarship 19(3):147, 1987.

Roberts SL: Nursing diagnosis and the critically ill patient, Norwalk, Conn, 1987, Appleton & Lange.

Roy Sr C: Introduction to nursing: an adaptation model, Englewood Cliffs, NJ, 1984, Prentice-Hall, Inc.

Sanford S: Administrative applications of nursing diagnosis, Heart Lung 16(6):600, 1987.

Satir V: Peoplemaking, Palo Alto, Calif, 1972, Science and Behavior Books.

Schlotfeldt RM: Defining nursing: a historic controversy, Nurs Res 36(1):64, 1987.

Shoemaker JK: Essential features of a nursing diagnosis. In Kim MJ et al: Classification of nursing diagnosis, St Louis, 1984, The CV Mosby Co.

Shortridge LM and Lee EJ: Introduction to nursing practice, New York, 1980, McGraw-Hill Book Co.

Sjoberg EL: Nursing diagnosis and the COPD patient, Am J Nurs 83:245, February 1983.

Smaldone A, Greenberg C, and Perez PW: Computer consult: nursing diagnosis: translate please!, Am J Nurs 88(3):363, 1988.

Spotts SJ: A nursing diagnosis taxonomy for quality assurance and reimbursement. In Duespohl TA, editor: Nursing in transition, Germantown, Md, 1983, Aspen Systems Corp.

Stanfield V: Perioperative documentation: integrating nursing diagnoses in the patient record, AORN J 46(4):699, 1987.

Stevenson JS: Issues and crises during middlescence, New York, 1977, Appleton-Century-Crofts.

Stolte K: A complementary view of nursing diagnosis, Pub Health Nurs 3(1):23, 1986.

Swehla MA: Nursing diagnosis as a standard: methodology for identifying and validating diagnoses in an ambulatory care setting, Nurs Admin Q 12(2):18, 1988.

Tinkham CW, Voorhies EF, and McCarthy NC: Community health nursing: evolution and process in the family and community, New York, 1984, Appleton-Century-Crofts.

Titler MG: Implementation of nursing diagnoses in nursing education, Nurs Clin North Am 22(4):987, 1987.

Townsend MC: Nursing diagnoses in psychiatric nursing: a pocket guide for care plan construction, Philadelphia, 1988, FA Davis Co.

Treu M and Brague J: Introducing nursing diagnosis throughout the hospital, Nurs Manage 18(4):94, 1987.

Turkoski BB: Nursing diagnosis in print, 1950-1985, Nurs Outlook 36(3):142, 1988.

Werley HH: Nursing diagnosis and the nursing minimum data set. In McLane AM: Classification of nursing diagnoses. Proceedings of the Seventh Conference, North American Nursing Diagnosis Association, St Louis, 1987, The CV Mosby Company.

Woods ME, editor: Nursing Diagnosis Newsletter 11:1, June 1984 (published by North American Nursing Diagnosis Association, St. Louis University School of Nursing, 3525 Caroline St., St Louis, Mo 63104).

Yura H and Walsh MB: The nursing process, ed 4, New York, 1983, Appleton-Century-Crofts.

# CHAPTER 9

# Planning: Priorities, Goals, and Objectives

PAULA J. CHRISTENSEN

## GENERAL CONSIDERATIONS

Plans for implementation are based on assessment and diagnosis of the client's health status, strengths, and concerns. After nursing diagnoses are validated, they provide direction for determining how to assist the client in resolving concerns related to the restoration, maintenance, and promotion of health. The descriptive and etiological clauses of the diagnosis help guide the nurse's development of the plan of care. The planning component involves judging priorities, establishing goals, developing objectives, identifying strategies, and specifying nursing orders for implementation.

Traditionally, planning for client care was done *by* the nurse *for* the client. Formerly, it was usually based on the medical diagnoses. The client was passive and followed without question what the nurse recommended. The client viewed the physician and the nurse as "knowing best," and accepted treatment accordingly. As clients' knowledge of health and illness increased and nurses assumed responsibility and accountability for care given, the traditional bases for care were no longer valid. Currently, nurses assess their clients' health status and formulate individual plans for care *with* their clients. Plans still reflect the client's *medical* problems, but now equally address *nursing* concerns: the client's *responses* to actual or potential health problems.

Planning, or determining how to assist the client in resolving health-related concerns, is through deliberate decision-making and problem-solving with each client. This mutual planning process holds nurses accountable and responsible to clients for the agreed-on actions and subsequent outcomes.

The nurse's level of proficiency affects the phases of the planning component. The novice or beginning nurse bases planning on empirical knowledge gained from basic education, other nurses' experiences, and his or her own limited experiences. Judgments about each phase are deliberate, conscious decisions. The new nurse may need to consult other nurses regarding which nursing diagnosis is the top priority or what is a realistic time frame for the client to achieve the goals and objectives. As the nurse's expertise develops, these judgments are made based on empirical and personal knowledge. Thus, the nurse's experience provides a foundation for clinical judgments. Decisions continue to be conscious ones, incorporating empirical knowledge; yet the nurse learns to trust clinical intuition, which is a part of personal knowledge.

Nursing care standards, guidelines, policies, procedures, laws, and regulations are used to influence planning. However, based on the nurse's assessment and diagnosis of the client's situation, an individualized approach to alleviate the client's health concerns is developed. Nurses may identify health concerns that call for interventions by other health professionals. Decisions regarding consultations, referrals, and collaborative approaches to care are included in the plan as well.

The nurse collaborates with others while developing the plan. Information and ideas are sought from the client, people directly involved with the client, other nurses, and health team members. A multidisciplinary approach to care is particularly important for clients with complex health concerns. Resource people for individual and family client plans include clinical nurse specialists, social workers, physicians, dietitians, activity therapists, nutritional support specialists, physical therapists, and chaplains. All these offer their own expertise to facilitate a comprehensive and effective plan. Resource people for a community client plan may include an organizational developer or trainer, a financial consultant and planner, a management educator, a long-range planning consultant, and a state representative. Goal-oriented group meetings of these and other experts often yield unique and varied ways to assist the client in attaining an optimal level of health and functioning. The ideas generated for the plan are then shared with the client to ensure mutuality of intent and accountability for action. The nurse must use professional judgment in choosing which plans to share in detail with the client. Some clients, because of their health status, limitations, and age, are not capable of being completely involved in the mutual planning process. However, decisions regarding which plans to use should involve the client as much as possible to increase the client's sense of personal control and commitment to the plan.

This chapter focuses on the first three phases of planning: judging priorities, establishing goals, and developing objectives. Guidelines for these elements are as follows:

1. Prioritizing nursing diagnoses
   a. Actual or imminent life-threatening concerns are considered before actual or potential health-threatening concerns.
   b. Temporal, human, and material resources are examined deliberately.
   c. The client is involved in determining the priority of concerns.
   d. Scientific and practice principles provide rationale for decisions.
2. Establishing goals
   a. Goals are client-focused and reflect mutuality with the client.
   b. Goals are appropriate to their respective diagnosis.
   c. Goals are realistic, reflecting the capabilities and limitations of the client.
   d. Goals include broad or abstract indicators of performance.
   e. Scientific and practice principles guide the establishment of goals.
3. Developing objectives
   a. Objectives are client-focused and reflect mutuality with the client.
   b. Objectives are appropriate to their respective goal.
   c. Objectives are realistic, reflecting the capabilities and limitations of the client.
   d. Objectives include specific indicators of performance.

   e. Objectives are numbered in appropriate sequence to achieve the goal.
   f. Scientific and practice principles guide the development of objectives.

All phases of the planning component are necessary to give direction for quality nursing care. Identifying strategies and specifying nursing orders for implementation are discussed in Chapter 10. Individual, family, and community clients need effective planning to achieve desired outcomes.

## JUDGING PRIORITIES

The process of judging priorities begins with the list of nursing diagnoses. Arranging these diagnoses in priority involves deciding a preferential order of the client's concerns. Making this choice, however, does not mean that one concern must be totally resolved before another is considered. Usually several diagnoses are focused on concurrently.

The act of choosing one diagnosis as the most important is based on several factors. Threats to life and health; temporal, human, and material resources available; the client's involvement; and standards, guidelines, policies, procedures, laws, and regulations all play a part in judging priorities.

### Guidelines for Judging Priorities

1. *Actual or imminent life-threatening concerns are considered before actual or potential health-threatening concerns.* Diagnoses that involve life-threatening concerns, such as severe depletion or loss of function, should be considered first. Examples of life-threatening concerns for the individual, family, and community are

| | |
|---|---|
| *Individual:* | Loss of cardiac, respiratory, or mental function |
| *Family:* | Loss of parent(s), home, or job |
| *Community:* | Water pollution, hurricane, tornado, nuclear radiation accident |

Actual or potential health-threatening concerns are those that may impair functioning or growth and development if not corrected. Examples of health-threatening concerns for the individual, family, and community are

| | |
|---|---|
| *Individual:* | Increase in life stressors along with decreased ability to cope, acute illness |
| *Family:* | Addition of family member, long-term illness of family member |
| *Community:* | Loss of key health care facility, major industry, or tax base |

2. *Temporal, human, and material resources are examined deliberately.* The amount of time that the nurse has to work with the client affects the actual

and potential diagnoses chosen on which to focus. The client in particular benefits from a sense of accomplishment; therefore, diagnoses in which short-term gains can be achieved will be important at first. In regard to human resources, the nurse determines whether the number of people and their qualifications and skills are adequate to attend to the client's concern. Material resources such as money, equipment, and supplies also need to be sufficient for intervention to be successful. For example, the nurse working in a marginally funded inner city clinic for indigent clients has different resources from those of a nurse working for a wealthy suburban home health care agency. The nurse in the clinic may see the client on an infrequent and irregular basis. Thus, time with the client is limited, and usually only high-priority actual health concerns are dealt with. Staffing, equipment, and supplies may also be inadequate because of the lack of funds. Therefore, the people and materials would be scarce, and could negatively impact eventual attainment of goals.

3. *The client is involved in determining the priority of concerns.* The client's involvement is essential when arranging concerns in order of importance. Because nurses work mutually with clients, the nurse considers the client's: (1) understanding of the health concerns and related situation; (2) values, thoughts, and feelings about resolving health concerns; (3) general state of health; and (4) ability to solve problems. The client must have an adequate knowledge of the health concerns and the situation. The nurse is responsible for assessing the client's knowledge level and teaching the client relevant information on which to make informed decisions. The client's values, thoughts, and feelings about resolving health concerns have an impact on the client's cooperation with certain interventions. For example, an individual client who smokes two packs of cigarettes per day and knows the health-related hazards may choose to continue to smoke. Plans to help the client quit smoking will be unsuccessful so long as the client does not *value* health promotion, or does not *think* that facts will influence the decision to smoke. The client's general state of health influences the client's ability to be involved in judging health concerns. A client who is psychotic or unconscious will have little involvement compared with the client who is awake and oriented. In the former situation, the client and the client's family should be informed of the priorities set by the nurse. If appropriate, the client's family is included in setting priorities for concerns. The client's ability to solve problems also influences

how active the client will be in determining priorities. Severe anxiety, stress, and altered level of consciousness often impair a client's thinking process, leading to disorganization and inability to make decisions. If possible, the nurse facilitates improved problem solving by using the problem-solving strategy and clearly summarizing the specific problem so that the client can focus on it. Details of this strategy are given in Chapter 10. Individual, family, and community clients are involved in judging priorities.

4. *Scientific and practice principles provide rationale for decisions.* Judging priorities is facilitated by the use of theories, models, and principles. One model often used to evaluate the relative priority of diagnoses is Maslow's (1968) hierarchy of needs. Maslow identifies basic needs that all people share: air, food, safety, and love. Growth needs are not necessary for sustaining life but they promote self-growth, such as self-esteem and self-actualization. Basic needs are more important than growth needs; the individual must have basic needs met before focusing on growth needs. Using this model with a client who has unmet basic and growth needs, the nurse develops and implements plans for the unmet basic needs first.

Working with individual clients, physiological principles are also helpful in judging concerns. Consideration of these principles guides the nurse in giving immediate attention to life-threatening concerns. For example:

1. Knowledge that increased intracranial pressure can lead to changes in vital signs and to possible brain damage takes precedence over personal hygiene.
2. Knowledge that high blood pressure poses a threat to circulatory and cardiac status takes precedence over learning about borderline diabetes.

Isolated data and patterns of data give the nurse cues that aid in judging precedence. Examples of *isolated cues* that lead to immediate plans and interventions include vital sign readings significantly above or below general or client norms and sudden changes in behavior. Examples of *patterns observed over time* that indicate a need for plans and interventions include gradual changes in vital signs and subtle changes in how the client relates to others. Table 9-1 provides an example of client's prioritized health concerns, using this rationale.

Standards, guidelines, policies, procedures, laws, and regulations influence the nurse's decision-making regarding priorities. They give direction—in varying capacity and degree—to nursing practice issues ranging from an authoritative prin-

**Table 9-1** An Appropriate Sequence of Priorities

| Nursing diagnosis | Sequence of priorities | Rationale |
| --- | --- | --- |
| Inadequate nutrition related to lack of knowledge of balanced diet | 3 | Latent health concern that can be dealt with somewhat concurrently with 2 |
| Alteration in circulatory status related to high blood pressure | 1 | Most life-threatening concern at this time |
| Increased anxiety related to first pregnancy and fear of the unknown | 2 | Threatening mental health and potential threat to physical health |

ciple or rule to suggested advice. Generally, though, nurses still use their own judgment along with these sources to individualize the client's priorities.

## CLIENT OUTCOMES: GOALS AND OBJECTIVES

Client outcomes are labeled as goals (long-term outcomes) and objectives (short-term outcomes). Achievement of goals results in the resolution of the health concerns indicated by the nursing diagnoses. Attainment of objectives leads to the achievement of their respective goals. The time frame of goals and objectives is related to the nature of the health concern, the availability of resources, the type of agency in which the care is being provided, and the characteristics of the clients.

For example, consider a male client who recently experienced a myocardial infarction and is still in an acute care setting. This person has a nursing diagnosis of "alteration in nutrition related to inadequate dietary intake." A goal for this client is to improve nutritional habits and adhere to recommended dietary guidelines (on his own volition). This goal is beyond the time limits of his anticipated stay at this setting. Some objectives that are needed to achieve the goal are well within the time and resources available. The client is able to learn about food groups, dietary guidelines, and food preparation, and to adhere to the recommended diet as prepared by the institution. In this situation, then, the goal reaches into the future, even past the client's discharge from the agency, and beyond the constraints of the immediate situation. The objectives focus on current means to alleviate the concern and to develop the client's knowledge, skills, and abilities in order to attain the goal. Continuity of care is facilitated through planning for both short-term and long-term resolutions to health concerns. Nurses work with clients to promote, maintain, and restore their optimal level of health through enhancing the achievement of goals and objectives.

## ESTABLISHING GOALS

After priorities have been determined, the nurse establishes goals. Goals flow directly from the nursing diagnosis, especially the descriptive clause. Goals are statements that reflect a client outcome, leading to alleviation of the concern indicated by the diagnosis. A goal is a statement describing a broad or abstract intent, state, or condition that reflects an outcome (Mager, 1984).

Because goals are long-term outcomes, they often reach beyond the time a client is in direct care or service within an institution. These outcomes lead to the client altering physiological and psychological responses, attaining psychomotor skills, increasing knowledge, and developing abilities. Because a goal describes a *client's* outcome, the statement is used as one basis to evaluate progress. If the nursing diagnoses reflect specific client concerns, then only one goal is needed per diagnosis. However, diagnoses stated in broad terms usually require more than one goal statement.

**Example**

| | |
| --- | --- |
| *Nursing diagnosis (specific):* | Inadequate exercise related to lack of frequency per week |
| *Goal:* | The client will increase frequency of exercise within 1 month. |
| *Nursing diagnosis (general):* | Alteration in metabolism related to inadequate insulin production |
| *Goal:* | The client will stabilize metabolism within 1 week. |
| *Goal:* | The client will decrease susceptibility to altered metabolism within 1 month. |

## Nature of Goals

The nature of the goal depends on the diagnosis: goals reflect health restoration, maintenance, or promotion. *Health restoration goals* are appropriate when a client's internal or external resources are inadequate or diminished.

**Example**

| | |
|---|---|
| *Nursing diagnosis:* | Depleted nutritional state related to anorexia |
| *Goal:* | The client will develop an adequate nutritional state within 1 month. |

*Health maintenance goals* are appropriate when the client wants to increase the existing internal or external resources or continue using those resources.

**Example**

| | |
|---|---|
| *Nursing diagnosis:* | Decreased use of open communication skills related to busy schedule |
| *Goal:* | The client will increase use of open communication skills within 2 weeks. |

*Health promotion goals* reflect a desire to function at a higher level of health, to grow beyond merely maintaining health.

**Example**

| | |
|---|---|
| *Nursing diagnosis:* | Increased concern regarding lack of knowledge of parenting skills for adolescence |
| *Goal:* | The client will increase knowledge of parenting skills for adolescence within 3 weeks. |

Goals need to be realistic so that the client can achieve them. Therefore, in determining the nature of the goal, the nurse assesses the client's available internal and external resources. If resources are not readily available to achieve the goal, the goal may need to reflect resource development first and include modification to realistically align the goal to available resources.

Differences and similarities between client goals and nurse-expected client goals must be considered. The nurse may have a greater knowledge base than the client, which could help the client understand the nature of the identified diagnoses; the client can help the nurse understand the client's own concerns and motivation. The nurse is responsible for establishing client goals that are mutually acceptable to both the client and the nurse.

### Relationship to Theories, Models, and Principles

The models used in the analysis/synthesis of data provide direction for establishing goals. Theories and principles describe norms of behavior and functioning, and determine the rationale for the goal.

Satir's (1967) model, for example, discusses healthy communication, describing in detail the concepts of functional and dysfunctional communication. This information assists the nurse in establishing a goal for a client with dysfunctional communication.

**Example**

| | |
|---|---|
| *Nursing diagnosis:* | Dysfunctional interpersonal communication related to the use of blaming and projection |
| *Goal:* | The client will use functional (leveling) communication with the family within 3 months. |

Immobility is an example of a physiological concept with principles that gives direction to goal development. Most nursing texts elaborate on the concept of immobility and its effects on body functions as well as on the psyche. That baseline knowledge about the concept and its related principles guides the client and nurse in planning to reduce the effects of immobility.

**Example**

| | |
|---|---|
| *Nursing diagnosis:* | Potential hazards of immobility related to prolonged bed rest |
| *Goal:* | The client will decrease susceptibility to hazards of immobility within 6 days. |

Any reliable source that describes norms of behavior can be used to assist the nurse in developing client goals. Table 9-2 gives examples of goals for different clients and shows how a variety of sources is used in establishing the goals.

### DEVELOPING OBJECTIVES

After goals are established for the diagnoses, objectives are developed to specify client performances, outcomes, and behaviors related to the goal. Whereas goals are derived from the descriptive clause of the nursing diagnosis, objectives flow from the etiological clause. Objectives are short term in nature and are usually achievable while the client is in the direct care or service of an institution. An objective describes an intended result of a particular action, not the process of the action itself (Mager, 1984). Usually three to six objectives are needed for each goal.

Mager states three reasons for developing objectives. First, objectives *give direction* for selecting or designing nursing strategies and orders. Next, a properly stated objective *implies* the content of, potential materials needed for, and method of the strategy or order. Last, objectives provide a *means* for the nurse and client to *organize effort*. Objectives are therefore useful tools in the design, implementation, and evaluation of client care.

**Table 9-2**   Goals with Different Theoretical Bases

| Client | Nursing diagnoses | Goals | Theoretical bases |
|--------|-------------------|-------|-------------------|
| Individual | Inadequate exercise related to low motivation | The client will exercise adequately within 1 month | Diekelmann (1977) |
| Family | Impaired affective functioning related to lack of separateness | The family will demonstrate affective functioning within 6 months | Friedman (1986) |
| Community | Inadequate decision-making related to use of coercion | The client will develop a democratic form of decision making within 1 year | Hart and Herriott (1985) |

## Characteristics of Objectives

Three characteristics of objectives that communicate their intent are performance, conditions, and criterion (Mager, 1984).

### Performance

A performance or outcome is any activity engaged in by the client. It can be an activity that is directly observable or not directly observable but assessable. Overt client performances are those that can be directly seen or heard. Verbs that indicate overt performances, which are directly observable behaviors, include recite, list, sort, verbalize, demonstrate, name, select, and state.

Covert performances are mental—invisible or cognitive—but have a direct way of being assessed. Verbs that indicate covert performances include identify, solve, use, compare, and determine. Whenever the performance stated in an objective is covert (such as identify), an indicator behavior (such as state) needs to be added to the objective.

**Example**

| | |
|---|---|
| *Overt verb:* | The client will demonstrate proper insulin administration according to the American Diabetic Association within 1 week. |
| *Covert verb (with indicator behavior):* | The client will identify (state) three complications of bed rest within 2 days. |

The objective creates a picture of what is expected of the client, communicating its intent to the client and those reading it. Each important outcome or performance is written in a separate objective. Therefore, each objective contains only one performance verb.

### Conditions

An objective may indicate the conditions under which the client is to complete the performance.

Conditions may include the experiences that the client is expected to have had before completing the objective, the resources available for use during the performance of the objective, and the environmental conditions under which the client will carry out the performance. The conditions are included if they are essential to meeting the objective. Conditions need not be included if the performance clearly states what is expected.

**Example**

| | |
|---|---|
| *Objective with clear expectations:* | The client will state three barriers to effective communication within 1 week. |

Below are examples of the three ways that conditions may be stated in an objective.

| Condition | Example |
|-----------|---------|
| 1. The experiences before completing the objective | *After attending* two group sessions of diabetic classes, the client will name two major types of diabetes. |
| 2. The resources available during the performance of the objective | *Given a menu* of a variety of foods, the client will circle the foods composing a 2000-calorie intake for 1 day. |
| 3. The environmental conditions during the performance | *When at home* the client will maintain a 2000-calorie diet according to the American Diabetic Association. |

### Criterion

The criterion is the standard by which a performance is evaluated (Mager, 1984). Criteria within the objective may be stated in one of four ways:

1. *Speed:* Set a time limit that is reasonable, given the client's health state and the client's and nurse's capabilities and limitations.

2. *Accuracy:* Identify a specific degree of performance quantitatively.

3. *Quality:* Indicate the standard that is expected in terms of given acceptable procedures.

4. *Criterion-referenced:* Use a book, pamphlet, or other resources as a guide. Criteria give direction to nursing orders for meeting the objective. They also provide a measure to evaluate the achievement of the objective.

Below are examples of the four ways of stating criteria in objectives.

| Criterion | Example |
|---|---|
| 1. Speed | The client will name four complications of bed rest *within 3 days.* |
| 2. Accuracy | The client will list *four of five* symptoms of highblood sugar. |
| 3. Quality | The client will catheterize self using *aseptic technique.* |
| 4. Criterion referenced | The client will describe (state) three components of the self-breast examination *according to* the American Cancer Society. |

## Domains of Objectives

Objectives related to client learning situations can be classified into three domains, which provide direction for selecting and individualizing the strategies and orders. This is a classification of the *intended* behaviors, or the way people are expected to *think, feel,* or *act* as a result of participating in given learning experiences.

The three identified domains are cognitive, affective, and psychomotor (Bloom, 1956). *Cognitive objectives* are associated with changes in knowledge or intellectual abilities and skills. A hierarchy of six major classes within this domain vary from simple recall of material to complex mental processes, such as analysis, synthesis, and evaluation of ideas. The six classes are:

1. *Knowledge:* ability to remember and recall specific bits of information as well as major schemes and patterns; the ability to organize, study, judge, and criticize

2. *Comprehension:* ability to make use of material or information without understanding its full implications

3. *Application:* ability to use abstractions in particular and concrete situations

4. *Analysis:* ability to clearly differentiate elements of a whole and their relationships

5. *Synthesis:* ability to constitute a pattern or structure not clearly there before; to create a whole out of its elements

6. *Evaluation:* ability to judge the value of material or methods for given purposes based on a standard of appraisal

Each class within this hierarchy requires achievement of behaviors within the preceding classes. As the behavior becomes more complex, the person is more aware of its existence. The nurse determines the level of understanding expected by the client in a learning situation, to help determine what is necessary to accomplish the objective identified.

*Affective objectives* emphasize changes in interests, beliefs, attitudes, values, or feelings, and may be expressed by adjustments or behavioral changes (Krathwohl and others, 1964). They include a degree of acceptance or rejection on the part of the participant. The hierarchy of five major affective categories reflects levels of internalization of an interest, belief, attitude, and so on. The categories range from minimal awareness of a value, for example, to the commitment to that value that guides or controls the person's behavior. These categories are described as:

1. *Receiving* (attending): being aware of and willing to receive or attend to the existence of certain phenomena and stimuli (for example, values, beliefs, attitudes, feelings)

2. *Responding:* having a low level of commitment or interest in the phenomena and stimuli to receiving a sense of pleasure or satisfaction accompanying the behavior

3. *Valuing:* being motivated by a value to display behavior consistently with held value; displaying loyalty and conviction to a value

4. *Organization:* determining interrelationships among values for self and establishing those that are most important

5. *Characterization by a value or value complex:* acting consistently in accordance with internalized values; integrating beliefs, ideas, and attitudes to one's own philosophy or world view

The person eventually makes adjustments or changes in behavior based on the interests, beliefs, attitudes, values, and feelings as they are increasingly internalized. Clients usually state their acceptance of a new value or attitude prior to acting on it. Working with clients in the affective domain is highly subjective and personal. The nurse exercises discretion, showing respect for the client's choices while providing necessary information and care to promote the client's optimal level of health. Affective objectives, in particular, include the performance (verb), condition, *and* criterion—or evaluation criteria—in order to evaluate the client's achievement.

*Psychomotor objectives* focus on developing the ability to perform a manipulative or motor skill. These skills are usually achieved in a complex combination with cognitive and affective abilities (Singer, 1972). The seven major levels vary from a basic awareness of senses involved to creating new motor acts. Simpson (1966) and Urbach (1970) classified the psychomotor skills as:

1. *Perception:* awareness of objects, qualities, or relations through the use of the senses; knowing what is essential to the act being performed
2. *Set:* mental, physical, and emotional readiness for an experience or action
3. *Guided response:* experience or action is attempted on the part of an individual under the guidance of an instructor or self using imitation or trial and error; performance is judged using a model or example
4. *Mechanism:* some confidence and proficiency is gained by performing the action; the learned response has become habitual
5. *Complex overt response:* smooth, efficient, and automatic performance, with minimal expenditure of time and energy
6. *Adaptation:* ability to master the challenge of a problem situation requiring adjustment of learned response
7. *Origination:* ability to create new motor acts based on previously acquired awareness, performance, and psychomotor skills

Psychomotor objectives are appropriate when the client needs to learn a particular technique or skill. The level of proficiency expected is determined by the client's health status, functional ability of the senses, previously learned (related) skills, dexterity, motivation and interest, cognitive abilities, biophysical strengths and limitations, sociocultural influences, environment, nurse-client relationship, and the nurse's knowledge and expertise as a teacher.

Cognitive, affective, and psychomotor domains are separated for purposes of categorizing behaviors, yet they are not mutually exclusive. People usually do not think without feeling, act without thinking, or feel without acting. When developing educational objectives related to a learning situation, the nurse identifies the domain of each objective to facilitate selecting strategies and orders. However, the nurse must be aware of the interplay among the cognitive, affective, and psychomotor aspects of the client. Therefore, more than one domain may be involved in the achievement of an objective or goal.

The following are examples of objectives in three domains that each meet one goal.

**Example**

| | |
|---|---|
| *Nursing diagnosis:* | Alteration in nutrition (more than body requirements) related to imbalance and excess eating of four basic food groups |
| *Goal:* | The client will consume an adequate nutritional diet following the recommended daily allowances of the four basic food groups within 3 weeks. |
| *Objectives:* | 1. The client will state the four food groups and recommended servings within 3 days (cognitive). |
| | 2. The client will identify (state) the importance of a balanced diet within 1 week (affective and cognitive). |
| | 3. The client will incorporate the recommended American Diabetic Association diet into eating patterns within 2 weeks (psychomotor and cognitive). |

Different verbs indicate client behaviors within each of the domains. These action verbs help differentiate the expected outcomes of the client. Below are lists of verbs that represent the three domains:

| Cognitive | Affective | Psychomotor |
|---|---|---|
| Recall | Accept | Show |
| Inform | Appreciate | Imitate |
| List | Enjoy | Demonstrate |
| Discuss | Desire | Practice |
| Interpret | Listen | Assist |
| Distinguish | Relate | Perform |
| Apply | Regard | Master |
| Compare | Participate | Adapt |
| Evaluate | Judge | Create |

## Relationship to Theories, Models, and Principles

The specific performances included in objectives are based on the same theories, models, and principles used in establishing goals. When objectives are developed, an in-depth understanding of the approach is necessary. The following example shows how the nurse's knowledge of the concept of immobility, related principles, hazards, and ways to prevent complications influences the development of objectives.

**Example**

| | |
|---|---|
| *Nursing diagnosis:* | Increased susceptibility to hazards of immobility related to decreased mobility |

*Goal:* The client will decrease susceptibility to hazards of immobility while hospitalized.

*Objectives:*
1. The client will participate in four preventive measures four times a day within 1 day.
2. The client will verbalize four hazards of immobility within 2 days.
3. The client will identify (state) one way to decrease susceptibility to each hazard within 2 days.
4. The client will incorporate at least three preventive measures into daily routine four times a day within 4 days on client's own volition.

The specifics of range of motion, skin care, deep breathing, and turning could be included in the objectives themselves or referred to in the nursing orders.

Below is another example of a goal and objectives, based on Satir's (1967) model. This example demonstrates the use of specific information about the importance of functional communication, barriers to it, and techniques of it. The examples of objectives show varying degrees of specificity.

**Example**

*Nursing diagnosis:* Dysfunctional communication related to the use of blaming and projecting.

*Goal:* The client will increase functional communication within 1 month.

*Objectives:*
1. The client will describe why functional communication is important, according to Satir, within 2 days.
2. The client will state three barriers to functional communication within 1 week.
3. The client will identify (state) two verbal and three nonverbal functional communication techniques within 1 week.
4. The client will use three functional communication techniques while talking to family within 3 weeks.

## GUIDELINES FOR WRITING GOALS AND OBJECTIVES

1. *Goals and objectives are client-focused and reflect mutuality with the client.* The goals and objectives are worded in *client* terms. Beginning each goal and objective with the terms "the client will" facili-

tates client focus. Mutuality is attained through communication with the client and involved persons about identified health concerns and strengths. The nurse discusses nursing diagnoses and related goals with the client to determine whether the client also recognizes the strength or concern and is willing to direct energy toward supporting, diminishing, or alleviating the conditions identified in the diagnoses.

Situations can arise when individual clients are unable to agree with goals and objectives because of an alteration in health status or age. The nurse is then responsible for including the client's family in decision-making. The goals and objectives still need to be worded in client terms.

**Example**

*Nursing diagnosis:* Altered sensory perception related to decreased level of consciousness

*Goal:* The client will maintain or improve present level of consciousness indefinitely.

*Objectives:*
1. The client will participate in the assessment of level of consciousness daily.
2. The client will accept auditory and tactile stimuli provided by the nurse at least every 2 hours.

2. *Goals are appropriate to their respective diagnosis, and objectives are appropriate to their respective goal.* The nursing diagnosis is the basis for each respective goal. Therefore, goals should clearly relate to the nursing diagnosis. Completion of the goal supports the strengths or diminishes or alleviates the concerns identified by the nursing diagnosis.

**Example**

*Nursing diagnosis:* Alteration in nutrition (less than body requirements) related to inadequate food intake

*Goal:* The client will consume an adequate nutritional diet within 1 month (goal clearly relates to diagnosis).

*Goal:* The client will learn about adequate nutrition within 1 month (goal has limited relationship to diagnosis).

Learning about adequate nutrition does not necessarily lead to better nutrition. The first goal clearly states that the client will consume an adequate nutritional diet. The goal is the basis for its respective objectives. Achievement of the objectives should be sufficient for the attainment of the goal.

3. *Goals and objectives are realistic, reflecting the capabilities and limitations of the client.* The client must perceive the goals and objectives as realistic in order to be motivated to achieve them. Being realistic involves developing goals and objectives that reflect the client's capabilities and limitations of internal and external resources. Examples of external resources to consider are time, money, family support, social agencies, personnel, and equipment. Examples of internal resources to consider are biophysical status, mental health, and coping patterns.

Inasmuch as health is a relative term, not all goals can reflect a maximum health state. Each client has an optimum potential for health that is reflected in the goals.

**Example**

| | |
|---|---|
| *Client:* | 40-year-old recently divorced man |
| *Nursing diagnosis:* | Lack of socialization related to recent divorce |
| *Goal:* | The client will develop a social support system within 6 months. |

**Example**

| | |
|---|---|
| *Client:* | 20-year-old single, mentally retarded woman |
| *Nursing diagnosis:* | Lack of socialization related to overprotection from family |
| *Goal:* | The client will increase participation in activities involving people other than family within 3 months. |

4. *Goals include broad or abstract indicators of performance.* Because a goal is broad or abstract by nature, the use of verbs such as improve, decrease, increase, maintain, promote, develop, and restore is appropriate. General criteria can be included in a goal to give more direction to strategies and nursing orders.

**Example**

| | |
|---|---|
| *Nursing diagnosis:* | Decrease in neighborhood safety related to poor lighting and limited patrols |
| *Goal:* | The client will increase neighborhood safety within 6 months (goal without general criterion). |
| *Goal:* | The client will improve neighborhood safety by increasing street lights and patrols within 6 months (goal with general criterion). |

Either goal is correct; both are client-focused and give a general direction for further plans.

Another aspect of stating goals is their reference to a time element. The length of time is determined by considering the client's health status and available resources. The resources include both the client's and nurse's capabilities and limitations.

5. *Objectives include specific indicators of performance.* Objectives need to be more specific than goals, referring to observable and measurable outcomes to meet the goal. Each objective statement includes the person, the performance, and a specific criterion. Conditions may be added to clarify the meaning. The performance needs to be assessable, and the criterion for assessment can be stated in terms of time, accuracy, quality, or reference. Time is usually included in all objectives, because it gives the client and the nurse a guideline for pacing activities realistically. Refer to p. 187 for examples of objectives with a variety of specific performances and criteria. These specific indicators of performance serve as a basis for evaluating the client's progress toward the goal.

6. *Objectives are numbered in the appropriate sequence to achieve the goal.* Proper sequencing, or time ordering, of objectives gives direction and understanding of what is expected. Communicating this sequence helps the client recognize success in movement toward goal achievement.

7. *Scientific and practice principles guide the establishment of goals and the development of objectives.* Goals and objectives are based on norms of behavior and functioning indicated in biophysical, psychological, sociocultural, and spiritual sciences. Theories, models, and principles from nursing and other practice disciplines provide the rationale for the goals and objectives. Standards of nursing care such as those developed by the American Nurses' Association (1973) and specialty nursing organizations also give direction for client outcomes. In addition, state nurse practice acts define the scope of nursing practice, and health care institutions develop standards and mores of practice.

## SUMMARY

The planning component of the nursing process is based on a sound assessment and diagnosis of the client's health status, strengths, and concerns. Judging priorities, establishing goals, and developing objectives constitute the first three phases of planning for implementation. Goals are broad, abstract, and long term; objectives reflect specific outcomes and a shorter time for achievement. Identifying strategies and specifying nursing orders for implementation are the last two phases of planning. These elements are discussed in Chapter 10.

Each phase of planning is based on the nurse's

knowledge of theories, models, and principles. Sources describing norms of behavior and functioning serve as the rationale for planning. To ensure client motivation and cooperation, the client must be involved in decision-making regarding priorities, goals, and objectives.

## REFERENCES AND READINGS

American Nurses' Association: Standards: nursing practice, Kansas City, Mo, 1973, The Association.

Atkinson L and Murray M: Understanding the nursing process, ed 3, New York, 1986, Macmillan, Inc.

Bloom B, ed.: Taxonomy of educational objectives: the classification of educational goals. Handbook I: cognitive domain, New York, 1956, David McKay Co, Inc.

Bower FL: The process of planning nursing care: nursing practice models, ed 3, St Louis, 1982, The CV Mosby Co.

Carnevali D: Nursing care planning: diagnosis and management, ed 3, Philadelphia, 1983, JB Lippincott Co.

Carpenito LJ: Nursing diagnosis: application to clinical practice, ed 2, Philadelphia, 1987, JB Lippincott Co.

Curtin L: Six step model for analyzing ethical problems. In Freebairn J and Gwinup K: Ethics, values, and health, Irvine, Calif, 1980, Concept Media.

Diekelmann N: Primary health care of the well adult, New York, 1977, McGraw-Hill Book Co.

Friedman MM: Family nursing: theory and assessment, ed 2, Norwalk, Conn, 1986, Appleton-Century-Crofts.

Hart SK and Herriott PR: Components of nursing practice: a systems approach. In Hall J and Weaver B, editors: Distributive nursing practice: a systems approach to community health, ed 2, Philadelphia, 1985, JB Lippincott Co.

Krathwohl D, Bloom B, and Masia B: Taxonomy of educational objectives: the classification of educational goals. Handbook II: affective domain, New York, 1964, David McKay Co, Inc.

Mager R: Goal analysis, ed 2, Belmont, Calif, 1984, Pitman Learning.

Maslow AH: Toward a psychology of being, New York, 1968, D Van Nostrand Co.

Maslow AH: Motivation and personality, ed 2, New York, 1970, Harper & Row, Publishers, Inc.

Mayers M: A systematic approach to the nursing care plan, ed 3, New York, 1983, Appleton-Century-Crofts.

Peplau HE: Interpersonal relations in nursing, New York, 1952, GP Putnam's Sons.

Reilly D: Behavioral objectives in nursing: evaluation in nursing, ed 2, New York, 1980, Appleton-Century-Crofts.

Satir V: Conjoint family therapy, rev ed, Palo Alto, Calif, 1967, Science and Behavior Books.

Simpson EJ: The classification of educational objectives: psychomotor domain, Urbana, Ill, 1966, University of Illinois Press.

Singer, RN, editor: The psychomotor domain: movement and behavior, Philadelphia, 1972, Lea & Febiger.

Singer RN: The learning of motor skills, New York, 1982, Macmillan, Inc.

Urbach F, editor: The psychomotor domain of learning. Papers presented at Teaching Research, Salishan Oregon, 1970, The Department of Higher Education, Monmouth, Oregon.

# chapter 10

# Planning: Strategies and Nursing Orders

ELIZABETH S. FAYRAM
PAULA J. CHRISTENSEN

## GENERAL CONSIDERATIONS

The identification of strategies and specification of nursing orders are the last two phases of the planning component. These phases build on the priorities, goals, and objectives, becoming even more specific in determining how to assist the client in resolving health-related concerns.

Strategies and nursing orders are prescriptive in nature. That is, the *nurse* determines which actions are most appropriate, based on the nurse's knowledge base, experience, and familiarity with the client situation. The nurse considers the autonomy and individuality of the client when choosing actions; yet the client now, more than ever, depends on the nurse to provide direction and support.

After goals are established and objectives developed, the nurse decides which strategies and nursing orders will facilitate the client's achievement of the objectives. Similar to goals and objectives, the strategies and nursing orders are directly related to the nursing diagnosis. A strategy is an overall method or approach that serves as a guide for individual nursing orders. Strategies are accepted methods and approaches that stem from many science and practice disciplines. Examples of strategies discussed in this chapter include teaching and learning, therapeutic use of self, contracting, and principles of nursing practice.

Nursing orders are individualized prescribed behaviors that flow from the strategies identified and lead to predictable client outcomes. The client as well as the nurse is included in the actions, along with others needed to achieve the desired goals and objectives.

This chapter focuses on the description of various strategies, how to choose strategies, and impli-

cations for their use. Nursing orders are discussed in terms of specific actions relating to the client's unique situation. Nursing care plans and Kardexes are addressed as tools that facilitate implementation of goals, objectives, strategies, and nursing orders. The guidelines emphasized are as follows:

1. Strategies
   a. Major strategies for implementation are identified.
   b. Strategies are appropriate to their respective goal and objectives.
   c. Strategies are based on scientific rationale.
2. Nursing orders
   a. Nursing orders are appropriate to their respective goal, objective, and strategy.
   b. Scientific and practice principles provide rationale for orders.
   c. Nursing orders incorporate the autonomy and individuality of the client.
   d. Nursing orders indicate specific intended behaviors, giving direction to the nurse, client, and others.
   e. Nursing orders reflect consideration of human, temporal, and material resources.
   f. Nursing orders are numbered in sequence to achieve the objective.
   g. Nursing orders are dated and include the signature of the responsible nurse.
   h. Nursing orders are kept current and are revised as indicated.
   i. Nursing orders include plans for termination of nursing services.

## STRATEGIES

An important part of the planning component is the selection of strategies. As discussed previously, a *strategy* is an overall method or approach that serves as a guide for individual nursing orders. Strategies arise from the science and practice disciplines, including psychology, sociology, education, and nursing.

Strategies are selected based on the model incorporated into the nursing process as well as on the nursing diagnosis, goals, and objectives that have been formulated. The model and its concepts provide guidance to the nurse in the selection of strategies. When using Orem's Self-Care model (1985), the nurse considers strategies fostering self-care such as teaching and learning, contracting, and problem solving. Neuman's Health-Care Systems model (1982), with its emphasis on stressors, reaction to stress, and levels of nursing interventions, guides the nurse in the selection of strategies such as stress management and teaching and learning.

More than one strategy may be appropriate to achieve the goals and objectives for a given client. The nurse selects the strategy most appropriate at that particular time based on the client situation, age of the client, and the nurse's expertise with the various strategies. When selecting strategies, the nurse considers the client's strengths such as the ability to problem solve and to communicate; the client's limitations, such as health problems; and the client's internal and external resources, such as coping patterns and support from family members. Several strategies could be considered for a client with the nursing diagnosis of "alteration in nutrition, more than body requirements," for example—teaching and learning, contracting, and behavior modification. Based on client variables, such as the client's knowledge of the four basic food groups and cognitive development, the nurse selects the strategy (or strategies) best suited for the situation. Having a variety of strategies to choose from provides the nurse with additional choices if revision of the plan is necessary.

Many situations are appropriate for client participation in the selection of strategies. An example is the client who desires to try a behavior modification program in an attempt to lose weight. The nurse, however, has the expertise concerning the strategies and is best able to determine which strategy is likely to be successful based on the nursing diagnosis, goals, and objectives. The nurse educates the client and explains the rationale for the choice of the strategy, especially if it differs from the one the client chose. Then, a mutual decision regarding which strategy to use is made.

Strategies discussed in the following section are: (1) teaching and learning, (2) problem solving, (3) therapeutic use of self, (4) caring, (5) stress management, (6) behavior modification, (7) contracting, (8) group process, and (9) principles of nursing practice. Guidelines, principles, or steps are presented whenever possible to direct the nurse with specific nursing orders when using the selected strategy.

## Teaching and Learning

The teaching and learning process is a strategy frequently used by professional nurses in a variety of settings and with various types of clients: individuals, families, and communities. The teaching and learning process is useful when dealing with health promotion goals and objectives as well as with health maintenance or restoration. Examples of when the teaching and learning process is appropriate are: (1) a community group learning the benefits of and foods included in a high-fiber diet (health promotion); (2) an individual client with newly diagnosed diabetes mellitus learning the symptoms of hyperglycemia and the appropriate actions to take (health maintenance); and (3) a spouse learning to care for the client's ulcerated lesion (health restoration).

Bloom (1956) identified three domains of learning: cognitive, affective, and psychomotor. The cognitive domain deals with intellectual ability such as recall or recognition; the affective domain deals with changes in attitudes and values; the psychomotor domain involves skill or motor development. The teaching and learning process is an appropriate strategy for use with all three domains of learning.

The nurse, as teacher, becomes the facilitator of learning. The nurse involves the client in the teaching and learning process, including assessment of the need for learning, planning learning experiences, implementing the learning experiences, and evaluating learning outcomes.

The teaching and learning process is integrated into the nursing process based on the goals and objectives that have been formulated. Principles of teaching and learning are used to facilitate learning. These principles are presented according to the components of the nursing process (Pohl, 1981; Redman, 1988; Rorden, 1987).

### Assessment

The nurse may find it necessary to return to the assessment component when the strategy of teaching and learning has been selected.

*Learning needs of the client must be determined.* Before a teaching plan is developed and implemented, the client's learning needs must be assessed. The client's learning needs vary based on previous knowledge and experience and the present situation.

*Perception of the need to learn by the learner facilitates learning.* Perceived needs for learning and priorities placed on learning by the client influence whether learning occurs. Perception of the need to learn is influenced by the person's beliefs and values as well as previous experiences.

*Physical and mental readiness are necessary for learning.* A learner must have the physical and mental ability to learn. Physical readiness is related to developmental level and physical health status; mental readiness refers to the cognitive abilities to understand, assimilate, and apply. The nurse considers the effect of developmental levels and health status on the client's physical and mental readiness. The level of readiness is evaluated in relation to the level of learning to be accomplished. When the client is not physically or mentally ready to learn, the nurse includes significant others in the learning situation.

*A client must be motivated in order to learn.* For learning to occur, the client must have a willingness or desire to learn or change. A client may be motivated for numerous reasons, such as need, status, fear, and achievement. Motivation may be constant or temporary, strong or weak, and will be directed toward the most pressing concern at the time. Frequently the nurse is involved in stimulating the client's motivation to learn. This may be accomplished by helping the learner to know what is to be learned and the reason for the learning. Providing incentives to learn, such as benefits of learning, and dealing with other more pressing concerns first, such as anxiety or discomfort, also facilitate motivation.

*The emotional climate affects learning.* The client's emotions have a strong influence on ability to learn. The nurse examines the client's feelings about the topic and his or her current emotional state. When intense emotions are present in the learner, such as extreme anxiety or fear, very little learning can occur. Through effective communication techniques, the nurse helps the client deal with the emotions before attempting teaching and learning.

*Knowledge of the client's cultural-ethnic patterns is essential.* The health practices and beliefs of clients based on cultural diversity must be identified. To individualize the learning situation requires knowledge of the cultural pattern of the various groups that the nurse most frequently encounters.

### Diagnosis

Following analysis and synthesis of the assessment data, a nursing diagnosis is formulated for which the teaching and learning process is the selected strategy. Examples of nursing diagnostic statements are:

Knowledge deficit (parenting skills) related to lack of experience as a parent and lack of role models

Ineffective individual coping related to lack of knowledge of effective stress management (eg, relaxation techniques)

### Planning

The planning component for the teaching and learning process includes formulating goals and objectives related to learning and selecting learning activities with suitable materials and techniques.

*Goals and objectives serve as guides in planning teaching-learning experiences.* The client and nurse determine what learning needs are to be accomplished and establish goals and objectives that state precisely and clearly the outcomes to be achieved. The goals and objectives serve as criteria for evaluating achievement of learning.

*New learning must be based on previous knowledge and experience.* Building upon previous knowledge and experience increases the effectiveness and efficiency of the teaching and learning process. Determining the client's current level of knowledge and experience about a topic before providing new information reduces the chance of misunderstanding by the client who lacks specific information or is misinformed. The nurse can also avoid repeating information the client is already familiar with, a repetition that might hinder the client's interest in learning.

*Learning is a sequential process that proceeds from simple to complex.* The nurse determines nursing orders to achieve the goals and objectives, being aware of the sequencing of content and experiences. For example, a client learning new nutritional habits may read about foods included and excluded in the diet and the reasons for the nutritional change, discuss with the nurse how great a change this would require in the client's nutritional pattern, plan a 3-day food plan incorporating the guidelines, and prepare food at home for a week based on the new nutritional guidelines.

*Teaching/learning techniques and materials are selected based on client needs.* A variety of teaching/learning techniques are available, such as explanation, discussion, demonstration-practice, and experiences such as role playing. In addition, teaching/learning sessions may occur on a one-to-one basis or in group sessions. The objectives, the domain of learning (cognitive, affective, psychomotor), and the specific client (developmental level, learning style) determine the techniques used. For example, a 4-year-old client learning about the surgical experience is provided a role-playing situation with real equipment such as masks and IV equipment. Written and audiovisual materials are selected to facilitate and reinforce learning. They are used in combination with the interactive techniques. Written materials are reviewed for accuracy, content, the ability to meet the objectives, and the appropriateness of the material for the client. Learning is aided by involving as many of the learner's senses as possible.

## Implementation

Implementation of the teaching and learning process occurs through active involvement of the client and significant others when appropriate. The nurse's ability to develop an effective nurse-client relationship is an important factor in the effectiveness of the teaching and learning.

*An effective nurse-client relationship is important for learning.* A positive interpersonal relationship enhances learning. Client learning is facilitated when the nurse and the client have a relationship that is trusting, cooperative, comfortable, and caring.

*Effective learning requires active participation.* Active involvement on the part of the learner through participation in the teaching and learning process facilitates learning. The client (and significant others as appropriate) is an active participant during identification of learning needs and the planning, implementation, and evaluation of learning experiences. During implementation, active participation may involve a variety of activities, such as using the senses (eg, sight and hearing), performing a physical activity, and using cognitive processes. The nurse provides opportunities for participation and encourages the client to ask questions. The more actively the client participates, the more effective the learning.

*Teaching and learning require effective communication.* New information is learned through effective verbal and visual communication techniques. Effective communication is accomplished when the listener grasps the meaning conveyed by the speaker. The nurse uses feedback from the client to validate that the client understands the information correctly.

*Effective teaching and learning require time.* First, the nurse sets aside time to develop an effective teaching plan. Second, the nurse collaborates with the client to find the most appropriate time for implementing the teaching plan.

*Control of the environment is an aspect of teaching.* The nurse considers personal and environmental factors that influence client learning. The comfort of the client and elimination of distracting interrup-

tions are important factors that promote an effective learning environment.

*Repetition strengthens learning.* Continued practice enhances the learner's retention of new information and the formation of new behavior patterns. Different clients need varying numbers of repetitions for effective learning, depending on the complexity of the content to be learned and the client's abilities to learn.

*Reinforcement influences learning.* When a person receives satisfaction in learning new behaviors, these new behaviors will be retained longer. Personal pride in accomplishment is a strong incentive for learning and retaining new skills. The nurse considers both internal (personal) and external (reward or praise) factors that facilitate client satisfaction in learning.

## Evaluation

Evaluation involves evaluating the outcomes, client responses to the learning, and the nurse's ability to use the teaching and learning process.

*Goals and objectives serve as the basis for evaluation of learning.* The fact that the nurse "taught" the client does not mean the client has learned. The client exhibits achievement of the learning objectives to validate having achieved the newly learned behaviors. Various evaluation methods are used, such as verbal statements and return demonstrations. Revision of the plan may be necessary to achieve the desired outcomes.

*The nurse evaluates his or her own ability to use the teaching and learning process.* The nurse identifies his or her own strengths and limitations in applying the principles of the teaching and learning process and ways to improve in that ability.

The basic principles presented describe methods of learning and factors that the nurse considers when facilitating client learning. Many of these principles provide the scientific rationale for nursing orders when implementing the teaching and learning process.

## Problem Solving

The use of the problem-solving process as a strategy involves assisting clients in identifying a specific problem, generating alternative solutions, analyzing consequences, and making a rational decision regarding an identified concern. The nurse, as in the teaching and learning process, is the facilitator. The nurse guides the client toward making a decision and supports the client in the process.

For the client to participate in the problem-solving process, several factors are necessary. The client must have the authority to participate in the problem-solving process and to make the decision.

The client's ability and desire to generate and analyze alternatives as well as the client's beliefs and preferences are also factors. Last, the client must accept participation in the problem-solving process and in making the decision.

The problem-solving process consists of the following steps:

1. Identification of the problem and purpose/goal of the problem-solving process
2. Development of alternative solutions to the problem
3. Consideration of consequences for each of the alternatives
4. Selection of a specific alternative
5. Implementation of the decision
6. Evaluation of the effectiveness of the problem-solving process

When using problem solving as a strategy, the *first step* is to ensure that all involved have accurately identified the problem (nursing diagnosis) and factors influencing the problem. Those involved also need to understand the purpose of the problem-solving process and the goal to be achieved by implementation of the decision.

The *second step* is to explore possible alternatives to resolve the problem. The client, from previous knowledge and experience, may be able to generate alternatives. Additional alternatives also may be generated from the nurse's knowledge and experiences as well as from other health team members and resource material (eg, community resources).

Factors identified by Bower (1982) as influencing the generation of alternatives are (1) the number of alternatives being considered at one time, (2) the number of people participating in the problem-solving process, and (3) the amount of time available in which to make the decision. Creativity, such as the use of brainstorming techniques, is another factor that influences the generation of alternatives (Gillies, 1989).

Usually two to four alternatives are generated. More than four becomes confusing and consumes more time when the consequences of each alternative are considered. If too much time is spent generating alternatives and making the decision, then action to deal with the problem is delayed. When generating alternatives, resources and constraints are considered, including finances, people, equipment, policies, and procedures.

The *third step* is to consider the consequences of the various alternatives. Each alternative is analyzed to determine whether it could achieve the goal and also analyzed for cost and risk. Cost factors not only include financial support necessary but also time, energy, equipment, and people. Risk

includes consideration of safety, comfort, and side-effects. Feasibility is also deliberated, including policy considerations and the protection of the rights of others. Acceptance of the alternative by those affected must also be weighed. The nurse plays an important role in helping the client analyze the various options.

Selection by the client of a specific alternative is the *fourth step*. The chosen alternative should be one that will meet the stated goal and have the most desirable consequences. The *fifth step* involves implementation of the decision as agreed on by the nurse and client. Evaluation is the *final step* of the problem-solving process. Evaluation methods are considered and planned before the decision is implemented. Evaluation of the decision includes the determination of goal attainment, the consequences that have occurred, and the need to reconsider the alternative that was selected.

Bailey and Claus (1975) have identified several *obstacles* to effective problem solving. One such obstacle is *failing to specify purposes and goals*. If the goal is unclear, then appropriate alternatives may not be considered. *Plunging into action* occurs when a decision is made before considering relevant alternatives. *Jumping to conclusions* may occur when the cause of the concern is incorrectly identified and the decision may or may not solve the concern. *Failing to look at probable consequences* means not considering the costs or risks adequately; thus undesirable consequences may occur. The nurse, who facilitates problem solving by the client, can minimize these obstacles to effective problem solving.

Problem solving is an appropriate strategy to use with clients in a variety of situations. For example, the problem-solving process could be used by the individual client who must make a decision regarding living arrangements following discharge from an acute care facility or by the community client in deciding about the distribution of health care services. The strategy requires active participation on the part of the client. The greater the involvement by the client, the greater the client's commitment to the decision and the greater likelihood of follow-through. This promotes feelings of independence and esteem and provides problem-solving skills for future use.

## Therapeutic Use of Self

Nurses, in considering strategies to use with clients, may consider using their own personalities. This strategy is known as therapeutic use of self and is the conscious effort by the nurse to use his or her personality for the purpose of benefitting the client. In a therapeutic nurse-client relationship, the client's identity is maintained and self-esteem is enhanced (Sundeen et al, 1989).

Therapeutic use of self is appropriate when clients need to express feelings, enhance their self-esteem, or clarify values. This strategy may be useful with a client who has recently undergone body changes, whether from trauma, illness, surgery, or growth, and needs to adjust to a change in body image. Using this strategy, the nurse assists the client to express feelings about body changes and what they mean to the client. This strategy may also be useful with family members, such as parents of a child with a chronic illness. Other examples include a new mother who lacks self-esteem regarding parenting abilities or a pregnant teenager clarifying her values.

Values clarification facilitates a person's identification of meaningful values and the priorities of these values (Stuart and Sundeen, 1987). Exploration of the relationship of a person's values with the decisions made and actions taken occurs through the values clarification process (Steele and Harmon, 1983). This process is facilitated by a therapeutic nurse-client relationship. The values clarification process identifies what is meaningful to the client, fosters the client's ability to make choices regarding significant values, and aids in understanding self. The nurse assists the client in realizing conflicting values and making decisions for the reestablishment of values and their priorities. An example involves a nurse, who through a therapeutic nurse-client relationship, facilitates a 21-year-old spinal cord–injured client's clarification of values in terms of sexuality and self-care.

The nurse, to be effective in therapeutic use of self, must develop in four areas: self-awareness, use of facilitative communication techniques, ability to develop a nurse-client relationship, and acceptance of others.

*Self-awareness* is the understanding of oneself. Nurses need to understand themselves before understanding others. This involves questioning one's own feelings and actions, maximizing one's strengths, minimizing limitations, and accepting self. Four aspects of the personality are considered in the process of self-awareness (Sundeen et al, 1989): body image (how one feels about one's body), self-ideal (who one wants to be), self-concept (what one is), and self-esteem (judgment of one's own worth). The more one's self-ideal and self-concept are similar, the greater will be one's self-esteem. These four aspects of personality influence the nurse's actions and interactions and are therefore an important aspect of self-awareness.

*Using facilitative communication techniques* includes congruent verbal and nonverbal communication, which fosters the client's sharing of feelings or information. Facilitative techniques include sitting down with a client, using open-ended questions and encouragement for the client to express feelings, seeking clarification, respecting that the client may not want to interact at a particular point in time, actively listening, using silence, and touch appropriately.

In therapeutic use of self the nurse develops a *collaborative relationship* with a client for the client's benefit. Characteristics of a nurse-client relationship include trust, empathy, caring, autonomy, and mutuality (Sundeen et al, 1989). *Trust* develops when the nurse is consistent and reliable. *Empathy* involves accurate perception of the client's feelings. *Caring* is demonstrated by showing respect and concern for the client. *Autonomy* involves recognition of the client's need for control. *Mutuality* is the active participation by the client to the extent possible.

Last, therapeutic use of self involves *acceptance of the client* and the client's values. Accepting the client's feelings, respecting differing values, and being responsive to individual differences are examples of nurse behaviors in accepting the client.

Characteristics of nurses who use therapeutic use of self include stable self-concept and positive self-esteem, the ability to face the reality of situations, effective use of verbal and nonverbal communication techniques, relating to clients in a natural, congruent manner, and functioning as a role model. The nurse who uses therapeutic use of self is able to assist clients to face reality and to promote their own self-acceptance.

## Caring

Caring is a crucial element for health, human development, and human relationships (Leininger, 1984). Professional nursing care, with an emphasis on personalized caring, involves cognitive and culturally learned behaviors that enable an individual, family, or community to improve or maintain health status.

One dimension of caring is that it is an integral part of nurse-client relationships. A client's health status is influenced by the relationship that the nurse establishes and maintains. Clients themselves indicate that person-to-person communication is an important ingredient of the caring behavior (Leininger, 1984). Watson (1985) states that caring is effectively demonstrated interpersonally and that the quality of the nurse-client relationship is the most significant element. Characteristics of this relationship include congruence, empathy, and nonpossessive warmth.

Another dimension of caring builds and expands on the first. This second dimension is concerned with helping the client to grow and develop (Mayeroff, 1971). This aspect of caring develops over time and enhances the quality of the client's life. It is selected as a strategy for use with a particular client based on the client's concerns. An example involves a nurse and the caring relationship that forms with a teen-aged client who has few social supports. The teenager has been sexually abused by a relative but is not believed by other family members. The nurse forms a long-term relationship with the client, providing support and guidance as the client gives birth to a child and completes high school.

Second-dimension caring activities are intentional activities by the nurse to bring about a positive change in the client (Gaut, 1984). Effective caring accepts who the person is and who that person may become (Watson, 1985). An important activity involves gaining knowledge. The nurse obtains knowledge of the client, including the client's needs, strengths, and limitations, and how to respond to those needs. Caring activities also include setting goals related to the identified need, planning, and implementing care to meet the goal, which results in a positive change for the client. By using the nursing process effectively, the nurse demonstrates caring activities.

Leininger (1984:49), in studying caring behaviors in a variety of cultures, identified more than 30 components of care, including:

| Comfort | Touch | Restoration |
|---------|-------|-------------|
| Support | Protection | Tenderness |
| Attention | Surveillance | Trust |
| Compassion | Personalized help | Instruction |
| Empathy | Presence | Direct assistance |

These components of caring have been classified into four general areas (Ray, 1984:104-108):
1. *Psychological*
     Affective: empathy, compassion, patience
     Cognitive: teaching, observation, decision-making
2. *Practical*
     Organization: time, coordination, safety
     Technical: skill, equipment
3. *Interactional*
     Physical: comfort, touch
     Social: communication, listening, reassurance, support

4. *Philosophical*
     Spiritual: spiritual concern, faith
     Ethical: attitude, trust, individualized care, respect
     Cultural: understanding of cultural care

This framework provides the nurse with a means of categorizing caring behaviors. Thus, the nurse has several means of exhibiting caring toward clients.

Second-dimension caring makes a significant difference in the health of individuals, families, and communities. It involves deliberate, individualized actions on the part of the nurse, with a sense of commitment to assisting the client to resolve concerns and meet goals.

## Stress Management

Stress management is a strategy that facilitates the client's ability to deal effectively with the stress confronting people in contemporary society. As a strategy, it emphasizes active participation by the client to develop skills to manage stress. Stress management involves identifying the stressors present, evaluating the effectiveness of existing coping mechanisms, and developing more effective coping mechanisms.

An important aspect of stress management is the client's ability to cope. Coping is the effort to master a situation that is perceived as being harmful, threatening, conflicting, or challenging (Monat and Lazarus, 1977). The ability of a client to cope with a particular situation is influenced by (1) personal characteristics, (2) resources available, (3) the situation, and (4) coping patterns the client has developed.

*Personal characteristics* that influence coping include stage of development, personal values and goals, beliefs about self, roles, and responsibilities. The client's perception of the situation and past experiences in coping with similar situations are also individual characteristics that influence coping.

*Resources available* to the client include both internal and external resources, such as health status, time and energy available, financial status, and an interpersonal support system.

The *situation* may be short- or long-term, and is classified as physical, psychological/intellectual, social, or environmental. A physical situation may be an illness, surgery, overwork, or physical danger. Psychological or intellectual situations include overstimulation, striving for success, lack of defined goals, and boredom. Social situations include multiple role demands, pressure to conform, change in employment, and isolation. Environmen-

---

### Examples of Indirect Coping Patterns

| Physical | Psycho/intellectual | Social | Spiritual |
|---|---|---|---|
| Walking | Meditation | Social clubs | Prayer |
| Swimming | Woodworking, | Recreation with others | Attend religious |
| Biking | crafts, painting | Attend social | services |
| Relaxation | Fantasy | gatherings | Read spiritual books |
| techniques | Positive self-talk | Talk with friends | Talk with clergy |

---

tal situations involve the weather, crowded living conditions, and pollution.

*Coping patterns* are individualized and develop to assist the individual in dealing with harmful, threatening, conflicting, or challenging situations. Coping patterns are described as direct or indirect (Pines and Aronson, 1981). Indirect coping patterns are actions to reduce anxiety caused by a particular situation, with no alteration of the situation. Direct coping patterns are actions that deal with the specific situation. Both types of coping patterns are useful. However, indirect coping patterns are more temporary and do not change the situation in the long run. Examples of each type are shown in the boxes on this page.

Physical coping patterns include using relaxation techniques or regular exercise. Psychological/intellectual indirect actions include meditation and creative activities such as painting or writing. Social actions include talking with others. Through talking with friends, support and advice are often obtained. Spiritual activities also offer ways to cope for individuals who find prayer or meditation helpful. These indirect coping patterns help the client to reduce the anxiety associated with a stressful situation.

Direct coping patterns indicate that positive action is being undertaken to resolve the situation. Problem-solving skills can be used to identify various actions and outcomes and to choose the best action. A person may need additional information on direct actions to deal with a situation. For example, a mother who is returning to work obtains information about licensed day care centers for her toddler. This information aids in the choice by providing direction and information. Setting limits on time and energy is another direct coping pattern. It may involve spending a specified time on an activity or interactions. Changing the situation is also a direct coping pattern. For example, a family living in crowded living conditions may look for a new apartment.

---

### Examples of Direct Coping Patterns

Use problem-solving skills to resolve the situation
Seek information and use it to act
Set limits on self or others
Use assertive techniques
Change or modify the situation

---

Some coping patterns are healthier and more effective than others. For example, the client who copes with a stressful job situation by consuming alcoholic beverages and withdrawing from others exhibits unhealthy coping, compared with the client who uses assertive communication techniques and exercise to cope with a similar situation. Coping patterns are considered to be *effective* when the uncomfortable feeling is reduced, the integrity of the individual is preserved, the client functions adequately in relationships and roles, and a positive self-concept is maintained (Miller, 1983).

Individuals usually have a variety of established coping patterns, and do not frequently change patterns. They may adopt different coping patterns when they recognize that their present coping patterns do not alleviate their anxiety or that their patterns cost too much time, energy, or self-esteem.

The goals of stress management (Mitchell and Betrus, 1987) are:

Developing an awareness of stress (eg, stressors)

Recognizing own response to stress (eg, coping patterns)

Developing and supporting effective coping behaviors

Using stress management techniques in everyday life

Consideration of the goals of stress management is part of the nurse's role in the restoration, maintenance, and promotion of client health. Nurses assist clients to assess their coping patterns and to identify which situations require additional coping efforts. When effective coping patterns are used, the nurse's role consists of providing support. If the client wishes to increase available coping patterns or to develop more effective coping patterns, the nurse's role is to provide knowledge and direction on how to use new coping behaviors. For example, if the nurse and client choose to use a more direct approach, such as problem solving, to deal with a situation, then the nurse assists the client in the problem-solving process. Or, the client may choose to learn assertive communication techniques, requiring the teaching/learning process and role playing. Relaxation techniques are indirect actions that help the client handle feelings that occur before, during, or after a stressful situation. For clients who have difficulty organizing their time, time management principles are appropriate interventions to include in a plan. Clients are also encouraged to use the resources available to them, such as support and self-help groups.

Another important aspect of stress management is clarification of values and goals. People need to sort out what is most important to them in a given situation. For example, a woman who is wife, mother, and career woman may find that she must reconsider her goal of a spotlessly clean house. Or, a man overwhelmed by a variety of roles may find that increasing organizational skills, such as planning tasks on a daily basis, is beneficial to stress management.

Nurses can use a variety of interventions to assist clients to develop or strengthen their coping patterns and to manage stress. The type of intervention depends on the client and the situation. Together, the nurse and client work to establish effective coping patterns.

**Behavior Modification**

Behavior modification is a strategy to assist clients to either increase desirable behaviors or decrease undesirable behaviors. Behavior modification attempts to structure the effect of the environment on human behavior.

*Behavior* has been defined as any "observable, recordable, and measurable act, movement, or response of the individual" (Peddicord, 1987:803). Two theories of conditioning are used to explain the effect of controlling the environment on behavior: classical conditioning and operant conditioning (Johnson, 1986). *Classical conditioning* refers to the stimulus-response theory, in which an antecedent event (stimulus) influences behavior (response). For example, whenever a man has a cup of coffee (stimulus), he lights up a cigarette (response). *Op-*

*erant conditioning* stresses that behavior is influenced by the consequence that follows the behavior. *Reinforcements* (positive or negative) are consequences that tend to increase behavior, and *punishments* are consequences that tend to decrease behavior. An example of operant conditioning involves a dieter who stops eating desserts and snacks (behavior) and loses weight (consequence). Assumptions of the operant conditioning theory are that people tend to repeat behaviors that lead to pleasant consequences and stop behaviors that lead to unpleasant consequences.

Behavior modification applies the principles of classical conditioning and operant conditioning to change behavior. The antecedent event *or* the consequence can be changed to increase or decrease behavior. *Increasing a desired behavior* may be accomplished by either (1) changing the antecedent event to one that will elicit the desired behavior or (2) following the desired behavior with a positive or negative reinforcer. An example of the use of a positive reinforcer involves a pregnant client who desires to practice breathing exercises daily. She enjoys watching the evening news, and agrees to spend 10 minutes exercising (behavior) before watching the news (consequence).

*Decreasing an undesirable behavior* may be accomplished by (1) changing the antecedent event to one that will decrease the behavior or (2) using a punishment, such as ignoring the behavior, time out, loss of something valued, or adding an unpleasant consequence. In most nursing situations, the first three types of punishments should be used before considering an unpleasant consequence. An example of the loss of something valued involves a child on a pediatric unit who refuses to eat. The child likes time in the playroom; therefore, playroom time is suspended if the child does not eat half of the food at each meal.

Often situations call for decreasing an undesirable behavior while at the same time increasing a desirable behavior. Therefore, a combination of reinforcers and punishments are used.

The following steps are implemented in a behavior modification program:

1. *Assessment of the client's behavior pattern.* The behavior is defined accurately, is observable and measurable, and does not consist of inferences or personal interpretations. The phrase "fights all the time" needs further clarification. The antecedent events and the consequences of the behavior are identified. A record is kept of the baseline behavior patterns of the client, the antecedent events, the frequency of the behavior, and events

that reinforce or punish the behavior after it has occurred.

2. *Formation of a nursing diagnosis regarding the behavior problem.* The nursing diagnosis must clearly state the specific behavior to be changed. Examples are inadequate weekly exercise, irregular contraceptive use or excessive intake of between-meal snacks.

3. *Develop the behavior modification plan.* Whenever possible, the plan regarding the behavior to be changed is mutually agreed on by the nurse and client. The method used and the type and frequency of reinforcement or punishment are discussed by the client and the nurse.

When the plan is being developed, methods to increase desirable behavior or decrease undesirable behavior are identified. If antecedent events can be altered, alternative events preceding the behavior are identified. For example, if the person usually eats a snack while watching evening TV, the person might give up watching TV and try reading or another hobby at that time.

Reinforcers are determined with the client and are of importance to the client. Examples of reinforcers are socializing with others, seeing a movie, and buying new clothes. The reinforcer must be available and realistic. A reinforcer that is dependent on someone else, such as the nurse or family member, needs to be identified as such.

Punishment, to be effective, has to be valued by the client as well. For example, loss of watching TV may not be important to a client who does not like TV and enjoys reading. Punishment must not deprive persons of basic human needs, such as a meal or the attention of a parent or loved one. Punishments that impair the health of the client must be avoided.

The speed with which the reinforcer or punishment follows the behavior is considered and depends on the client's age, the behavior to be changed, and the situation. The schedule of the reinforcer or punishment is also determined. Reinforcement or punishment can occur each time the behavior occurs (continuous) or on an intermittent basis. In early stages of behavior change and with young children, reinforcers and punishments should follow soon after the behavior occurs and each time the behavior occurs.

The plan must be communicated to significant others and to other health team members. Family members can support the client, provide reinforcement or punishment, or alter the antecedent events.

4. *Implement the plan as specified.* Either by changing the antecedent event or providing reinforcement or punishment, implementing the plan *as written* is crucial to its success or failure. Consistency is necessary to determine whether the plan is working. Inconsistent application of the behavior modification plan undermines the situation, and the desired change in behavior will probably not occur.

5. *Evaluate the effectiveness of the plan in changing the client's behavior.* Compare the baseline behavior frequency with the frequency of the "new" behavior. If there is no change or only minimal change, the antecedent events, reinforcers, or punishments may not be effective. Modify the plan as needed by changing the antecedent events, reinforcers, or punishments or by breaking the desired behavior change into smaller units to be accomplished.

Self-modification programs are an adaptation of behavior modification in which clients actively participate and develop their own behavior modification programs. The client voluntarily selects a behavior to develop or change, such as a change in lifestyle (Pender, 1987). The behaviors are usually health promotion or health maintenance activities (eg, cessation of smoking, weight loss).

The nurse's role is to facilitate the client's self-modification of behavior through use of the steps of the behavior modification program. The nurse assists the client to assess the behavior pattern, the reasons for the behavior change, the knowledge and skills to be used, the perceived benefits of the new behavior, and the support for the new behavior in the client's social and physical environment (Pender, 1987). The nurse also supports the client's use of the principles of classical and operant conditioning.

A behavior modification program is a useful strategy when a change in a client's behavior is desired. Clients can actually set up their own self-modification programs with encouragement and support by the nurse or they can participate in programs set up by the nurse and other health professionals.

## Contracting

Establishing contracts between a nurse and client may be beneficial when the client wants to change complex behaviors to adhere to the health care regimen. Contracts may also be considered for clients who want to maximize their health potential.

Contracting provides a systematic method of increasing desirable behavior. The nurse and client explicitly identify the desired behavior and the responsibilities of both client and nurse. The specific

## Sample Contract

I, _____(client)_____ , would like to achieve the following objective:
1 Walk three times per week for 30 minutes.

To achieve this objective, I, _____(client)_____ , agree to the following responsibilities:
1 Arrange my weekly schedule to provide 30 minutes three times per week for walking.
2 Record dates and times spent walking.
3 Bring the record of the walking schedule to the next clinic appointment in 1 month.
4 Meet with the nurse monthly for counseling, support, and encouragement.
5 Reward myself for achieving the objective on a weekly basis by treating myself to a paperback book, movie, or long distance telephone call to a friend or relative.

Signature: _____(client)_____     Date: _____

I, _____(nurse)_____ , agree to assist _____(client)_____ with the objective of walking 30 minutes three times per week. My responsibilities include:
1 Meet with _____(client)_____ on a monthly basis for 1 hour.
2 Review the walking record monthly.
3 Monitor _____(client's)_____ blood pressure on a monthly basis.
4 Listen to the achievement and/or disappointment in the accomplishment of the objective. Offer support and encouragement and assist in problem solving during monthly meetings.

Signature: _____(nurse)_____     Date: _____

Date of evaluation: _____
Results/Revisions:
Record brought to appointment. Thirty minutes of walking three or four times per week recorded. Walking time established as after work. Rewarded self with book or telephone call after achievement of weekly objective. BP 152/90. Nurse and client agree to continue the contract and reevaluate in 1 month.

behaviors and responsibilities of each are outlined. The desired behavior must be measurable and specific. Contingency contracting adds the element of reinforcement. Some form of reinforcement is provided in return for the performance of the specified behavior (Steckel, 1982).

Contracts may be either written or verbal. An advantage of a written contract is that it signifies a more formal agreement between the nurse and the client. There is a greater chance for communication to be clearly understood (eg, responsibilities) when the contract is written. The use of written contracts has been shown to be beneficial in a variety of situations, such as with clients desiring to modify diet (calories, cholesterol, sodium, fluids), reduce smoking, establish an exercise regimen, cough and deep breathe, and ambulate after surgery (Jensen, 1985). It is particularly useful with clients experiencing long-term solutions to health problems or concerns that necessitate changes in lifestyle. Examples for individual, family, and community clients include:

**Examples**

*Individual:*   Learn relaxation techniques
Establish a social support system
Adjust to a chronic illness

*Family:*   Develop new communication styles
Improve parenting skills
Use seatbelts

*Community:*   Develop a neighborhood "watch" program
Adhere to a new health regulation
Incorporate problem solving into meetings

As can be seen, contracting is useful with health promotion activities as well as with health restoration and maintenance. Contracting is a strategy that strongly encourages client adherence to a new health care practice.

Contracting uses many of the principles of behavior modification and problem solving. Elements of the contracting process are as follows:
1. The client is an active participant in the process.

2. The behavior must be clearly identified and measurable by the nurse and the client.
3. The behavior may need to be broken into smaller, more manageable steps.
4. Responsibilities of both the client and the nurse are identified.
5. Time for evaluation is specified.
6. A reinforcer is identified by the client if contingency contracting is used.
7. Signatures of both the client and the nurse are obtained.
8. Both the client and the nurse receive a copy of the written contract (if written).
9. The contract is evaluated and revised as necessary (Brykcznski, 1982; Steckel, 1982).

An example of this process (shown in the box on p. 200) involves a man who wants to control his blood pressure. This behavior needs to be broken down into more measurable and achievable steps. After discussing the variety of measures to control his blood pressure, the client chooses to establish a regular exercise regimen as a first step. It is important for the client to choose the behavior, because this will increase the potential for adherence. A written contract is formulated to establish an exercise regimen including the behavior to be achieved, the responsibilities of the nurse and client, and the time frame in which the behavior should occur.

It is important to note that the results include whether the responsibilities of nurse and client were met. Reinforcement such as praise should be given on achievement of the objective and responsibilities. Note that the nurse is unable to evaluate whether the client walked 30 minutes three times a week, but is able to evaluate whether the client recorded the information.

There are many benefits in using contracting as a strategy. Contracting enables the client to actively plan and carry out changes in behavior. Through active participation, the client becomes more responsible for the behavior change, is given needed support and reinforcement, and is more likely to adhere to the desired behavior change. Through open communication between the nurse and client, expectations are clarified and feedback provided. Emphasis is placed on accountability of the nurse and the outcomes of the contracting process. The client is also provided with a strategy that can be used in future situations.

## Group Process

Group process is a strategy that is useful when two or more people have a common goal or purpose. Types of groups frequently used within nursing are community, family, therapeutic, and psychotherapy groups (Gardner and LaSalle, 1987). Examples of therapeutic groups are self-help groups such as Alcoholics Anonymous, and the educational group, "I Can Cope," for clients who are experiencing cancer and their families.

Groups used in nursing practice are planned gatherings of persons designed to accomplish a common goal. Examples are a group of older women from a community health center wanting to discuss mutual health concerns or teenagers wanting support or information about parental divorce. Clients experiencing a stressful situation (eg, heart problems, new parents, rehabilitation) may find it useful to be involved in a group with other members experiencing similar situations and concerns.

Examples of nursing diagnoses in which group process could be considered include:
Alteration in family process
Alteration in parenting
Anxiety
Disturbance in self-concept
Grieving
Knowledge deficit
Powerlessness
Rape-trauma syndrome
Social isolation
Factors to consider prior to setting up or referring a client to a group (Kinney et al, 1985) include:
- Type, purpose of the group in relation to the client's concern
- Client's perception of need
- Group leadership
- Location and cost
- Duration, frequency, and timing of meetings

The nurse, when effectively using and leading groups, considers the following factors of group process:

*Stage of development of the group.* Groups develop in stages: orientation, working, and termination phases. Being aware of behaviors of group members and tasks within each stage is beneficial to nurses working with groups.

*Structure.* Structure includes the size, membership, communication within the group, decision-making, and roles. Effective groups consist of 5 to 15 members, have a cooperative rather than a competitive spirit, have a cohesive membership, and are meeting the purposes/goals of the group.

*Leadership.* A nurse who is in a leadership role within the group needs additional knowledge of leadership styles and strategies and their effect on the group. Functions of leaders within the group include obtaining and receiving information, helping to develop the group's goals, facilitating communication, helping to integrate various perspectives and possible alternatives, and evaluating proposals and decisions (Sampson and Marthas, 1981).

Effective interpersonal skills are essential to effective group leadership. The specific skills used, such as support, confrontation, summarizing, and clarification, are based on the goals of the group and the needs of its members.

Group process is an effective strategy to use with clients when two or more have the same concern and goal.

## Principles of Nursing Practice

A strategy frequently used by nurses involves the principles of nursing practice. A principle is considered to be an accepted rule of action or a basis of conduct or operation. Principles are found in the form of standards, guidelines, policies, and procedures. Many principles of nursing practice are unique to nursing; others have been adapted by nurses from other disciplines for application to the nursing process. Principles of nursing practice provide the scientific base of nursing by guiding many of the nursing orders included in the plan of care. Principles of nursing practice have evolved from a variety of sources, including nursing specialties, professional organizations, and agencies and institutions.

A large number of the principles have evolved from nursing specialties such as gerontological, maternal-child, mental health, family, community health, and oncology nursing. The principles, often in the form of guidelines, are developed by nurses with knowledge and expertise in the care of clients who have concerns related to that specialty. Guidelines are found in nursing textbooks as well as journal and research articles. An example involves the planning of nursing care with a client with recently diagnosed chronic obstructive pulmonary disease. The nurse selects nursing orders related to activity tolerance, breathing exercises, and precautions from guidelines developed by nurses experienced in the care of clients with respiratory concerns.

Principles of nursing practice have been developed by nurses in professional organizations such as the American Nurses' Association and the American Association of Critical Care Nurses. For example, the ANA developed the Standards of Nursing Practice (1973) and Standards of Psychiatric Mental Health Nursing Practice (1973).

Agencies and institutions have also developed principles of nursing practice, which are often in the form of policies and procedures. Policies are statements of institutional standards. An example is the standard an institution establishes in regard to frequency of changing the site for intravenous administration of drugs or fluids. A procedure is a particular course or method of action formulated by the agency or institution. An example is the procedure to be used when a client is being discharged. These written policies and procedures should be based on nursing research and provide rationale and consistency for nursing care within agencies and institutions.

Examples of principles of nursing practice for an individual client, a family client, and a community client are provided.

*Examples of principles of nursing practice for the individual client:*

Guidelines for communicating with the hearing impaired

1. Talk directly to the person.
2. Speak slowly and articulate clearly, but not in an artificial manner.
3. Talk in a normal tone of voice; do not shout.
4. Speak toward the ear that has the best hearing.
5. Restate with different words when not understood.
6. Provide visual cues to augment communication (Phipps et al, 1987).

*Examples of principles of nursing practice for the family client:*

Principles of family health practice

1. Work with the family collectively.
2. Begin where the family is.
3. Plan nursing interventions based on the family's stage of development.
4. Recognize the validity of family structural variations.
5. Emphasize family strengths (Spradley, 1985).

*Example of principles of nursing practice for the community client:*

Guidelines for occupational health nursing practice

1. Assess health needs of employees and promote and maintain their health.
2. Analyze factors in the work environment that are hazardous to employee health and minimize their impact or prevent their occurrence.
3. Provide early diagnosis and prompt treatment for injury or illness on the job.

4. Provide programs for employees with disease or disability aimed at restoring and maintaining their maximum level of functioning (Spradley, 1985).

Many principles of nursing practice are based on medical diagnoses, such as myocardial infarction and fractured hip. Principles of nursing practice are currently being developed in relation to specific nursing diagnoses, such as self-care deficit and spiritual distress. Nursing research is being conducted to substantiate and expand the principles of nursing practice, which will increase the scientific base of nursing, help direct nursing care, and add to the predictability within nursing practice. Opportunities are also available for nurses to communicate principles to other nurses. Nurses have the responsibility for being knowledgeable in regard to the principles of nursing practice that involve the concerns of clients with whom they interact. These principles are valuable when dealing with care plans for health maintenance, restoration, or promotion.

## Guidelines for Strategies

1. *Major strategies for implementation are identified.* At least one strategy is identified for each goal and its subsequent objectives. One strategy or a combination of strategies provides direction to nursing orders. For example, the strategies of teaching/learning and problem solving help the client to learn about community resources and decide which services to use. The teaching/learning strategy gives suggestions for nursing orders through principles. Application of this strategy facilitates the client's increased knowledge regarding available and pertinent community resources. Identifying the exact problem or need for community resources, generating alternatives, and analyzing and choosing from alternatives are promoted through problem solving.

2. *Strategies are appropriate to their respective goal and objectives.* The strategy is directly related to the goal and its objectives. Inasmuch as the goal and objectives are mutually established with the client, the nurse has determined the client's willingness to achieve the outcomes. Different methods or approaches are used to achieve the outcomes. The nurse's knowledge of the client and the situation guides the choice of strategies that can truly facilitate the achievement of goals and objectives without the use of trial and error.

An example is that of a client who is experiencing a biophysical crisis of alteration in respiration related to a partially obstructed airway and who

also has anxiety. The nurse prioritizes diagnoses, determines that the altered respiratory status is the more life-threatening, and sets a goal that the client will improve respiratory function by clearing the airway. The principles of respiratory nursing practice or guidelines from the American Heart Association (basic life support choking procedure) facilitate specific nursing orders and actions. Second, the nurse deals with the goal of decreasing anxiety based on the strategy of principles of mental health nursing practice. In this situation one strategy cannot be interchanged for the other; each is specific to its respective goal.

More subtle differences among diagnoses, goals, objectives, and client situations call for more discretion on the part of the nurse. Two community neighborhood clients may have the same goal and objectives relating to improvement of street conditions and sidewalks. One neighborhood group has already looked into the different kinds of materials that could be used and their costs. Therefore, the decision-making step of the problem-solving strategy would probably be the place to start. The other neighborhood needs to explore the materials and options before making a decision about them. In this case, the nurse would start the problem-solving strategy at the second step of determining possible solutions.

3. *Strategies are based on scientific rationale.* Strategies themselves stem from the science and practice disciplines. Theories, models, concepts, and principles provide rationale for some of the strategies. Others have their foundation in accepted methods or approaches determined by long-standing practice. Research findings and current literature may reveal new strategies, or substantiate the use of identified strategies. Nurses need to recognize the scientific bases of all strategies used in their practice. Knowledge of scientific rationale for strategies facilitates nurses' own self-confidence, increases their ability to justify methods or approaches to care, and establishes accountability for nursing practice.

## NURSING ORDERS

Nursing orders represent the independent function of the professional nurse: specifying the intended behaviors of the nurse, client, and others to achieve the desired outcomes. Nursing orders are directly related to their respective objective and the content area of the goal or objective (eg, grieving). The specific nursing orders are also determined by the selected strategy. Strategies provide steps, principles, concepts, guidelines, and rules that serve as a basis for choosing appropriate nursing actions. The nurse individualizes care to the client's unique situation: the personal human responses to actual or potential health problems and concerns. The nurse considers the client's strengths and limitations, and internal and external resources available. The unique way in which the client integrates psychological, developmental, biophysical, spiritual, and sociocultural aspects influences the nursing orders. In addition to specifying nursing orders for independent nursing actions, the nurse also develops nursing orders related to the client's biomedical health concerns. The nurse uses clinical judgment and critical thinking when planning nursing orders related to collaborative actions. For example, the nurse considers the physician's order for an intravenous diuretic when planning nursing orders for a client experiencing chronic heart failure.

The nurse uses decision-making skills of deliberation, judgment, and choice (Schaefer, 1974) to determine which nursing orders are most likely to achieve the objective. Either alone or with other nurses and health team members, the nurse considers the available options, using knowledge of nursing practice and other disciplines. Then the nurse forms an opinion and chooses among the options. During this process the nurse must consider the feasibility of the actions in relation to the client situation, the risks and costs involved, temporal, material, and human resources, and the skills and knowledge of the practitioners.

## Guidelines for Nursing Orders

1. *Nursing orders are appropriate to their respective goal, objective, and strategy.* The nature of the goal, and hence the objective, leads to the nature of the orders. The orders reflect health maintenance, promotion, or restoration, depending on the focus of the goal and objective.

### Examples

*Maintenance:* Turn client every 2 hours during the day and night, maintaining proper body alignment of the client.

*Promotion:* Teach client basic nutrition patterns, explaining the basic food groups with the use of pamphlets and pictures; use the dietitian or nutritionist as a resource person.

*Restoration:* Assist client with range of motion exercises for the affected leg and hand every 2 hours during the day; maintain the limbs in a position of use and in good alignment during the night by using pillows and splints.

The content area of the goal or objective also needs to be addressed in the nursing orders to reflect internal consistency. For example, if the goal or objective addresses use of open communication (content area), the orders need to include reference to achievement of open communication.

The strategy gives direction to the order specified through principles, concepts, guidelines, and rules. Therefore, if the nurse uses principles of mental health nursing practice and teaching/learning as strategies to promote the use of open communication, nursing orders will reflect those principles. Examples of the use of strategies are provided on pp. 207 to 209.

An adequate number of nursing orders is needed to achieve the given objective. Usually two to six orders are sufficient. To determine "adequacy," question whether the actions named in the nursing orders will achieve the respective objective.

2. *Scientific and practice principles provide rationale for orders.* Theories, concepts, models, and principles are the scientific bases for nursing orders. Current literature and research findings from nursing and other disciplines give direction to actions. The nurse needs to have a broad scientific knowledge base to justify a wide variety of nursing orders.

There are two major types of rationale for nursing orders: strategy-oriented and content-oriented. Strategies provide rationale for some nursing orders. Statements reflecting the strategy's principles, guidelines, steps, rules, and concepts are used as rationale for the *strategy-oriented nursing orders.* Rationale for the content area must also be included. *Content-oriented nursing orders* refer to the topic or focus of the objectives and goal. The content area is identified for each objective. The content area can be the same for all objectives, leading to some goals that are more specific. The objectives for more general goals probably have a varied content. Statements citing rationale from each content area provide a scientific basis for those nursing orders.

For example, if a client is to name the four basic food groups as the first objective in attaining the goal of improved nutritional status, nursing orders and rationale statements for teaching and learning (*strategy*) and nutrition (*content*) must be included. Therefore, the scientific rationale statements for nursing orders include reference to the strategy identified and to the content of the order itself.

Using this scientific base deliberately leads to predictability in nursing practice. Through purposeful nursing actions, the nurse determines which orders are more successful in achieving projected client outcomes.

The scientific basis for orders is not usually documented in nursing practice settings. Documentation of the rationale along with the orders may be important if other health team members need to understand the rationale in order to follow through. For example, a psychiatric/mental health facility may place all teenagers in a behavior management program. In a client situation in which the therapeutic effect of this program is counterproductive, the nurse postpones and recommends not using the behavior management approach with a particular client. It would be helpful to communicate the scientific rationale for that decision in writing to other members of the health care team. Whether the rationale is written or not, the nurse should be prepared to state the rationale for nursing orders and defend decisions made regarding nursing practice.

3. *Nursing orders incorporate the autonomy and individuality of the client.* The uniqueness of the individual is reflected in the nursing orders. Based on a comprehensive and multifocal assessment, the nurse has identified the client's strengths, limitations, and internal and external resources. This information helps the nurse decide what is realistic to expect from the client. Nurses encourage clients' participation and responsibility to increase their sense of personal control and esteem. However, the client's strengths determine the level of participation and amount of responsibility that can be expected. For example, the client's cognitive level determines the extent of material and the manner in which the nurse presents information in a learning situation. Cultural and developmental aspects are also considered in specifying nursing orders. Historical information regarding patterns of behavior give direction for individualizing the approach to care.

Whenever nursing orders are based on the client's unique situation, a rationale statement supporting the nursing order is provided or readily available. These rationale statements indicating *individuality* may come from previously collected data or from literature and research citing differences among people based on culture or development.

4. *Nursing orders indicate specific intended behaviors, giving direction to the nurse, client, and others.* Nursing orders are detailed statements of *who* is to do *what* and *when* (within a given time frame). Each nursing order includes a subject, verb, and conditions or criterion for completion (see Chapter 9).

Each order indicates the anticipated date of implementation.

**Examples**

*Specific nursing orders:*  1. The client will use walker to ambulate 50 feet four times a day, beginning 2/7/89.
2. The nurse will accompany the client during ambulation to provide verbal support and monitor safety and response to ambulation.

These examples state who is to perform what and under what conditions or purpose. The statements are concise and clear. Depending on the setting and expertise of the practitioners, one might explicitly define "verbal support" and "monitor safety and response to ambulation." Based on a professional nurse's education and the practice of the institution, agency, or practice, those phrases would have definable interpretations.

Nursing orders reflect behavior of all people involved in the client's care, that is, the nurse, client, family members, and other health team members. When appropriate, referrals, consultation, and collaborative approaches to care are given. For example, if the nurse writes an order for social service referral, the order should specify the intent of the referral. This clarity of intent gives direction to the social worker and facilitates accuracy and efficiency of service.

**Example**

*Specific nursing order for referral:*   Social service referral to provide family support and evaluate home care needs in conjunction with primary nurse.

The use of audio and visual aids is specifically indicated. Pamphlets, tapes, brochures, and books are used to facilitate understanding and increase the client's participation in care. These aids are named to give direction to the appropriate health team members and to inform others of the intended content and level of material being addressed.

5. *Nursing orders reflect consideration of human, temporal, and material resources available.* The assessment of available resources is necessary before specifying nursing orders. As in judging priorities, many variables are considered to determine realistic means to the client's achievement of the goal and objectives. The nurse considers human resources, or people who can participate in the client's care. The number and type of services, employees, staff, and family members and their quali-

fications and expertise are analyzed. Also, abilities, motivation, and willingness to be involved influences follow-through.

Temporal resources, or time available for objective achievement, influence nursing orders. In general, acute care settings for individual clients mandate shorter term achievements than do community settings. Some types of client outcomes and their related nursing orders take much more time than others. When outcomes and nursing orders involve many people or alteration of long-standing patterns of behavior, more time is needed, and the nurse can anticipate some resistance. People who seek out health care services or consultation are usually looking for guidance and direction to solve problems and concerns. Even with this motivation, if the guidance and direction involves a change in behavior (which it usually does), there will probably be resistance at some level. Anticipating this resistance helps the nurse set realistic expectations while writing nursing orders.

Material resources such as money, equipment, and supplies are also important to evaluate. The options from which the nurse chooses actions vary with the amount and types of material resources. The costs, risks, and benefits of using certain services, equipment, and supplies affect the choice. The source of funds may determine the actions chosen. For individual and family clients, local, state, federal and private payers and services are all involved. For community clients, funding and services sources include grants, special-project funding, property tax income, and community programs.

After consideration of human, temporal, and material resources for nursing orders, the nurse may reassess the achievability of the client outcomes. Modification of the outcomes is necessary if they are not aligned with resources available.

6. *Nursing orders are numbered in the appropriate sequence to achieve the objective.* Listing the nursing orders in recommended succession gives direction to the nurse, client, and others. Similar to the proper sequencing of objectives to reach a goal, the nursing orders should be in sequence to meet their respective objective. This sequence is used by the nurse to review with the client progress toward objective achievement.

Some strategies guide the sequencing of nursing orders. For example, the strategies of behavior modification, problem solving, and contracting follow a recommended order of events. Principles of nursing practice based on procedures usually provide a step-by-step process to follow. Other strategies, such as teaching/learning, imply a sequence. Stating that the client must show readiness to learn

implies that the nurse assesses readiness before actually teaching.

Sequencing of orders also promotes predictability in nursing practice. Through experience and knowledge, nurses learn prescriptions of events that lead to expected client outcomes. Studying and communicating these prescriptions adds to the scientific base of the discipline of nursing.

7. *Nursing orders are dated and include the signature of the responsible nurse.* Dating the nursing orders when written provides the nurse and others with a point of reference for the actions prescribed. The nurse uses the date while reviewing, modifying, updating, and evaluating the effectiveness and realistic nature of the nursing orders. Certain orders are discontinued and others initiated based on progress or lack of progress toward objective and goal achievement. By knowing when orders were initiated, the nurse determines whether the stated approach has had sufficient time to effect change.

The signature of the responsible nurse is necessary to determine accountability for the orders written. The nurse's signature is a personal and professional statement of responsibility. Other health team members will know who to contact with questions regarding the orders, recommended changes, and positive feedback. The client's responses to the actions prescribed are communicated accordingly. Individual nurses are increasingly determining their own case loads of clients in a variety of settings. The nurse's signature on orders indicates responsibility and accountability to clients and to others.

8. *Nursing orders are kept current, and are revised as indicated.* Nursing orders reflect a client's concerns, strengths, and limitations at a given moment in a given situation. Inasmuch as health is a dynamic pattern of behavior and functioning, those patterns can and do change. The nurse is sensitive to those changes through ongoing assessment and evaluation of the client's situation and progress. The nurse recognizes when a given order is no longer appropriate and a revision is indicated. This may take place before the intended achievement of an objective. The need for a revision in orders does not necessarily reflect on the validity of the original orders or competence of the practitioner. Many variables affect the client; some are anticipated and expected, others are not. Through evaluation and self-reflection, the nurse determines whether the variables causing a change in the situation could have been (or were) predicted. An in-depth review of the previous components of the nursing process can explain the change and subsequent need to modify the orders.

---

## Example of Individual Client Plan

---

*Situation:* The client, a 58-year-old woman with diabetes, receives health care in a storefront clinic. Her diabetes was diagnosed 3 years ago, and she visits the clinic infrequently. She is able to give herself insulin, but the nurse, on assessment, has discovered that the client has been giving herself the injections in the thighs only. The client remembers being taught "something" about other "places" for injection, but has since forgotten them and does not realize the importance of rotating sites. She says that if it is important she will use other sites, if she knows what they are. The nurse recognizes the client's need to learn about and use other areas appropriate for insulin injection.

*Nursing model:*     Orem's Self-Care model (1985) is selected because the client is responsible for carrying out insulin injections. The client, being in the supportive-educative nursing system, influences the selection of strategy and development of goals, objectives, and nursing orders.

*Nursing diagnosis:*   Knowledge deficit (insulin injection sites) related to lack of recognized need (12/6/89).

*Goal:*     Client will increase knowledge of insulin injection sites by 12/13/89.

*Objective 1:*     Client will list three appropriate sites for insulin administration by 12/6/89.

**Nursing orders**

1 Nurse and client will discuss reasons for rotating sites on 12/6/89.

2 Nurse and client will discuss alternate injection sites and a rotation schedule, using pictures and pamphlets on 12/6/89.

**Rationale**

*Strategy:* Teaching and learning
*Content:* Insulin administration
Development of concepts is part of learning (strategy) (Pohl, 1981). Insulin, if given in the same site over time, causes scarring and decreased absorption (content) (Phipps, 1987).

Teaching requires effective communication; repetition strengthens learning (strategy) (Rorden, 1987). Audiovisual aids appropriate to client situation promote communication and repetition.

*Objective 2:*     Client will demonstrate administration of insulin using three sites by 12/13/89.

**Nursing orders**

1 Nurse will demonstrate how to give an injection in the abdomen, arms, and buttocks on 12/13/89.

2 Client will demonstrate injection into three areas without puncturing the skin on 12/13/89.

**Rationale**

Learning occurs through demonstration-practice (strategy) (Redman, 1988). Variety of sites decreases scarring and increases absorption (content) (Phipps).

Effective learning requires active participation of the learner; evaluation is an integral part of teaching (strategy) (Redman).

---

Nursing orders are reviewed on a regular basis to determine the need for modification and updating. At a minimum, the orders are reviewed on the expected dates of order implementation and objective achievement. In acute care settings, that probably indicates review at least every 24 hours. In long-term care settings, review is less frequent, and determined by expected implementation and outcome dates. Family and community client orders involve many people and tend to be long-term. Therefore, a minimum review guideline is the dates of the implementation and the projected outcomes.

9. *Nursing orders include plans for termination of nursing services.* Plans for termination of nursing services are included for clients with health promotion, maintenance, or restoration goals. From the inception of services, the nurse and client consider the time frame for goal and objective achievement in terms of continuation of care. Nursing orders reflect anticipation of the need for education, referrals, special instructions, follow-up, and community linkage. This anticipation facilitates the transition to the client's increased independence and self-reliance. Whether clients receive residential, overnight, clinic, day care, home care, or consultation services, goals, objectives, and nursing orders reflecting the period after service are often necessary.

Guidelines for writing goals, objectives, and nursing orders were used to develop the examples of plans for implementation for the individual, family, and community client given on pages 207 to 209.

## Example of Family Client Plan

*Situation:* In June 1989, the home health care nurse began seeing a family with two children, a 3-year-old boy (John) and a 4-month-old boy (Adam). Both parents live at home, and both work outside the home during the day. The 3-year-old was toilet trained, but has been wetting his pants intermittently for the past few months and is starting to act out (fighting, arguing with others) at the day care center. The nurse was referred to the family by the day care center to assess the home situation and to recommend/implement actions as appropriate. After two home family visits, the nurse concludes that John's behavior is a symptom of the recent change in family dynamics with the addition of Adam in the home.

*Nursing model:*     Friedman's Structural/Functional Family model (1981) is selected for its focus on interaction among family members.

*Nursing diagnosis:*  Alteration in family processes related to John's reaction to a new family member (Adam) (6/23/89).

*Goal:*             Family will adjust to Adam's presence within 3 months, by 9/30/89.

*Objective 1:*       Family will name at least three ways that Adam has influenced their lifestyle by 7/1/89.

| **Nursing orders** | **Rationale** |
|---|---|
| 1 Nurse will establish rapport with the family using facilitative communication techniques on 7/1/89. | *Strategy:* Therapeutic use of self<br>*Content:* Sibling rivalry<br>Effective use of communication techniques promotes development of the nurse-client relationship (strategy) (Sundeen, 1989). |
| 2 Nurse and family will discuss the changes in family interactions that have occurred since Adam's birth and their feelings about the changes on 7/1/89. | Verbalization of the event and responses to it promotes understanding and decreases anxiety (strategy) (Stuart and Sundeen, 1987). |
| 3 Parents will state how they relate to John and his behavior since Adam's birth on 7/1/89. | Changes in a child's behavior (daytime/nighttime wetting "accidents"; aggressive/quarrelsome) can be the result of decreased attention from parents and child's own fears (content) (individuality) (Whaley and Wong, 1987). |

*Objective 2:*       Parents and day care center will use a behavior modification approach to decrease John's acting out by 8/1/89.

| **Nursing orders** | **Rationale** |
|---|---|
| 1 Parents, teacher, and nurse will record baseline of incidents and preceding situations that led to John's acting out behaviors by 7/8/89. | *Strategy:* Behavior modification and therapeutic use of self<br>Identification of behavior pattern is necessary before determining approach: all key people need to be involved in developing the plan (strategy) (individuality) (Peddicord, 1987). |
| 2 Nurse will assist the parents and teacher in naming potential reinforcements/punishments that are realistic and valued by John by 7/8/89. | Reinforcements/punishments need to be valued and appropriate to the client and situation (strategy) (content) (individuality) (Peddicord). Facilitative communication techniques promote expression of thoughts and feelings (strategy) (Sundeen). |
| 3 Parents and teacher will develop a plan to decrease John's undesirable behaviors using identified reinforcers/punishers by 7/15/89. | People implementing the plan need to be a part of developing it (strategy) (Peddicord). |
| 4 Parents, teacher, and nurse will determine implementation and evaluation dates for plan on 7/15/89. | Consistent implementation and evaluation are essential to successful behavior modification (strategy) (Johnson, 1986). |

## Example of Community Client Plan

*Situation:* A women's community organization became concerned about single mothers who could not afford health care services. Through various community contacts and an informal survey, the organization ascertained that services were provided to the poor and unemployed as well as the middle- and upper-income people. However, a certain group of employed, low-income single mothers could not afford health care services. This assessed need was taken to the organization's board, which decided to investigate the potential of solving this problem. With board approval, a task force was formed, and a nurse consultant contracted to develop a plan to meet this community need. Based on the information presented, the nurse concluded that lack of services in the community was creating inadequate health care to low-income single mothers.

*Nursing model:*  Neuman's Health-Care Systems model (1982) is selected for its systems orientation and nursing focus on primary, secondary, and tertiary prevention.

*Nursing diagnosis:*  Insufficient health care to low-income single mothers related to lack of services in community (1/15/89).

*Goal:*  Community will develop health care services for low-income single mothers within 1 year (1/15/90).

*Objective 1:*  Organization board will accept a written plan for health care services to low-income single mothers within 6 months using recommendations from the task force and nurse consultant.

| Nursing orders | Rationale |
|---|---|
| 1 Nurse and task force will review the community's health care situation, problem, organization's board commitment, and identified goal. These issues will be discussed and clarified on 2/1/89. | *Strategy:* Problem solving<br>*Content:* Adequate health care services<br>People involved need to understand the situation (strategy) (Sullivan and Decker, 1988). |
| 2 Task force will determine four potential alternative solutions to the situation with nurse's guidance by 2/30/89. | Potential solutions need to be generated by the people concerned to provide anticipated resolution to the unique situation. Options are limited to focus group on goal attainment (strategy) (individuality) (Bower, 1982). |
| 3 Task force and nurse will examine the risks and costs of each alternative by 3/30/89. | Consequences of alternatives are analyzed prior to selecting one (strategy) (Sullivan and Decker, 1988). |
| 4 Task force will choose one alternative to recommend to the organization board for approval by 4/15/89. | Client (organization task force) needs to choose an alternative most likely to achieve intended goal (strategy) (Sullivan and Decker, 1988). |

(Another objective is needed regarding implementation and evaluation of the alternative chosen.)

## Nursing Care Plan

The nursing care plan is the tool for documenting and communicating the client's nursing diagnoses, expected outcomes, strategies, nursing orders, and evaluation (Fig. 10-1). The care plan serves as the key vehicle to promote an individualized and consistent approach to client care. Through documentation of the client's major concerns and plans to alleviate or modify the concerns, the nurse facilitates coordination of all the members of the health care team. If the plans are written according to recommended guidelines, goals and objectives provide the intended direction for care and an eventual basis for evaluation. Also, the strategies and nursing orders guide and coordinate the client, nurse, and others in their actions to promote goal and objective achievement. A completed care plan needs to be *used* to fulfill its purposes. A well-developed plan can prevent the use of time-consuming trial and error, avoid duplication of effort, and alleviate costly and timely omissions of care.

The professional nurse is responsible and accountable for developing the nursing care plan. Ideally, the primary nurse, case manager, or nurse responsible for the ongoing care of the client, completes the care plan. Many implications are made in developing a plan. An accurate and multifocal assessment is the necessary basis for the plan. Nursing diagnoses evolve from data analysis and synthesis, which requires a comprehensive knowledge base. The diagnoses are put into order of priority, goals established, objectives developed, strategies identified, and nursing orders specified using

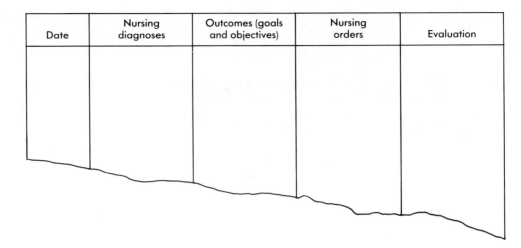

| Date | Nursing diagnoses | Outcomes (goals and objectives) | Nursing orders | Evaluation |
|------|-------------------|--------------------------------|----------------|------------|
|      |                   |                                |                |            |

Fig. 10-1. Components of nursing care plan.

scientific rationale. Other health team members may have input and feedback regarding the approach to the client, but the professional nurse is responsible for the care plan's development.

The care plan is initiated on the inception of nursing services. After an initial assessment of the client's situation is completed, the nurse consolidates that information for current and future use. Even if more data are needed to verify nursing diagnoses, the nurse records inferences of diagnoses and recommended approaches to those concerns. Subsequent data collection may lead to alteration or validation of the nurse's initial judgment. The goals, objectives, strategies, and nursing orders are modified accordingly.

Typically, the nursing care plan includes the *individualized* plan for a client's situation. Yet some actual or potential health problems and concerns create *common patterns of human responses* among people. These similarities of altered patterns of behavior and functioning usually call for similar approaches to care on the part of the nurse (eg, general postoperative nursing care, elements of cardiac rehabilitation programs). Nursing care guidelines, policies, procedures, and standards are developed by various nursing organizations, institutions, agencies, and practices. These approaches are based on scientific and practice principles and are intended for use in predictable circumstances. Advantages of using routinized approaches in select situations are that they provide standards of care and criteria for evaluation of care, increase predictability in nursing practice, and save the nurse's time by decreasing repetitive documentation. Reference to these approaches on the care plan is appropriate *only* in terms of the *commonalities* with which clients are treated for *similar patterns* of hu-

man responses. *Individualized* nursing diagnoses and related plans that reflect the client's unique situation are still needed. All nursing care guidelines, policies, procedures, and standards should be kept current and readily available as a reference for nurses while writing nursing care plans.

The nursing care plan, the key vehicle for nursing care, needs to be a part of the client's permanent record. Therefore, the care plan is completed in ink and follows the guidelines suggested in this and other chapters regarding the nursing process components.

### Kardex

The Kardex is a working form usually used in the care of individual clients. Divided into compartments, the Kardex contains information regarding collaborative biomedical health concerns and interventions (such as diet, activity level, laboratory tests and x-ray studies, medical consultations) as well as select nursing orders reflecting the client's current health situation and independent nursing actions (such as assistance with activities of daily living, nursing consultations, client's personal preferences, restriction of visitors). The Kardex is a fluid document subject to frequent change and thus is usually completed in pencil. It functions as a quick reference for many members of the health care team. As such, the Kardex must be kept current and accessible for use.

### SUMMARY

Strategies and nursing orders are considered the *prescriptive* elements of the planning component. The nursing model, nursing diagnoses, goals, and objectives form the basis for choosing strategies and nursing orders. Several strategies exist that stem from scientific and practice disciplines. The principles of nursing practice include those strategies unique to the nursing profession.

Nursing orders are specified to give direction to the nurse, client, and others to achieve the outcomes identified. Nursing orders address the client's unique situation as well as similar patterns of human responses. The nursing care plan is the tool used for documenting all plans for implementation.

Implementation, or the act of carrying out the nursing care plan, is addressed in Chapter 11. The importance of following the plan as written is stressed.

## REFERENCES AND READINGS

American Nurses' Association: Standards of nursing practice, Kansas City, Mo, 1973, The Association.

American Nurses' Association: Standards: psychiatric-mental health nursing practice, Kansas City, Mo, 1973, The Association.

Bailey JT and Claus KE: Decision making in nursing: tools for change, St Louis, 1975, The CV Mosby Co.

Benner P and Wrubel J: The primacy of caring: stress and coping in health and illness, Redwood City, Calif, 1989, Addison-Wesley Nursing.

Bloom B: Taxonomy of educational objectives: the classification of educational goals. Handbook I: cognitive domain, New York, 1956, David McKay Co, Inc.

Bower FL: The process of planning nursing care: nursing practice models, St Louis, 1982, The CV Mosby Co.

Bradley JC and Edinberg MA: Communication in the nursing context, New York, 1986, Appleton-Century-Crofts.

Brykcznski K: Health contracting, Nurse Pract 7(5):27, 1982.

Bulechek GM and McCloskey JC: Nursing interventions: treatments for nursing diagnoses, Philadelphia, 1985, WB Saunders Co.

Friedman MM: Family nursing: theories and assessment, New York, 1981, Appleton-Century-Crofts.

Gardner KG and LaSalle PC: Small groups and their therapeutic forces. In Stuart GW and Sundeen SJ, editors: Principles and practice of psychiatric nursing, St Louis, 1987, The CV Mosby Co.

Gaut D: A theoretical description of caring as action. In Leininger MM: Care: the essence of nursing and health, Thorofare, NJ, 1984, Charles B Slack, Inc.

Gillies DA: Nursing management: a systems approach, Philadelphia, 1989, WB Saunders Co.

Hamberger LK and Lohr JM: Stress and stress management: research and applications, New York, 1984, Springer Publishing Co, Inc.

Jensen DP: Patient contracting. In Bulechek GM and McCloskey JC, editors: Nursing interventions: treatments for nursing diagnoses, Philadelphia, 1985, WB Saunders Co.

Johnson SH: Nursing assessment and strategies for the family at risk: high-risk parenting, Philadelphia, 1986, JB Lippincott Co.

Kinney C et al: Support groups. In Bulechek, GM and McClos-key JC, editors: Nursing interventions: treatments for nursing diagnoses, Philadelphia, 1985, WB Saunders Co.

Leininger MM: Care: the essence of nursing and health, Thorofare, NJ, 1984, Charles B Slack, Inc.

Mayeroff M: On caring, New York, 1971, Harper & Row, Publishers, Inc.

Miller JF: Coping with chronic illness: overcoming powerlessness, Philadelphia, 1983, FA Davis Co.

Mitchell PH and Betrus PA: Adaptation, stress, coping, and stress management. In Phipps WJ et al, editors: Medical-surgical nursing, St Louis, 1987, The CV Mosby Co.

Monat A and Lazarus RS: Stress and coping: an anthology, New York, 1977, Columbia University Press.

Neuman B: The Neuman systems model, New York, 1982, Appleton-Century-Crofts.

Orem DE: Nursing concepts of practice, New York, 1985, Mc-Graw-Hill Book Co.

Peddicord HR: Behavior modification. In Stuart GW and Sundeen SJ: Principles and practice of psychiatric nursing, St Louis, 1987, The CV Mosby Co.

Pender NJ: Health promotion in nursing practice, Norwalk, Conn, 1987, Appleton & Lange.

Phipps WJ, Long BC, and Woods NF: Medical-surgical nursing: concepts and clinical practice, St Louis, 1987, The CV Mosby Co.

Pines AM and Aronson E: Burnout: from tedium to personal growth, New York, 1981, The Free Press.

Pohl ML: The teaching function of the nursing practitioner, Dubuque, 1981, Wm C Brown Co.

Ray MA: The development of a classification system of institutional caring. In Leininger MM, editor: Care: the essence of nursing and health, Thorofare, NJ, 1984, Charles B Slack, Inc.

Redman BK: The process of patient education, St Louis, 1988, The CV Mosby Co.

Rorden JW: Nurses as health teachers: a practical guide, Philadelphia, 1987, WB Saunders Co.

Sampson EE and Marthas MM: Group process for the health professions, New York, 1981, John Wiley & Sons, Inc.

Schaefer J: The interrelatedness of decision making and the nursing process, Am J Nurs 74:1852, 1974.

Spradley BW: Community health nursing: concepts and practice, Boston, 1985, Little, Brown & Co.

Steckel SB: Patient contracting, New York, 1982, Appleton-Century-Crofts.

Steele SM and Harmon VM: Values clarification in nursing, Norwalk, Conn, 1983, Appleton-Century-Crofts.

Stuart GW and Sundeen SJ: Principles and practice of psychiatric nursing, St Louis, 1987, The CV Mosby Co.

Sullivan EJ and Decker PJ: Effective management in nursing, Menlo Park, Calif, 1988, Addison-Wesley Publishers Co.

Sundeen SJ, Stuart GW, Rankin ED, and Cohen SA: Nurse-client interaction: implementing the nursing process, St Louis, 1989, The CV Mosby Co.

Watson J: Nursing: the philosophy and science of caring, Boulder, 1985, Colorado Association University Press.

Whaley LF and Wong DL: Nursing care of infants and children, St Louis, 1987, The CV Mosby Co.

Yura H and Walsh MB: The nursing process: assessing, planning, implementing, and evaluating, Norwalk, Conn, 1988, Appleton & Lange.

# Implementation

CHAPTER

11

ELIZABETH S. FAYRAM

---

## GENERAL CONSIDERATIONS

Implementation is the client and the nurse carrying out the plan of care. The nurse is responsible for client-focused, outcome-oriented nursing care as delineated in the plan. The primary focus of the implementation component is the provision of individualized, safe nursing care with a multifocal approach. Implementation of the plan involves completion of actions necessary to fulfill the goals and objectives as delineated in the plan. Actions may be carried out by the nurse, the client, family members, other health team members, or a combination of these. Implementation promotes client advocacy and coordination among team members.

This chapter begins with a discussion of the integration of previous components of the nursing process into the implementation component. Three categories of skills necessary for implementation are described. The three phases that comprise the implementation component are presented, including a description of nurse behaviors that occur in each phase. Documentation regarding the implementation component is explored. The guidelines for implementation are listed here and discussed at the end of the chapter.

1. The actions performed are consistent with the plan and occur after validation of the plan.
2. Interpersonal, intellectual, and technical skills are performed competently and efficiently in an appropriate environment.
3. The client's physical and psychological safety is protected.
4. Documentation of actions and client responses is evident in the health care record and care plan.

## INTEGRATION OF NURSING PROCESS COMPONENTS

The implementation component incorporates aspects of previous components of the nursing pro-

cess. Data collection continues, diagnoses are validated, and priorities and plans are reexamined. Assessment continues throughout the implementation component, providing further data about the concerns and strengths already identified or discovering new ones. Modifications of plans may be necessary before implementation proceeds. This is especially true when a period of time has elapsed between the nurse's contact with the client. For example, a nurse met one month ago with a single parent of a 6-week-old child. Before proceeding with the teaching plan regarding the need for immunizations that was agreed upon previously, the nurse reassesses the situation for changes that will make an impact on the implementation of the plan, such as the mother's concern about symptoms of a cold in the infant.

In other situations, such as in an emergency, the implementation component quickly follows the previous components (eg, assessment, diagnosis, planning). An adult with a history of atherosclerotic heart disease, who is complaining of chest pain, is quickly assessed. The concerns of "alteration in comfort: pain" and "potential alteration in tissue perfusion: cardiopulmonary" require the nurse to quickly implement a plan. Actions by the nurse, based on the nurse's level of proficiency and experience, are quickly initiated.

## IMPLEMENTATION SKILLS

The skills necessary to implement the plan are categorized as intellectual, interpersonal, and technical (Yura and Walsh, 1988). The nurse's ability to use these skills determines the success of the implementation of the plan. Nurses' levels of proficiency are based upon their knowledge, experience, and expertise (Benner, 1984). Novice practitioners need to attend to the steps or guidelines for these skills more specifically, whereas expert practitioners internalize the principles and can implement the skills with a more creative approach. In addition, clients' abilities to use these skills influence the extent of their participation and the outcome of the plan. Proficiency by other health team members in terms of these skills is also considered when involving others in the execution of the plan.

*Intellectual skills* involve the ability to reason and understand. These skills are used by the nurse in reviewing a currently existing plan as well as in determining how the plan is to be implemented. Decision-making is used as the nurse puts actions into order of priority or determines the timing of a procedure. The nurse's knowledge is used as the basis for scientific rationale for actions being implemented. Creativity and innovation are also intellectual skills used during this component of the nursing process. Observation skills are used by the nurse when collecting data regarding the client's reaction to implementation of the plan as well as when assessing actual and potential concerns of the client. The client's ability to reason and understand are also considered when the nurse is actively involved in implementing strategies such as teaching/learning and problem solving.

*Interpersonal skills* are used during the implementation component by the nurse while communicating with the client and while collaborating with other health team members or members of other agencies, for example, in making a referral. Interpersonal skills involve verbal and nonverbal communication techniques including active listening, the provision of clear explanations, and support as feelings are expressed. These techniques convey a concern and respect for the client and are consistent with the purpose of the interaction. The nurse's ability to develop therapeutic nurse-client relationships influences the success of the implementation component. The client's interpersonal skills are considered and used, for example, in family dynamics or in consultation with health professionals.

*Technical skills* involve performing a procedure competently and safely. The focus in performing technical skills is usually with the individual client, such as in the provision of skin care or performance of passive range of motion exercises. Technical skills are also used while implementing a plan with a family or community. An example is the nurse assisting parents to learn the correct procedure to attach their infant to an apnea monitor. Technical skills the nurse uses with community clients include demonstrating cardiopulmonary resuscitation to a group and running a film projector to show a film to a community group. Clients' technical skills are often being developed during the implementation component, such as self-administering an insulin injection and drawing blood from a Hickman catheter by a mother whose son is receiving chemotherapy.

Technical skills cannot be separated from intellectual and interpersonal skills. Intellectual skills related to technical skills include the nurse's knowledge of the principles and steps of the procedure, the expected outcomes, the possible complications, and the legal and ethical aspects of the procedure. The nurse uses decision-making when determining the appropriateness of modifications to the procedure.

Interpersonal skills related to technical skills are used to offer support and instructions to the client as well as to obtain data regarding the client's reactions. For example, prior to performing range of motion exercises, the nurse, through interaction, informs the client of the following:

1. Purpose of the action
2. Expected outcomes of the action
3. Client's role and responsibilities during the procedure
4. Equipment needed
5. Length of time the procedure will last
6. Sensations to be anticipated during the procedure
7. Amount of privacy that will be provided (Yura and Walsh, 1988)

## ACTIONS

Whether the nurse uses intellectual, interpersonal, or technical skills while implementing the plan, *actions* are being executed. The nurse is action oriented in teaching a family parenting skills, in supporting a client as the client ventilates feelings about adjustments in life after amputation of a leg or in assisting a community with the planning process regarding home health services.

The actions of the nurse as well as those of the client are based on the model incorporated, the strategies selected, and the nursing orders developed as part of the plan. The model, through its concepts relating to client, health, nursing, and environment, provides guidance to the nurse on roles and actions used with clients in relation to their health.

Orem (1985) describes three nursing systems: wholly compensatory, partly compensatory, and supportive-educative. Nurse and client actions are influenced by which system is necessary at a particular point in time. A client requiring the supportive-educative system needs assistance in decision-making, behavior control, or acquiring knowledge or skills. Actions used with this nursing system may include support, counseling, and teaching/learning, with active participation on the part of the client.

Strategies selected and the nursing orders included in the plan also influence the actions of the nurse and client. For example, when problem solving is the strategy selected with a group of adolescents, then actions taken by the group and the nurse are relevant to this strategy. The nurse facilitates problem solving by assisting the group to analyze the problem or to develop alternative solutions.

The model, strategies, and nursing orders also influence who carries out the actions of the plan. As described previously, the actions may be performed by the client, nurse, family members, or other health team members. During development of the plan, consideration is given to the skills necessary to carry out the actions, in terms of the client, the client's family members, other health team members, and the nurse. During implementation, this consideration continues. The nurse determines when the client or the family members are ready to carry out the actions. The nurse still remains accountable for the actions carried out by the client and the family members and facilitates the actions carried out by others.

## PHASES OF IMPLEMENTATION

Implementation occurs in three phases: preparation, implementation, and postimplementation. The nurse's responsibilities for each phase are delineated below.

### Preparation

The preparation phase of implementation involves preparing for the actual implementation of the plan. This phase consists of the following:

Knowledge of the plan
Validation of the plan
Knowledge and skills to implement the plan
Preparation of the client
Preparation of the environment

The nurse first becomes familiar with the established plan. The nurse may be familiar with the plan if he or she was involved in its development. The nurse can become familiar with the plan by listening to a verbal report or reading the written plan.

The plan is validated with the client and other health team members. By reviewing client records and using knowledge and experiences, the nurse determines whether the plan is still viable. Following are questions to consider regarding validity:

1. Is the plan relevant based on the client's status and concerns at this point in time?
2. Have priorities changed or remained the same?
3. Is the plan safe and based on sound rationale, including legal and ethical aspects?
4. Is the plan individualized?

Based on input from the client, other health team members, the client's record, and the nurse's knowledge and experiences, the nurse may determine that the plan needs to be revised. Modifications may be *temporary*, such as revising the time for implementation of the plan. A situation requiring temporary modification of the plan includes postponement of a teaching session when the client receives an unexpected visitor from out of town. A client's discomfort may also temporarily change priorities. Modifications to the plan may be *permanent*, for example, when the method of a procedure such as a dressing change is revised. In addition to time and method, modifications may include who is to implement the plan and where. If an elderly couple decides to have Meals on Wheels instead of going to the senior community center, validating the plan requires the nurse to be flexible enough to make the necessary changes when needed.

Another aspect of the preparation phase involves development of the nurse's knowledge and skills needed to implement the plan. If the nurse lacks the specific knowledge or skill, several options are available. The nurse may refer the plan to someone else, receive assistance from another nurse, read about the necessary knowledge or skill, or observe another nurse carry out the actions. The nurse should not attempt to implement actions without assistance when the nurse is inadequately prepared in knowledge and skill.

The nurse prepares the client for what will occur during implementation of the plan. The nurse explains the actions as well as the purpose, the expected sensations, the client's responsibilities, and the expected outcomes. Preparation of the client also involves providing privacy, preparing the client physically if necessary, such as positioning, and ensuring protection of the client's sense of modesty.

Prior to implementation of the plan, the nurse also prepares the environment. The nurse obtains the resources necessary to carry out the plan. The nurse assembles the equipment needed for procedures and the audiovisual material for learning purposes, and gathers other members of the health team to assist with implementing the plan, if necessary. Other aspects of preparing the environment involve ensuring adequate lighting, consideration of seating arrangements, and minimizing distractions and interruptions by shutting doors, informing others where and how long the nurse will be involved with the client, turning down the volume of televisions or radios, and finding a quiet room for a group meeting.

## Implementation

On completion of the preparation phase, the nurse carries out the plan with the client. The nursing care is client-focused and outcome-oriented, and meets the physical and psychological safety needs of the client. Skillful and efficient implementation of the plan enhances the provision of competent care. The nurse uses intellectual, interpersonal, and technical skills when providing nursing care.

*Client-focused* nursing care consists of being aware of the bio-psycho-social-spiritual aspects of the client and individualizing care. Examples are explaining a procedure thoroughly the first time the client experiences it, varying communication approaches according to age or cognitive level of the client, and allowing a newly formed group the time necessary to develop into the working phase of group development. Client-focused nursing care also involves the nurse acting in the role of client advocate, providing for active participation of the client, protecting client rights, and collaborating with other health care professionals.

Implementation of the plan is *outcome-oriented*. Actions are consistent with the goals and objectives of the plan. For example, the nurse implements the teaching and learning process as specified for counseling a pregnant teenager about nutrition. When appropriate, it is possible to meet several goals or objectives simultaneously. While assisting the client with a self-care deficit such as bathing or dressing, the nurse may also implement part of a teaching and learning plan. This uses time efficiently and focuses on the needs of the client.

The nurse provides for the *physical and psychological safety* of the client. Physical safety occurs when aseptic techniques are used, when assistance is obtained if necessary, and when the client is placed in a safe environment. Psychological safety and comfort are accomplished through interpersonal skills, for example, by explaining what is going to happen, holding an anxious client's hand during a procedure, and reinforcing the client's progress.

The nurse performs care *skillfully and efficiently*. Whether the actions involve intellectual, interper-sonal, or technical skills, the nurse performs them competently. The competent nurse is more likely to enhance the client's progress toward the goals and objectives of the plan. Efficiency in implementing the plan by using time management techniques allows more time for the nurse and client to interact or accomplish other objectives. When the nurse performs actions skillfully and efficiently, the client's trust and confidence in the nurse's competence are enhanced, furthering the nurse-client relationship.

Through the development of the plan and its validation in the preparation phase, the client's role in carrying out the plan has been established. When the client is actively involved in implementing part of the plan, the nurse's role shifts from provider of competent care to facilitator. The nurse ensures that safe and outcome-oriented care is provided. This is accomplished by adequate preparation, including thorough preparation of the client, and by being available to assist and support the client during the implementation of the plan.

An important responsibility during implementation is the collection of data regarding the client's reactions to the execution of the plan. These reactions include physical, psychological, social, and spiritual responses. The nurse uses the methods of observation, measurement, and interaction. During implementation of the plan, the nurse focuses on the client as well as on the specific procedure or the teaching plan being implemented. For example, the nurse notes when a client is becoming tired, when family members show improved verbal communication with each other, and when group members react to alternative solutions to problems. These client responses may indicate the client's readiness to progress further with implementation of the plan or the need to modify the plan.

## Postimplementation

When nursing actions are completed, the post-implementation phase begins. The first part of post-implementation involves closure between the nurse and client on the aspect of the plan being implemented. This includes summarizing what actions took place, clarifying information, answering questions, indicating follow-up with the client for evaluation or the implementation of other parts of the plan, and identifying the client's response to the implementation of the plan.

Following implementation of the plan, the nurse leaves the client in a safe, comfortable environment. For example, the siderails are raised, curtains opened, and bedside table and call button are placed within easy reach. Any equipment or teaching aid that the nurse and client used is removed and disposed of properly. The nurse is then responsible for the documentation of the actions implemented and the client's response to the actions as well as verbal communication to appropriate health team members to provide continuity and coordination of care.

## PROFESSIONAL NURSING ROLES

The nurse assumes a variety of roles during the implementation of the plan. As described in Chapter 1, professional nursing roles are practitioner, educator, researcher, collaborator, advocate, role model, evaluator, and leader/manager. The plan, strategies, nursing orders, and model integrated into the nursing process influence the roles used by the nurse during the implementation component. The nurse's own philosophy, such as willingness to incorporate research findings into nursing practice, also determine the roles used.

A professional nursing role often used during the implementation component is that of educator, which is enacted when the teaching/learning strategy has been selected. The role of practitioner is also used frequently, for example, when the principles of nursing practice are being implemented. Role modeling may be enacted when using therapeutic use of self as a strategy. Several roles may overlap and be enacted simultaneously, such as practitioner and advocate or collaborator, along with the role of leader/manager.

An important role of the nurse that is used during the implementation component is that of client advocate. Being an advocate for a client involves a nurse-client relationship based on mutuality and respect. The client is an active participant in relation to health needs. The nurse, as a client advocate, protects client rights and keeps the client first in priority (Leddy and Pepper, 1985). It also involves speaking on behalf of a client and forming collaborative relationships with others in the health care system so that health needs of a client are met.

In the role of leader/manager during the implementation component, the nurse is involved in coordination and also delegation of client care. Coordination is a leadership activity that the nurse performs during the implementation component as well as during other components of the nursing process such as planning. The nurse is the one health professional who focuses on the client's whole response to the health situation. Therefore, the nurse is responsible for coordinating the client's nursing care as well as other aspects of care needed, such as occupational therapy or counsel-

ing services in the community. While coordinating care, the nurse ensures that individuality is maintained, such as the scheduling of physical therapy to coincide with pain relief measures or referring to agencies with a sliding scale fee for those with limited income.

Coordination of care avoids duplication of effort and provides organized care so that the client's goals and objectives can be achieved. In providing effective client care, coordination requires frequent exchange of information among the nurse, client, and other health care members. Collaborative relationships and assertive communication techniques are used by the nurse when coordinating client care.

Delegation is another aspect of the role of leader/manager during the implementation component. *Delegation* is sharing responsibility, authority, and accountability with another health team member for actions performed with a client. At times it is necessary for the professional nurse to delegate certain actions to another health care member such as another professional nurse or a licensed practical nurse or to delegate from a primary nurse to an associate nurse.

The other health team member needs to be legally qualified to safely perform the actions. State laws, policies, job descriptions, educational preparation, and the health team member's strengths and limitations are used to guide the nurse regarding delegation of actions to another health team member. When a therapeutic nurse-client relationship is needed to accomplish the actions of the plan, delegation is not recommended. For example, clients who need to verbalize feelings or would benefit from encouragement and emotional support need a consistent professional caregiver.

Delegation works best if the actions are well defined. The nurse who is delegating to others provides the following:

- Clear objectives and instructions
- Checkpoints and follow-up
- An empathetic ear if problems arise (Vestal, 1987)

Guidelines to effective delegation involve selecting the right person to perform the actions and providing the health team member with sufficient instructions to carry out the actions with the client. Delegation requires an investment of time in preparing the health care member to perform the action. Instructions are to be as specific as possible. The other health care members need to know their exact responsibilities. The nurse also needs to develop an effective means of communication involving such things as feedback, problem solving, and client responses when delegation is occurring (Kron and Gray, 1987).

The nurse realizes that the actions done by another may not be performed exactly the same way. Proper selection and instructions can minimize inconsistency. The person to whom the action is delegated becomes accountable and responsible for the action. However, the nurse who delegates the action also retains responsibility and is accountable for the client's care (Sullivan and Decker, 1988).

Delegation allows the nurse to implement nursing care efficiently by using others to perform actions for which they are qualified. This provides the professional nurse with additional time for implementing other actions and accomplishing other components of the nursing process.

## DOCUMENTATION

Documentation of the implementation component involves the use of written records—the health care record and the care plan. The care plan is actually becoming a permanent part of the health care record in many agencies. Documentation describes the actions implemented by the nurse, client, or others in terms of the nursing diagnoses. The client's response to the implementation of the plan is also recorded. Responses consist of physical, psychological, social, and spiritual behaviors. The progress the client is making toward meeting the goals and objectives is noted on the care plan to provide continuity of care with other health team members. Documentation also includes a description of the actions that were not implemented and why, such as when priorities change.

Recording in the client's health care record guides future care by providing additional data and a reference point for changes that may take place. Documentation also fosters greater individualization of care and reduction in the duplication of efforts. The health care record improves the quality of care when it is used as an evaluation tool to determine what actions were effective and could be used again in similar situations. In addition, the health care record provides the legal proof that care was or was not given (Brill and Kilts, 1986).

To meet the purposes of documentation, various types of record systems have been formulated. In the traditional narrative or source format, nurses write notes for a given period of time or after each client contact. This format has been found to be ineffective because the narrative is usually unsystematic and includes information about several areas of concern in one paragraph. It becomes difficult to follow the progression of a concern during the course of the client's care.

To counteract the disadvantages of the unorganized narrative format, Weed (1970) developed the problem-oriented record. This multidisciplinary system consists of the following components:

Data base → Problem list → Plans → Progress notes

The data base consists of a history, physical examination, and laboratory data. The problem list is numbered and dated and is the first page of the client's health record. A plan for each problem is formulated and is numbered and titled according to the number and title in the problem list. The progress notes are the mechanism for follow-up on each problem. Progress notes consist of structured narrative notes, flow sheets, and a discharge summary. The narrative notes are structured using the SOAP format: subjective data, objective data, assessment, and plan (Berni and Readey, 1978).

The problem-oriented record has been modified to incorporate the components of the nursing process. The nursing diagnoses give direction to the planning, implementation, and evaluation of nursing care and therefore are used in the recording system. Each relevant nursing diagnosis appears in the problem list or a separate nursing diagnosis list and is addressed in the care plan. The progress notes address a specific nursing diagnosis and include the actions implemented, the client's reactions, and any additional data pertinent to that particular nursing diagnosis. The status of the concerns, goals, and objectives as well as recommendations for continuation or modification of the original plan is also recorded in the progress notes.

One format for writing progress notes oriented toward the nursing process is the SOAPIER method (Kron and Gray, 1987). It involves the following:

S Subjective data — Client statements/interactions
O Objective data — Nurse's observations and measurements
A Analysis — Status of nursing diagnosis
P Plan of care — Objectives and actions planned
I Implementation — Actions implemented
E Evaluation — Client responses to actions/outcomes
R Revision — Changes in plan when necessary

The entire format does not have to be used in every recording. An example of the SOAPIER method follows:

2/18/89 *Nursing diagnosis:* alteration in nutrition (more than body requirements)

**S:** I've lost 3 pounds. That's great! I really tried to watch the salt and I did my walking.

**O:** 3-lb wt loss in 2 weeks.

**A:** Remains 19% over ideal wt.

**P:** 1. Client will lose 1–2 lb per week until ideal wt reached.
   a. Continue with 1450 calorie, low-sodium diet.
   b. Weigh self 1/wk.
   c. Complete a 3-day food diary for next clinic visit in 1 month.
   2. Client will continue walking program at least 3×/wk for 30 min.

**I:** Discussed difficulties with diet.

**E:** Realizes that new nutritional patterns will be lifelong. Plans to continue with the 1450-calorie, low-sodium diet.

The type of record forms and method of charting are determined by the agency. Nurses often have input into the design of chart forms and the method of charting used in the agency. The method chosen should foster efficiency and be oriented toward the client's concerns and the nursing process.

An increasing number of nursing organizations are using computer systems to facilitate documentation in terms of care planning and recording actions and client responses. Automated care plans and progress notes benefit the nurse and the client by decreasing the time spent in documenting nursing care and revising care plans, increasing the accuracy and legibility of recordings, allowing immediate availability of the client record to other health team members, and providing efficient retrieval of information for the evaluation of care (Gillies, 1989).

When documenting implementation of the plan, the recording of actions and responses is done systematically, clearly, and accurately, no matter what type of record is used. Descriptions of behavior rather than labels are recorded. Attempts are made to avoid duplication of recording. Recording in a systematic, clear fashion benefits the client as well as the health care team.

## GUIDELINES FOR IMPLEMENTATION

The guidelines describe the important elements necessary for the implementation component.

1. *The actions performed are consistent with the plan and occur after validation of the plan.* Before actions are implemented, the plan is validated. Validation determines whether the plan is still relevant, of immediate concern, based on sound rationale, and in-

dividualized. The nurse ensures that the actions being implemented, whether by the client, nurse, or others, are purposeful and outcome oriented. The actions during implementation are directed toward meeting the plan.

2. *Interpersonal, intellectual, and technical skills are performed competently and efficiently in an appropriate environment.* Nursing actions during implementation consist of interpersonal, intellectual, and technical skills. The nurse needs to be competent and able to efficiently perform these skills to carry out the plan. The nurse's self-awareness of strengths and limitations contributes to providing competent and efficient care while enacting the professional nursing roles.

3. *The client's physical and psychological safety is protected.* During execution of the plan, the client's physical and psychological safety is ensured by adequately preparing the client, performing skillful and efficient nursing care, applying sound principles, individualizing actions, and supporting the client during the actions. A caring attitude and protection of client rights also are aspects of psychological safety.

4. *Documentation of actions and client response is provided in the health care record and care plan.* Documentation in the health care record consists of a description of the actions implemented and the client's response to the actions. Actions not implemented are also recorded, as well as the reason. In addition, documentation occurs on the care plan to provide continuity of care and to note the client's progress in meeting the goals and objectives.

## SUMMARY

Implementation involves client, nurse, and others in carrying out the plan. Other components of the nursing process, such as assessment and planning, continue during this component. The nurse's ability to perform interpersonal, intellectual, and technical skills influences the effectiveness of the actions provided. The implementation component consists of three phases: preparation, implementation, and postimplementation. In this chapter, the responsibilities and roles of the nurse, including client advocacy, coordination, delegation, and documentation during each phase of the implementation component were described.

## REFERENCES AND READINGS

Alfaro R: Application of nursing process: a step-by-step guide, Philadelphia, 1986, JB Lippincott Co.

American Nurses' Association: Standards of nursing practice, Kansas City, Mo, 1973, The Association.

Benner P: From novice to expert: excellence and power in clinical nursing practice, Menlo Park, Calif, 1984, Addison-Wesley Publishing Co.

Berni R and Readey H: Problem-oriented medical record implementation, St Louis, 1978, The CV Mosby Co.

Bradley JC and Edinberg MA: Communication in the nursing context, Norwalk, Conn, 1986, Appleton-Century-Crofts.

Brill EL and Kilts DF: Foundations for nursing, Norwalk, Conn, 1986, Appleton-Century-Crofts.

Bulechek GM and McCloskey JC: Nursing interventions: treatments for nursing diagnoses, Philadelphia, 1985, WB Saunders Co.

Gillies DA: Nursing management: a systems approach, Philadelphia, 1989, WB Saunders Co.

Iyer PW, Taptich BJ, and Bernocchi-Losey D: Nursing process and nursing diagnosis, Philadelphia, 1986, WB Saunders Co.

Kron T and Gray A: The management of patient care, Philadelphia, 1987, WB Saunders Co.

LaMonica E: The humanistic nursing process, Monterey, Calif, 1985, Wadsworth Health Sciences Division.

Leddy S and Pepper JM: Conceptual bases for professional nursing, Philadelphia, 1985, JB Lippincott Co.

Orem DE: Nursing: concepts of practice, New York, 1985, McGraw-Hill Book Co.

Peplau H: Interpersonal relations in nursing, New York, 1952, GP Putnam's Sons.

Roy Sr C: Introduction to nursing: an adaptation model, Englewood Cliffs, NJ, 1984, Prentice-Hall, Inc.

Soontit E: Installing the first operational bedside nursing computer system, Nurs Management 18:39, July 1987.

Sorenson KC and Luckmann J: Basic nursing: a psychophysiologic approach, Philadelphia, 1986, WB Saunders Co.

Sullivan EJ and Decker PJ: Effective management in nursing, Menlo Park, Calif, 1988, Addison-Wesley Publishing Co.

Sundeen SJ, Stuart GW, Rankin E et al: Nurse-client interaction: implementing the nursing process, St Louis, 1989, The CV Mosby Co.

Vestal KW: Management concepts for the new nurse, Philadelphia, 1987, JB Lippincott Co.

Weed LL: Medical records, medical education, and patient care, Cleveland, 1970, Case Western Reserve University Press.

Yura H and Walsh MB: The nursing process: assessing, planning, implementing, and evaluating, Norwalk, Conn, 1988, Appleton & Lange.

# Evaluation

JANET W. KENNEY

## GENERAL CONSIDERATIONS

Evaluation is a planned, systematic comparison of the client's health status with the desired expected outcomes. It is an ongoing, continuous, deliberate activity, which involves the client, nurse, and other health care team members. Knowledge of health, pathophysiology, and evaluation methods is required for an effective evaluation.

Evaluation serves several purposes. The major purpose is to determine the client's progress in meeting specified goals and objectives. Another important purpose is to judge the effectiveness of the nursing process components as they have been used. Nurses are accountable for designing effective care plans, implementing appropriate nursing actions, and judging the effectiveness of their nursing interventions. Unfortunately, systematic evaluation is often the most neglected part of the nursing process.

Ideally, evaluation is an integral part of each component of the nursing process, beginning with the initial assessment. The client's initial assessment serves as a baseline with which to compare changes in human responses and to determine the client's progress. The nursing diagnosis identifies the client's health concerns and directs the areas that will be evaluated. Client goals and objectives are the criteria for the client's improved health status. The client's current health behaviors are compared with the goals and objectives to determine the client's progress. During nursing implementation, the nurse appraises the client's response to the nursing orders and judges whether the plans are facilitating the client's progress. Based on the client's progress, the nurse may maintain, modify, or change the nursing care plan.

Both the client's progress and the nursing actions are considered in evaluation. In measuring the client's progress toward meeting the desired outcomes, the nurse also judges the effectiveness

of the nursing care plan and the quality of care, and identifies ways to promote attainment of goals and objectives. These actions demonstrate accountability for nursing actions and practice. Accountability implies responsibility for one's behavior; it requires the ability to define, explain, and measure the results of nursing actions. Evaluation helps the nurse identify nursing actions that are effective or ineffective, and also enhances the scientific foundation of professional nursing practice. Personal, experiential, and empirical knowledge increases through evaluation and serves as the basis for one's own practice.

This chapter begins with a brief history of the development of evaluation in nursing. The difference between the use of criteria and standards in evaluation is explained. Three major forms of evaluation, structure, process, and outcome, each are described and illustrated, along with the differences between concurrent and retrospective evaluation. General characteristics of evaluation are presented, including who should evaluate, what should be evaluated, and when evaluation should occur. Broad guidelines for the evaluation component of the nursing process are listed below and discussed later in the chapter.

### Guidelines for Evaluation

1. The nurse continuously monitors, appraises, and reassesses the client's response to nursing actions.
2. The client's response to nursing implementation is compared with the client's objectives to determine the extent to which the objectives have been achieved (formative evaluation).
3. The client's progress or lack of progress toward goal attainment is determined (summative evaluation).
4. The nursing care plan is revised to reflect changes in the client's condition or when the

goals or objectives have not been adequately met.

## HISTORICAL PERSPECTIVE

In the last two decades, evaluation of health care delivery has changed hands and focus, sparked by the concerns of consumers and the government over increasing costs and inadequate services. In health care agencies client evaluation was formerly the prerogative of physicians. With new legislation and interest among all health care providers, evaluation is now performed by each profession. In the 1970s the federal government created professional standard review organizations (PSROs) to monitor costs of health services, and the Joint Commission on the Accreditation of Hospitals (JCAH; 1985) developed guidelines to evaluate hospital services.

Traditionally nurses were evaluated by their supervisors. Characteristics such as clinical skills, organization, leadership, dependability, and punctuality were judged. These evaluations did not consider the effectiveness of nursing care or improvement in the client's health status. As the responsibility for evaluation was dispersed among health care professionals and agencies, nurses recognized the need to change their focus and improve their methods. Currently, professional nurses have established standards of quality care and measure their ability to meet those standards. This involves evaluating delivery of nursing care to both individual clients and agencies. Agency evaluation is usually called *quality assurance,* and may involve nursing audits with standard guidelines.

Evaluation of nursing care is a complex task, because it is extremely difficult to separate the unique contributions of nurses to client care from the overlapping functions of other team members. This difficulty in distinguishing nurses' unique activities makes it hard to evaluate the results of nursing actions. The activities unique to nursing must be identified and the results of nursing interventions evaluated. The profession continues to address these issues.

## CRITERIA AND STANDARDS

Although the terms criteria and standards are often used interchangeably in evaluation, they have very different meanings. *Criteria* are measurable qualities, attributes, or characteristics that specify skills, knowledge, or health status. They describe acceptable levels of performance by stating the expected behaviors of the client or nurse in the objectives or nursing orders. *Criteria are written by individual nurses in care plans:* they are *not* specified by an agency, institution, or professional nursing organization.

*Standards* represent acceptable, expected levels of performance by nursing staff or other health team members. *Standards are established by authority, custom, or general consent.* Professions, such as nursing, have developed standards to improve the level of practice. In 1973, the American Nurses' Association (ANA, 1974) established the Standards of Nursing Practice, which describe eight essential actions in the nursing process. These standards are broad, general statements that describe nursing practice. Most clinical specialty groups within the ANA have adopted and modified these standards to reflect clinical practice and teaching within the specialty. The standards provide a frame of reference for judging the quality of nursing care.

## FORMS OF EVALUATION

Evaluation has been categorized according to *what* is to be judged and *when.* Three major types of evaluation describe what is to be evaluated: structure, process, and outcome. Each is defined below.

Structure—the physical facilities, equipment, services, and credentials of employees

Process —the *nursing actions* within each component of the nursing process, which include:
- *Adequacy*—the amount and quality
- *Appropriateness*—relevance to each component and the client situation
- *Effectiveness*—ability to facilitate client goals and objectives
- *Efficiency*—conservation of time, energy and resources of client, health team, and agency

Outcome—the changes in the *client's behaviors,* which include:
- *Physiological responses*—temperature, wound healing, neurological responses
- *Psychological responses*—appropriate affect, congruent verbal and nonverbal behaviors
- *Psychomotor skills*—infant care, wound dressing, colostomy irrigation, crutch walking
- *Knowledge*—about illness, including drugs, treatments, diet, and prevention
- *Abilities*—to resolve grief, perform activities of daily living, exercise

Within the process and outcome types of evaluation, there are two forms, based on *when* the evaluation occurs:

**Table 12-1** Evaluation Forms

| Structure | Process | Outcome |
|---|---|---|
| **Purpose** | | |
| Structure evaluation measures the existence and adequacy of facilities, equipment, procedures, policies, and staffing to meet the client's needs | Process evaluation measures the adequacy of the nurse's actions and activities in implementing each component of the nursing process | Outcome evaluation measures the changes in the client's behavior in comparison with the expected response or the client's written goals and objectives |
| **Tools or instruments** | | |
| Joint Commission on the Accreditation of Health Organizations<br>Association of Operating Room Nurses nursing audit | Slater Nursing Competencies Rating Scale<br>Quality Patient Care Scale<br>Nursing audit | Wisconsin system<br>JCAHO performance evaluation procedure (PEP) partially |
| **Sources of data** | *Concurrent* | *Concurrent* |
| Procedure manuals<br>Policy statements<br>Position descriptions<br>Nursing care plans<br>Orientation plans and in-service programs<br>Staff educational level<br>Facilities and equipment available<br>Charting and Kardex | Nurse demonstrates knowledge and performance of skills<br>Chart contains evidence of nursing actions performed<br>*Retrospective*<br>Chart cites nursing procedures implemented, such as checking of vital signs and teaching | Client demonstrates new knowledge, skills, and physiological and psychosocial improvement in health status<br>*Restrospective*<br>Chart cites evidence of changes in clients behavior, skills, and knowledge |

Concurrent —*present*, ongoing evaluation as either nursing actions (process) or client behaviors (outcome) occur

Retrospective—*past* nursing actions or client behaviors that are evaluated *after* services to client have been discontinued

Each of the three major forms of evaluation is presented separately. Table 12-1 describes the different purposes, tools, and sources of data.

## Structure

The focus of structure evaluation is on the physical facilities, equipment, organizational pattern, services provided, and the employees' credentials for administrative and staff positions. The basic question addressed by this type of evaluation is: "Is the agency/institution able to provide the necessary services for the client population it serves?"

Most community agencies and organizations, including hospitals and health care centers, have established guidelines or policies describing the required facilities, equipment, administrative structure, and employee credentials and responsibilities. Also, the JCAH (1985) has specific standards that are used to evaluate hospitals periodically. Each state also has a Department of Public Health that establishes acceptable standards for hospitals,

health departments, long-term care facilities, and home health agencies.

## Process

Process evaluation focuses on the nurse's activities. These activities are judged by (1) observing the nurse's performance, (2) asking clients what the nurse did, and (3) reviewing the nurse's notes in the chart. Process evaluation looks at each component of the nursing process, and makes judgments about nursing care by asking the following questions:

Was the nursing care *adequate?*
Were nursing actions *appropriate?*
Were nursing strategies *effective?*
Were nursing actions accomplished *efficiently?*
There are two forms of process evaluation: concurrent (during the nursing action) and retrospective (after the client has been discharged).

*Concurrent process evaluation* judges nursing performance as it takes place. The nurse is observed during a client interaction, or the client may be asked what the nursing actions were. For example, a nurse may be evaluated while giving an injection on use of the appropriate technique, or after client instruction a nurse may be evaluated to determine whether specific topics were covered. The Slater

**Table 12-2** Methods of Process and Outcome Evaluation

| Process (Evaluation of Nurse) | Outcome (Evaluation of Client) |
| --- | --- |
| **Concurrent** | |
| *Client:* Ask the client about the actions performed by the nurse. | *Client:* Observe the client for changes toward improved health status through new knowledge, skills, or abilities. Observe the client's physiological status or psychosocial affect and behaviors for signs of improvement. |
| *Nurse:* Observe the nurse administering care, teaching, and examining client. | |
| *Chart:* Audit the client's chart for documentation of appropriate nursing action, plans, and evaluation while client is receiving service. | |
| **Retrospective** | |
| *Chart audit:* Look for documentation of nursing actions: nursing history, client goals and objectives, nursing plans, and actions implemented, such as vital signs, medications given, and teaching performed, after client has been discharged from the health service. | *Chart audit:* Look for documentation of changes in the client's health status, knowledge, abilities, or skills. Physiological and psychosocial behavioral changes toward improved health would also be appropriate evidence, after the client has been discharged from the health service. |

Nursing Competencies Rating Scale (Wandelt and Stewart, 1975) and the Quality Patient Care Scale (Wandelt and Ager, 1974) are examples of tools used for concurrent process evaluation. In addition, the client's chart may be reviewed while the client is receiving services in order to determine whether appropriate nursing actions are charted. Examples of concurrent process evaluation questions are:

- Does the nurse identify the client before giving medications?
- Is the consent form signed before the client's surgery?
- Are all procedures adequately explained to the client?
- Are all nursing actions properly performed?

*Retrospective process evaluation* judges nursing performance *after* services to the client have been discontinued. This evaluation, called a *nursing audit* or *chart review*, examines any aspect of nursing that should be documented in the client's chart and determines whether specific nursing actions were performed and documented. The audit is usually performed by trained clerks. Examples of tools for retrospective process evaluation include the Nursing Audit by Phaneuf (1972) and Monitoring Quality of Nursing Care forms developed by Jelinek and others (1974). The differences between concurrent and retrospective process evaluation are shown in Table 12-2. Examples of retrospective process evaluation questions are:

- Were the client's intake and output accurately recorded?
- Were a client history and nursing physical exam recorded?
- Were all medications and treatments signed?
- Were all relevant symptoms monitored on time?

**Outcome**

Outcome evaluation focuses on changes in client's health status and responses to his or her health concerns. Examples of these changes are altered physiological and psychological responses, acquired psychomotor skills, and increased knowledge and abilities. Outcome evaluation is based on the stated client outcomes and is directly related to efforts to promote, maintain, and restore the client's health. During nursing interventions, the nurse appraises the client's health status for changes that indicate progress toward the goals and objectives. Outcome evaluation, though difficult, is the most meaningful way to judge the effectiveness of nursing interventions. The client's progress toward meeting the expected outcomes is evaluated by asking these and other related questions:

- Have the client's *physiological* and *psychological responses* improved?
- What *psychomotor skills* can the client perform?
- What specific *knowledge* has the client acquired?
- What *abilities* has the client developed?

There are two forms of outcome evaluation: concurrent and retrospective.

*Concurrent outcome evaluation* judges the client's

*present* health status, skills, knowledge, and abilities *before* services to the client are discontinued. The nurse measures the client's progress by comparing the client's initial data base with the current health status in relation to the goals and objectives. This comparison can be done by observing the client directly or by examining the chart for documentation of client behaviors which indicate the client's health status, knowledge, or abilities.

The Wisconsin system, as reported by Hover and Zimmer (1978) illustrates a method of concurrent and retrospective outcome evaluation. Usually, outcome evaluations are individualized for each client; however, some hospitals have developed standardized expected client outcomes for specific diagnoses. Examples of concurrent outcome evaluation questions are:

- Can the client demonstrate crutch walking correctly?
- Does the client relate to others appropriately?
- Can the client prepare and administer insulin accurately?
- Are the client's vital signs stable?
- Is the client's surgical wound healing properly?

*Retrospective outcome evaluation* judges the client's health status and behaviors as documented in the chart *after* services to the client have been discontinued. The chart is examined for documentation of the client's progress toward meeting the goals and objectives, as a result of nursing intervention. The JCAH (1985) incorporated some aspects of retrospective outcome evaluation in their guidelines. The following are examples of retrospective outcome evaluation questions:

- Was the client able to demonstrate activities of daily living?
- Was the client's attitude positive upon discharge?
- Was the client able to plan a diabetic daily menu?
- Did the client demonstrate appropriate bonding behaviors?
- Was the client's caregiver able to perform physical care activities?

## CHARACTERISTICS OF EVALUATION

Three major aspects of evaluation need to be considered in the nursing process: *Who* participates in the evaluation? *What* should be evaluated? and *When* should evaluation occur? Evaluation always involves judgments based on knowledge and experience. The quality of health care is based on the values of those who participate in the evaluation.

They determine what is important to evaluate and when to evaluate. Therefore, the client, nurse, health team members, and agency all may be involved in evaluation.

*Who* participates in the evaluation? The ANA (1974) Standards of Nursing Practice has two standards related to the evaluation component of the nursing process. Standard VII states:

> The client's/patient's progress or lack of progress toward goal achievement is determined by the client/patient and the nurse.

This statement means that the client and nurse mutually evaluate the client's progress in achieving goals and objectives. Other health team members may also participate, but the nurse is responsible for writing the evaluation data in the client's chart.

*What* should be evaluated? Ultimately, the client's health behaviors, which indicate progress or lack of progress toward goal attainment, are evaluated. The nurse may focus solely on the client's progress and achievement of specific objectives, or the nurse may broaden the evaluation to include all aspects of the nursing process. In evaluating the nursing process each component that contributed to the client's behavioral changes and progress is examined. This broad, comprehensive process evaluation includes judging the *adequacy, appropriateness, effectiveness,* and *efficiency* of each component. This type of evaluation may be part of a quality assurance study in a health care organization.

Some questions that the nurse may use to evaluate the effect of the nursing process in facilitating the client's progress toward goal achievement follow.

### Assessment

*Adequacy*
- Was the data collection comprehensive and multifocal?
- Were sufficient data collected on the client's health concerns?
- Were data collected from a variety of sources?
- Was the client's record updated periodically?

*Appropriateness*
- Were appropriate methods used for data collection?
- Were the data relevant to the client's health concerns?
- Were relevant data verified by others?

*Effectiveness*
- Were there sufficient data to establish nursing diagnoses?

*Efficiency*
- Were data collected in a systematic, organized manner using a nursing model?

**Diagnoses**

*Adequacy*
- Were nursing diagnoses clear and concise?
- Were *all* nursing diagnoses client-centered, specific, and accurate?
- Did all nursing diagnoses include an etiological statement?
- Were all the client's health concerns identified?

*Appropriateness*
- Were the diagnoses relevant to the client and the agency?
- Were the diagnoses appropriate for nursing intervention?
- Were the diagnoses mutually agreed on by the client and the nurse?
- Were the diagnoses appropriate to the resources and the timetable?

*Effectiveness*
- Did the nursing diagnoses accurately reflect the data analysis?
- Did the nursing diagnoses guide client goals and objectives?
- Did the nursing diagnoses guide planning and interventions?

**Planning**

*Adequacy*
- Were the client objectives sufficient to achieve each goal?
- Were there sufficient nursing orders to achieve each objective?
- Did the strategy and nursing orders clearly guide nursing interventions?
- Were the nursing plans clearly documented?

*Appropriateness*
- Were client goals appropriate to their respective diagnoses?
- Were client goals and objectives prioritized appropriately?
- Were the objectives and nursing orders in a logical sequence?
- Were the plans realistic for the client, the setting, and the timetable?

*Effectiveness*
- Was the client agreeable to the plans?
- Did the plans facilitate the client's progress?
- Was the client satisfied with the plans and progress?

*Efficiency*
- Did the plans use resources and team members efficiently?

**Implementation**

*Adequacy*
- Were all the plans implemented accordingly?
- Were team members able to follow the plans?
- Were all resources available as needed?

*Appropriateness*
- Were nurses able to implement the nursing orders?

- Were the client's safety, privacy and confidentiality maintained?
- Were the nursing actions realistic to achieve client objectives?

*Effectiveness*
- How did the client respond to nursing actions?
- Did the nursing actions facilitate the client's progress?
- Were client's goals and objectives achieved within timetable?

*Efficiency*
- Were nursing actions performed efficiently?
- Were resources used economically?
- Was the client's energy expenditure minimized?

*When* should evaluation occur? Evaluation is an ongoing process and includes both formative and summative elements. Formative evaluation is the continuous judgment of the client's health status and progress in meeting the objectives. It begins with the initial assessment, during which baseline data are collected for comparison at a later time. In the planning component, client outcomes are identified for ongoing comparison with the client's health status. During interventions, the nurse monitors, appraises, and reassesses the client's response. As data accumulate, the nurse identifies the client's pattern or behavioral trend, and compares this with the initial data base and the stated client objectives and timetable. Then, the nurse judges the level of the client's progress toward achieving the objectives. As the plan is implemented, the nurse evaluates the client's response to determine the effectiveness of the plan or the need to change the plan.

*Formative evaluation* may be performed by the nurse as frequently as every few minutes in a life-threatening situation, every hour, during every change of shift, or daily or weekly. The frequency depends on the health status of the client, the types of client changes expected, and the unit or agency policies. For example, an unconscious client in an acute care unit may need to be checked every 15 minutes for signs of change, whereas a home health client with a chronic disability may be evaluated on a weekly schedule.

While implementing nursing care, the nurse evaluates the effects of the nursing actions in achieving the plan and the client's progress toward attaining the objectives. Formative evaluation compares the client's response with the actions in the plan and the client's progress toward achieving the objectives. This serves as a basis for continuing or changing the plans. For example, the nursing orders may state, "The client will discuss dietary likes and dislikes." The client's response, "Mr. Smith said he likes red meat and chicken, but won't eat liver or seafood," may be included in the formative evaluation by the nurse.

*Summative evaluation* occurs after the client has met several objectives. The nurse judges the client's progress or lack of progress toward goal attainment. The nurse writes a summary of how well or to what degree the client has progressed toward attaining each goal. Sometimes objectives or resources are insufficient to attain a goal, or the timetable for accomplishment is unrealistic. Occasionally, the objectives may be met, but the client has not achieved the goal. For example, the goal may state, "The client will modify his diet to lose weight." After achieving several objectives toward this goal, the nurse's summative evaluation may read, "The client can explain the reasons for weight loss and plan appropriate menus, but lacks motivation to stay on the diet. Further counseling is needed." The summative evaluation describes how well and to what degree the client has achieved the goals.

## REVISING THE NURSING CARE PLAN

After comparison of the client's progress toward achieving the objectives with progress toward goal attainment, the nurse is responsible for revising the nursing care plan. This responsibility is clearly stated in Standard VIII of the ANA (1974) Standards of Nursing Practice, which reads

> The client's/patient's progress or lack of progress toward goal achievement directs reassessment, reordering of priorities, new goal setting, and revision of the plan of nursing care.

During both formative and summative evaluation, the nurse judges the client's response to determine the effectiveness of the nursing care plan. The client may have achieved several objectives completely, partially, or not at all. The nurse compares the client's health status with the objectives and timetable and makes *one* of the following decisions:

1. Continue the plan as documented.
2. Reconsider the importance or priority of the objectives.
3. Modify the nursing actions, client objectives, goals or timetable.
4. Change the nursing diagnoses and care plan.

If the objectives were achieved, has the client met the goal? If the goal was met, has the nursing diagnosis been alleviated or resolved? If the client's health concern was alleviated, this is documented in the chart and further action is not required.

However, if the concern is temporarily resolved, the nurse would continue to monitor the client's progress. If the objectives are only partially met, or not met at all, the nurse must reassess the client and evaluate the nursing care plan to determine the reason for the client's lack of progress.

Following are some explanations for modifying or revising the nursing care plan:

The nursing diagnosis was inaccurate.

The client's condition changed or new diagnoses occurred.

The nursing orders were unrealistic (inadequate time or resources).

The nursing orders overestimated or underestimated the client's capabilities.

Additional data altered the client's health concern.

Resources were unavailable or became available.

Another nursing strategy may be more appropriate.

## GUIDELINES FOR EVALUATION

The guidelines describe the broad phases of the evaluation component. They presuppose the achievement of all the preceding components in the nursing process. Example of individual, family, and community evaluations are shown on pages 227 to 229. These reflect evaluations of selected objectives to meet designated goals.

1. *The nurse continuously monitors, appraises, and reassesses the client's response to nursing actions.* While implementing any nursing order, the nurse observes the client's current health status and response to the nursing intervention. The nurse also reviews the client's chart and notes changes in the client's condition as a result of nursing care. The results of blood studies, chest x-ray studies, urinalysis, and vital signs may be useful in evaluating the client's progress. The nurse also checks on the client's or family's compliance with the prescribed therapeutic regimen and tests. The client's understanding of information or care is also ascertained.

2. *The client's response to nursing implementation is compared with the client's objectives to determine the extent to which the objectives have been achieved (formative evaluation).* The nurse judges the appropriateness of the nursing actions and their intended and unintended effects on the client and family. The nurse compares what the client is able to do with the stated objectives. The effectiveness of the nursing orders is determined by changes in the client's behavior. The client's statements and behaviors, such as physiological and psychological responses, skills, knowledge, and abilities, are written in the

## Example of Individual Evaluation

*Nursing model:*    Orem's Self-Care model was chosen to guide the nursing process because the client required supportive education.

*Nursing diagnosis:*    Inadequate knowledge of diabetic diet.

*Client goal:*    The client will apply the American Diabetic Association (ADA) diabetic diet in menu planning and daily nutritional intake.

*Objective:*    The client will accurately plan his diabetic meals for 3 days by April 10, 1989.

*Strategy:*    The teaching-learning strategy is used in this example.

### Nursing orders

**1** The nutritionist will meet with the client and explain the ADA diabetic diet by 3/20/89.

**2** The nutritionist or nurse will provide the following literature on diabetic diets by 3/22/89. (List names of diabetic booklets.)

**3** The client and nurse will discuss the ADA diabetic diet by 3/23/89 to determine:
  **a** Client's comprehension.

  **b** Client's food preference.

  **c** Need for more teaching.
  **d** Need for family involvement.

**4** The client will write three daily menu plans that meet the ADA diabetic standards for him by 3/24/89.

**5** The client and nurse will discuss the client's three written menus by 3/26/89 in relation to:
  **a** Accuracy.

  **b** Preparation.

  **c** Food preference.

### Formative evaluation

On 3/18/89 Miss S., the nutritionist, met with Mr. G. and explained the diabetic diet. Mr. G. was receptive, asked relevant questions, and took notes.

On 3/19/89 Mr. G. was given three booklets on the diabetic diet. He read and highlighted them that evening.

Mr. G. correctly stated carbohydrate (CHO), protein, and fat intake for his diet.

Mr. G. stated that he will give up sweets, but will miss ice cream.

Mr. G. was unsure of how to calculate CHO intake.

Mr. G. asked if we would explain his diet to his daughter, who cooks for him.

Mr. G. wrote three daily menu plans, which included snacks. These plans were accurate in fat and protein but excessive in CHO on 2 days.

On 3/26/89 the client and nurse discussed Mr. G.'s three menu plans.

Mr. G. recognized his excess CHO intake and was able to correct it.

Mr. G. described how he or his daughter would prepare his diet.

Mr. G.'s three menus reflected his personal food preferences.

### Summative evaluation

Mr. G. has shown some progress toward goal achievement by writing three accurate daily diabetic menus. Continued supervision will be necessary. It is recommended that he continue writing menu plans and that his daughter meet with the nutritionist to receive instruction in diabetic menu planning. More objectives are needed to reach the goal.

# Example of Family Evaluation

*Nursing model:*    Friedman's Structural-Functional model was chosen for the nursing process since the client's safety hazards could be addressed in the *physical necessities and care* subconcept.

*Nursing diagnosis:*    Inadequate safety precautions in the home.

*Family goal:*    The family will eliminate safety hazards to children from their home (mutually established).

*Objective 1:*    The family will identify ways to remove safety hazards from their home by 6/5/89.

*Strategy:*    Counseling and teaching-learning strategies were used with this family.

| Nursing orders | Formative evaluation |
|---|---|
| 1 The nurse will write a checklist of safety factors that homes with small children should have. | On 4/30/89 the nurse, after consultation with the health department, wrote a safety checklist. |
| 2 The family and nurse will discuss the checklist and the family will complete the list by 5/15/89. | On 5/5/89 Mr. and Mrs. T. seemed enthusiastic in reading the checklist and agreed to fill it in during the next week. On 5/7/89 the nurse visited the family, but they had not completed the safety list. They promised to work on it. |
| 3 The family and nurse will discuss the results of the safety checklist by 5/20/89. | On 5/15/89 the checklist was completed and discussed with the family. Four areas were deficient, and the family agreed to work on improving safety in those areas. |
| 4 The family and nurse will explore ways to eliminate safety hazards in four areas by 5/25/89. | On 5/20/89 the family and nurse discussed several ways to remove each safety hazard. |

*Objective 2:*    The family will remove safety hazards from their home by 6/30/89.

| | |
|---|---|
| 1 The family will decide the best way to eliminate safety hazards in their home by 6/1/89. | The family discussed alternatives for eliminating each safety hazard and decided on a specific measure for each on 6/1/89. |
| 2 The family will implement each safety precaution they previously decided on by 6/21/89. | On 6/7/89 the family agreed to take the necessary measures but had not had time to do so yet. On 6/14/89, the family showed the nurse how they had corrected each safety hazard. The family seemed pleased by their action. |
| 3 The family and nurse will evaluate the results of their safety precautions by 6/30/89. | On 6/21/89 the family and nurse discussed the family's feelings about precautions, and the family expressed relief and gratitude to the nurse. |

## Summative evaluation

This family was able to identify and correct four safety hazards to their children in the home. The family took appropriate measures to eliminate safety hazards, and maintained these measures. The family goal was effectively met; no further action is deemed necessary at this time.

## Example of Community Evaluation

*Nursing model:*      The Community-as-Client model was chosen for this example because teenagers represent an aggregate core and the health concern could be analyzed in the eight subsystems.

*Nursing diagnosis:*  Increased incidence of venereal disease among teenagers in the community.

*Community goal:*     The community will reduce the incidence of venereal disease among teenagers by 9/30/89.

*Objective:*          Appropriate community officials will develop strategies to reduce venereal disease by 7/30/89.

*Strategy:*           Problem-solving and collaboration strategies were used to meet the objective.

**Nursing orders**

1 The nurse will meet with the public health department, county board of health, and high school personnel to discuss (1) the increased incidence of venereal disease, (2) complications of venereal disease, and (3) venereal disease control strategies by 6/20/89.

2 The nurse will develop a list of strategies for improving teenagers' knowledge of prevention and treatment of venereal disease from suggestions of community health members by 6/30/89.

**Formative evaluation**

On 6/5/89 the nurse and public health officials met and discussed the nursing order. Three of five members expressed an interest in developing improved educational services.

On 6/10/89 the nurse and 10 members of the county board of health met to discuss the nursing order. The board moved to increase educational services and publicity to reduce the incidence of venereal disease among teenagers.

On 6/18/89 the nurse met with six high school personnel to discuss the nursing order. They suggested having a special assembly program on venereal disease.

The nurse developed the following list of strategies from suggestions of community members contacted above: (1) radio and television messages, (2) venereal disease pamphlets distributed in high school, (3) high school assembly on venereal disease, and (4) posters with information on signs of venereal disease, and treatment clinics.

**Summative evaluation**

Community members from the public health department, the county board of health, and the high school met with the nurse during June 1989 to discuss the increased incidence of venereal disease among teenagers and to suggest strategies to reduce the incidence. Each group demonstrated an interest in reducing this community concern and offered several suggestions for improving education about venereal disease and trying to reduce the incidence. Community members are aware of the problem, but the nurse will follow up and facilitate community action to improve educational service and clinic information. Some progress has been made toward goal achievement, but follow-up is necessary. More objectives are needed to achieve the goal.

chart and in the evaluation column of the nursing care plan. Appropriate information from the family and health team members is also recorded. Then the nurse judges whether and to what extent the client has progressed in achieving the objectives. The nurse decides whether the objectives have been completely met, partially met, or not met at all. Based on this decision, the nurse also decides whether a change is needed in the plan of care.

3. *The client's progress or lack of progress toward goal attainment is determined (summative evaluation)*. The nurse evaluates the client's response in meeting the objectives and judges whether the client's behavior shows progress toward goal achievement. Is the client's response desirable and reasonable, considering the alloted time and situation? Have the client's needs, concerns, or potential concerns been resolved, and if so, to what extent? The nurse may gather evaluation data from the family, team members, and chart. The client's response, indicating progress or lack of progress toward goal achievement, is recorded in the chart and in the nursing care plan. Then the nurse determines whether there is a need to change the goals or to revise the objectives or nursing orders.

4. *The nursing care plan is revised to reflect changes in the client's condition or when the goals or objectives have not been adequately met*. Modification of the nursing orders, objectives, or goals is the last phase in the evaluation process. If the goals were easily met, perhaps the nursing care plan is moving too slowly or at just the right pace. The client's behavior may show little or no change or change in the wrong direction. If the goals and objectives were only partially met or not met at all, the nurse must gather more information to determine what happened. At this point, the nurse may need to examine the adequacy, appropriateness, effectiveness, and efficiency of each component of the nursing process. Relevant questions that may be addressed were listed earlier in this chapter. The nurse considers the possible reasons why the orders, objectives, or goals were not achieved and then decides whether to reassess the client or revise the care plan. New goals, objectives, or orders would be mutually established by the client and nurse and written in the Kardex or chart and the nursing care plan.

## SUMMARY

Evaluation is an ongoing, systematic, planned process of comparing the client's health status with the expected outcomes. Evaluation involves comparing the client's present responses with previous responses to determine the client's progress in

achieving the objectives and goals. Judgments about the client's progress are made from interactions, observations, and measurements by the nurse, client, family, and team members. If progress is insufficient toward attaining the objectives and goals, the client and nurse revise the plan of care.

## REFERENCES AND READINGS

Alfaro R: Application of nursing process: a step-by-step guide, Philadelphia, Pa, 1986, JB Lippincott Co.

American Nurses' Association: Standards of nursing practice, Am Nurse 6:11, July 1974.

Barba M, Bennet B, and Shaw WJ: The evaluation of patient care through use of ANA's standards of nursing practice, Superv Nurse 9:42, January 1978.

Deets C and Schmidt A: Process criteria based on standards, AORN J 26:685, 1977.

Deets C and Schmidt A: Outcome criteria based on standards, AORN J 27:657, 1978.

Dickson N: Quality assurance: do you measure up?, Nurs Times 83(44):25, 1987.

Foglesong D: Standards promote effective production, Nurs Manage 18(1):24, 1987.

Hegyvary ST and Haussmann RK: The relationship of nursing process and patient outcomes, NLN Pub 21-2194: 29, 1987.

Hover J and Zimmer M: Nursing quality assurance: the Wisconsin system, Nurs Outlook 26:242, 1978.

Iyer PW et al: Nursing process and nursing diagnosis, Philadelphia, 1986, WB Saunders Co.

Jelinek RC et al: A methodology for monitoring quality of nursing care, HEW Publication (HRA) 74-25, 1974.

Joint Commission on the Accreditation of Hospitals: Accreditation manual for hospitals, Chicago, 1985, The Commission.

Joint Commission on the Accreditation of Hospitals: Procedure for retrospective patient care audit in hospitals, nursing edition, Chicago, 1973, The Commission.

Kanar RJ: Standards of nursing practice assessed through the application of the nursing process, J Nurs Qual Assur 1(2):72, 1987.

Kemp N: Monitoring the nursing process, Nurs Focus 4(8):1, 1983

Law GM: Accountability in nursing: providing a framework, Nurs Times 79(40):34, 1983.

Lillesand KM et al: Nursing process evaluation: a quality assurance tool, Nurs Adm Q 7(3):9, 1983.

Machie LCR et al: Quality assurance audit for the nursing process, Nurs Times 78(42):1757, 1982.

Mehmert PA: A nursing information system: the outcome of implementing nursing diagnoses, Nurs Clin North Am 22(4):943, 1987.

Patterson CH: Standards of patient care: the Joint Commission focus on nursing quality assurance, Nurs Clin North Am 23(3):625, 1988.

Phaneuf M: The nursing audit: profile for excellence, New York, 1972, Appleton-Century-Crofts.

Pinnell NN: The nursing process: theory, application, and related processes, New York, 1986, Appleton-Century-Crofts.

Richards DA and Lambert P: The nursing process: the effect on patients' satisfaction with nursing care, J Adv Nurs 12(5):559, 1987.

Roeder MA: Patient care plans and the evaluation of nursing process, Superv Nurse 11:57, June 1980.

Roper N and others: Identifying the goals: the importance of assessment and evaluation in the nursing process, Nurs Mirror 156(24):22, 1983.

Runtz SE et al: Evaluating your practice via a nursing model: the Orem self-care model and the Peplau interpersonal process model, Nurse Pract 8(3):30, 1983.

Schmidt A and Deets C: Writing measurable nursing audit criteria, AORN J 26:495, 1977.

Schmidt A and Deets C: Responsibilities for audit criteria, AORN J 27:657, 1978.

Smeltzer CH, et al: Nursing quality assurance: a process, not a tool, J Nurs Adm 13(1):5, 1983.

Tucker SM et al: Patient care standards: nursing process, diagnosis, and outcome, St Louis, 1988, The CV Mosby Co.

Wandelt MA and Ager JW: Quality Patient Care Scale, New York, 1974, Appleton-Century-Crofts.

Wandelt MA and Stewart DS: Slater Nursing Competencies Rating Scale, New York, 1975, Appleton-Century-Crofts.

Watson A and Mayers M: Evaluating the quality of patient care through retrospective chart review, J Nurs Adm 6:17, March-April, 1976.

Zimmer MJ: Quality assurance for outcomes of patient care, Nurs Clin North Am 9:305, 1974a.

Zimmer MJ: Guidelines for development of outcome criteria, Nurs Clin North Am 9:317, 1974b.

SECTION

III

# Application of the Nursing Process to Practice

# Nursing Process of the Individual Client in the Hospital

LINDA J. DRIES
CATHY D. MEADE
PAULA J. CHRISTENSEN

The client in this case study is a 15-year-old female (C.L.) who is facing knee surgery. She is an active participant in school sports, on the track team, is an avid runner, and has many friends. Her academic work is above average and she hopes to get a college scholarship. She had a skiing accident that necessitates hospitalization and corrective surgery. She is concerned about activity limitations that the surgery will impose on her. In selecting a nursing model to guide the development of C.L.'s care plan, a critical analysis of the concepts of a model and its application to nursing practice are necessary. Recent emphasis has been placed on client participation and accountability for health care. A model that is congruent with this aspect of client participation is Orem's (1985) concepts of nursing practice, which provides a framework for self-care.

Orem's generalized model of nursing is comprised of three major concepts. First, the type of assistance that the nurse can provide to the client may be focused on universal, developmental, or health deviation self-care requisites. Second, self-care deficits determine the relationship that is established between client and nurse. The central idea is that clients can benefit from the nurse, either through support/education, partial assistance with deficits, or total assistance. A self-care limitation is present when self-care demands are not within the capability of the client, and the nursing domain can help meet these demands. Last, nurs-

The authors wish to thank Mary Linn Swanson, R.N., M.S.N. and Bonnie Zollman, R.N., B.S. (SwedishAmerican Hospital Rockford; IL) for their thoughtful review and suggestions about this case example.

ing systems identify the qualities and capabilities of the nurse that can assist the client in maximizing self-care. Inherent in Orem's model is the recognition that a variety of factors may influence the establishment of this relationship, such as gender, age of client, knowledge competencies, previous hospital experiences, and values placed on health (Orem, 1985).

The first type of requisite refers to conditions common to all individuals that are related to basic human structure and functioning. The six *universal* self-care requisites are maintenance and balance of air, water, intake of food; rest/activity; elimination; solitude/social interaction; prevention of hazards; and promotion of human functioning and development. In our case example, hospitalization and surgery necessitate incorporation of these requisites into a plan of nursing care for C.L. The second type of requisite refers to *human development* processes that occur during an individual's life span—in the case of C.L., adolescence. *Health deviation* self-care requisites are reflective of conditions that develop abnormally. Such requisites represent structural or functional deviations that may exist in persons who are ill or injured (eg, knee injury). When care is directed toward meeting these requisites, the likelihood for self-actualization and control over health is increased. All these requisites help initiate and foster the development of the nurse-client relationship (Orem, 1985). Self-care is the second major concept within Orem's model of nursing and delineates self-care activities as learned behaviors that may vary among individuals.

Featuring the client in a central focus with rights

and responsibilities makes Orem's model of nursing very appealing in a clinical setting. The concept of self-care implies that individuals can increase their competencies required for self-care in illness. Nurses have the responsibility and skills necessary in assisting clients to increase their self-care capabilities. At times, the nurse may provide and compensate totally for the client's self-care deficits, for example, immediately after surgery. In other instances, partially compensated care occurs when the nurse and client work together in increasing self-care abilities, such as, during the recovery period as C.L. learns ambulation. A third variation of nurse-client relationships may be based on the supportive-educative system. This situation occurs when the client needs assistance in performing required care activities; for example, the nurse provides teaching, guidance, and support to C.L. as she copes with body image changes.

The following case study is guided by Orem's model of nursing and specifically focuses on self-care deficits that emphasize that individuals can benefit from nursing because health limitations are predictive of nursing requirements. When a self-care deficit exists in the client's knowledge, motivation, or skill, for example, as related to knee sur-

gery, the nurse is uniquely qualified to assist in maximizing the client's self-care agency. The nursing goal in this case example is to maintain and assist C.L. in returning to her previous level of self-care activities. The nursing process described in this chapter reflects three consecutive days of contact with C.L., starting with the night before surgery.

The nursing process is organized into two sections. First, the nursing assessment, analysis/synthesis, and nursing diagnoses for each of the 3 consecutive days are presented. Then, the nursing plans, which include the goals, objectives, strategies, nursing orders, scientific rationale, and evaluation, are presented. Although plans for implementation are placed last, they are written after the initial assessment and are implemented and updated with each successive visit. The dates of each implementation are identified in the objectives, orders, and evaluations. The nursing plans—goals through evaluation—are written consecutively to show their interrelationship and sequence. They are placed at the end of the nursing process because they are ongoing and subject to revision and because they demonstrate the continuity of the care plan.

## DATA COLLECTION: Day 1—Preop 1/14/89

| Interactions | Observations | Measurements |
|---|---|---|
| | **From chart:** | **From chart:** |
| | Client's initials: C.L. | Age: 15 years |
| | Reason for admission: Rt anterior cruciate & medial collateral ligament repair; right medial meniscectomy 1/15/89. | Urinalysis: color—yellow; clarity—clear; sp gr—1.031; pH—5.0; protein—neg; glucose—neg; acetone—neg; Hb—neg; WBC—none; RBC—none. |
| | No previous health concerns noted. | Complete blood count: WBC—8.0; RBC—5.67; Hb—17.1; HCT—50.8; MCV—90; MCH—30.2; MCHC—33.7 (All within hospital norms) |
| | No known allergies. | |
| | Lives with parents. | |
| | Religious preference: Protestant. | Chest x-ray: WNL. |
| | Insurance: Blue Cross/Blue Shield. | Admission blood pressure: 110/70. |
| | Surgical consent signed by mother. | Admission TPR: 98.4°, 90, 20. |
| | Regular diet—no specific food preferences; drinks 8 glasses water or juice/day. | Height: 5'3". |
| | | Weight: 115 lb. |
| | NPO after midnight. | Preop medications: Reglan 10 mg, Zantac 150 mg, Valium 5 mg p.o. together on call. |

## DATA COLLECTION: Day 1—Preop 1/14/89—cont'd

| Interactions | Observations | Measurements |
|---|---|---|
| | **From client:** | |
| Hi! Yeah, I'm C.L. | Eye contact with nurse; smiles. | |
| My mother will be here later, | Lying supine in bed with head of | |
| Oh, pretty good. | bed up. | |
| Well, my right knee hurts a lot. | Rt leg is in an immobilizer. | |
| | Rt knee is swollen. | |
| | Head is resting on pillow. | |
| | Looks down toward bed, and then | |
| | up at nurse. | |
| | Flat facial expression. | |
| Yeah, I really like running. I like | **From client:** | |
| sports in general. I swim and bicy- | Maintains eye contact. | |
| cle, too. Then I like to watch foot- | | |
| ball and basketball games with my | | |
| friends. | | |
| I sure hope I'll be able to run again | | |
| after the surgery. I love to be in- | | |
| volved in sports. | | |
| No, I'm not too sure what's going to | Uncovers legs; looks at knee; smiles | Toes on both feet have capillary re- |
| happen tonight or tomorrow. | at nurse. | turn when blanched <5 sec. |
| Oh, OK. | | Flexes lt knee 0°-135°. |
| No, I think I understand now. | | Rt knee flexion unable to determine. |
| Sure. What do you want me to do? | | Pedal pulses 3+. |
| No, they (her feet and legs) don't | | Lungs clear to auscultation. |
| tingle or anything. | | System assessment WNL. |
| Yeah, it hurts a lot. | | |
| OK, I'll see you tomorrow night. | | |
| Thanks. Bye. | | |

## ANALYSIS/SYNTHESIS OF DATA: Day 1

When Orem's concepts related to self-care are used, each universal self-care requisite is addressed and appropriate data are referred to. Supporting theories and concepts are included when appropriate.

### Analysis/Synthesis

1. *Maintenance of sufficient intake of air:* The data indicate adequate circulation to C.L.'s legs. Capillary return on toes <5 seconds. Pedal pulses 3+ bilaterally. Whaley and Wong (1987) cite the following normal measurements: (1) average systolic blood pressure for 15-year-old, 120 mmHg; (2) pulse for a person over 4 years of age, 55-90 beats per minute; (3) respiration, 18-19 per minute. When these norms are compared with C.L.'s vital signs, a tentative inference can be made regarding adequate intake of air. More readings of vital signs, other circulatory data, and her history of smoking are data needed for a conclusion to be made. Due to immobility and the effects of anesthesia, C.L. may have inadequate air exchange after surgery.

2. *Maintenance of sufficient intake of water:* A very tentative inference can be made of adequate water intake. Adolescents should take in 50 cc of water/kg weight over a 24-hour period. C.L. should have approximately 2600 cc water/day (Whaley and Wong 1987). According to her history, C.L. consumes 1900 cc water from her fluid intake alone. More data are needed, such as observations of the skin and mucous membrane conditions (Whaley and Wong, 1987). C.L. may have an inadequate intake of water postop if intake decreases.

3. *Maintenance of sufficient intake of food:* Data were not collected about C.L.'s eating habits. She is on a regular diet with no dietary restrictions. After midnight she will be NPO,

which will alter her food intake. Her height and weight fall within the norms given by Malasanos and others (1986) for her age (height range: 59.5–68.1 inches; weight range: 89.5–150.5 lb). The calorie intake for C.L.'s age is 2000 to 2400 calories/day according to Whaley and Wong (1987). The sources of her nutrition are data gaps at this time.

4. *Adequate elimination processes and excrements:* Minimum data on elimination were obtained. The values of the urinalysis fell within the norms given by the hospital. Urinary excretion can be considered adequate, but data gaps exist about patterns of excretion as to difficulties experienced previously and bowel output.

5. *Maintenance of balance between activity and rest:* Exercise requirements vary according to the individual's health status and age. Sports help to contribute to growth and development by increasing heart rate, respirations, and muscle tone (Whaley and Wong, 1987). Data collected indicate that the client had regular exercise before her knee injury. Malasanos and others (1986) indicate that the normal range of motion of the knee is 0° to 135° flexion. However, due to leg immobility, flexion information on rt leg is not available. A tentative inference of inadequate exercise can be made at this time, especially in anticipation of upcoming surgery. No data were obtained regarding rest and sleep patterns. Teenagers vary in sleep and rest requirements.

6. *Maintenance of balance between solitude and social interaction:* The data obtained indicate that C.L. is involved in activities with other people. Orem discusses the importance of bonds of affection, love, and friendship; social warmth and closeness; and individual autonomy. More data need to be collected regarding C.L.'s family and friends in meeting these needs. C.L. is friendly and warm toward the nurse. Observations of the number of visitors, cards, and phone calls that C.L. has, as well as how she responds to these, are important data to obtain.

7. *Prevention of hazards to human life, functioning, and well-being:* Orem describes this requisite as including awareness of potential hazards and knowledge of preventive measures to avoid or minimize their effects. C.L. will have hazards to her functioning. One specific hazard is her lack of understanding of the events

surrounding her surgery and the outcome. She is also concerned about activity limitations.

8. *Promotion of human functioning and development within the individual's potential and desire to be normal:* Orem describes the elements of this requisite as having a realistic self-concept, fostering human development, and acting to maintain and promote the integrity of human structure and function. Some data indicate that the client is striving to maintain and promote her physical integrity. Data indicate that C.L. has been concerned about her health and tries to maintain a physical fitness level. She states she is involved in social activities with friends. Erikson (1968) discusses the developmental task of this age as identity versus identity confusion. The adolescent essentially restages each of the previous stages of development in reestablishing a separate autonomy. Much data are needed from C.L. to ascertain her stage of development and sense of identity. Sundeen and others (1989) describe self-concept as the aspects of the self that the individual is aware of. Self-concept includes the individual's feelings, values, and beliefs that influence behavior. Self-ideal is the standard by which one judges one's own behavior, including goals, aspirations, and values one would like to achieve. After surgery the nurse needs to explore the impact of surgery and its effects to better assess C.L.'s self-concept.

Considering the previous review of universal self-care requisites, the following strengths and health concerns are identified:

### Strengths
1. Adequate intake of air
2. Adequate urinary excretion
3. Desire to promote human functioning
4. Desire to be normal in relation to peer group

### Health concerns
1. Potential alteration of intake of air, water, and food
2. Inadequate activity
3. Hazards to human functioning
4. Decreased self-concept

Because of the concerns listed, C.L. has a therapeutic self-care demand and health-deviation self-care requisites. Her desire and ability to promote her own human functioning, plus assistance from health care professionals, place her in a supportive-educative nursing system at this time.

## NURSING DIAGNOSES: Day 1

| Date | Diagnoses | Priority |
|---|---|---|
| 1/14/89 | 1. Hazards to human functioning related to upcoming surgery and lack of knowledge concerning surgery | 1 |
| 1/14/89 | 2. Potential alteration of air, water, and food intake related to upcoming surgery | 2 |
| 1/14/89 | 3. Decreased self-concept related to alteration in role of active sportsperson | 3 |
| 1/14/89 | 4. Inadequate activity related to right knee injuries and upcoming surgery | 4 |

## DATA COLLECTION: Day 2—day of surgery 1/15/89

| Interactions | Observations | Measurements |
|---|---|---|
| **From 7-3 report from nurse:** | **From chart:** | |
| C.L. has been sleeping since she got back, until 1500. | Postop orders: | |
| She has been using PCA pump. | Clear liq as tolerated to soft diet. | |
| Circulation checks have been WNL: capillary return <5 seconds on toes of both feet; pedal pulses present bilaterally | I and O. Elevate rt leg on pillow. Ice on rt knee. Bed rest. | |
| Ice bag is on her rt knee. | Tylenol, gr X q4h prn for T 101° PO. | |
| Rt leg is in a bent long leg cast. | PCA order: 1 mg morphine sulfate with delay 10 minutes. Initiate basal rate of 1 mg/hr from 2200-0600. | |
| Vital signs are stable; next due at 1600. | Tylenol, tab #3 q4h PO pain, prn. | TPR: 98.4°, 76, 18 (preop) 99°, 72, 16 (postop) |
| She's been taking a little ice and 7-Up by mouth with no problem. | IV: D₅NS at 75 cc/hr. Vital signs q4h. | BP: 108/60 (preop) 110/68 (postop) |
| Yes, she has voided. | Preop med given per order at 0700 in holding area; to OR at 0730. | PCA pump: morphine 11 mg (7-3) |
| C.L. has been turned to lt side to help dry cast. Handled cast with palms of hand; no drainage noted on cast. | Returned from surgery at 1200. Client sleeping most of time since 1200. Tolerating cl liq PO sm amts. IV infusing according to schedule. | I and O (7-3): I: IV (surg): 500 cc IV (unit): 225 cc PO: 100 cc O: 500 cc (urine) |
| **From client:** | **From client:** | **From client:** |
| Hi, not so good right now. I've been pressing my PCA button. | Lying supine in bed with head of bed (HOB) up 15°. | Capillary return when rt toenails blanched <5 sec. |
| I had to use the bedpan a while ago, and that was hard to do—but I did go. | Rt leg elevated on two pillows. Bent long leg cast on rt leg. | Vital signs at 1600: BP: 106/66 |
| Uh-huh. I can feel it. OK (in response to telling C.L. to let me know if she has any tingling or numbness of rt leg). | No drainage noted through cast. Rt toes warm to touch. Wriggled rt toes when asked. Facial skin and arms warm, dry, and pinkish. | TPR: 99°, 76, 18 |
| I see (in response to telling C.L. about the possible postop complications of decreased sensation, discomfort, and decreased circulation, as related to surgery). | Lips pink and moist. Flat facial affect. Eye contact with nurse. | |
| Yeah, they showed me earlier (in response to nurse asking if she knew how to CDB). | Took five deep breaths and coughed (CDB) when nurse requested her to do so. | (Nonproductive cough) |

*Continued.*

**DATA COLLECTION: Day 2—day of surgery 1/15/89—cont'd**

| Interactions | Observations | Measurements |
| --- | --- | --- |
| I'll try (in response to nurse informing C.L. about the need to CDB q2h while she is on bedrest to increase air intake). <br> OK (in response to nurse encouraging her to rest now) | Environment: <br>   Mother at bedside. <br>   Call light within C.L.'s reach. <br>   Bedside table within reach. <br>   Glass of clear liquid and ice chips on bedside table. <br>   Television on low volume. <br>   Roommate in bed watching television. | |
| *Later:* <br> I need to use the bedpan again. <br> Thanks <br> I'm better now. It still hurts, but not as much. <br> Oh, that's enough. | Used trapeze with ease when bedpan was placed under buttocks. <br> Urine deep amber and clear. <br> IV infusing into lt hand at 75 cc/hr (D$_5$NS). <br> HOB up 30° for supper. <br> Drank all broth and juice and ate gelatin by herself. | Voided 350 cc urine |
| That's better. <br> When will I be able to get this thing out [referring to IV]? <br> Oh, OK (in response to "probably tomorrow" from nurse). | Mother assisted C.L. in reaching items on supper tray. Visited each other during meal. Overheard mother updating C.L. on dad's and brother's activities. C.L.'s facial expression indicated interest. <br> Pillows resituated to provide more support for rt leg. <br> New ice bag applied to rt knee for 24 hr. <br> CDB five times when nurse initiated. <br> Mother remained at bedside until 1900. | Oral intake: 575 cc (supper) |
| *Later:* <br> No, no tingling or numbness. <br> It's just a constant aching most of the time. Now it's starting to pound. <br> I can't get comfortable. <br> I'm going to press my button for pain. <br> Could I have some more 7-Up, too? | Rt toes warm to touch and move freely. C.L. grimaces. <br> HOB to 10° elevation. Turned to lt side. <br> Lungs clear to auscultation. <br> Skin on back moist and warm. <br> No redness on back or hips. <br> IV infusing on schedule. <br> CDB five times on request of nurse. Nonproductive coughs. <br> Skin warm and dry. | Vital signs at 2000: <br> BP: 110/70 <br> TPR: 98.6°, 72, 16. <br> Oral intake: 120cc 7-Up |
| *Later:* | C.L. lying supine with eyes closed. <br> Relaxed facial muscles. <br> Body in alignment. <br> Rt leg elevated with ice bag to rt knee. | PCA pump: morphine 15 mg (3-11) <br> I and O (3-11): <br>   I: 600 cc (IV) <br>      695 cc (PO) <br>   O: 350 cc urine |

## ANALYSIS/SYNTHESIS OF DATA: Day 2

Orem's concepts of universal self-care requisites are addressed individually.

### Analysis/Synthesis

1. *Maintenance of sufficient intake of air:* C.L.'s intake of air has been threatened because of surgery and immobility. Phipps and others (1987) state that the effects of both anesthesia and immobility impair adequate intake of air. According to the norms given by Malasanos and others (1986) and the implementation of preventive postoperative measures suggested by Phipps and others (1987), and by Ferrell (1986), data indicate that this self-care requisite is being met now but remains a potential health concern.

2. *Maintenance of sufficient intake of water:* Data indicate that intake of water has been threatened because of surgery and inability to take fluids in volume by mouth. Phipps and others (1987) state that fluid volume depletion manifests itself with the following symptoms: poor skin turgor, dry mucous membranes, low blood pressure, tachycardia, increased respiration, decreased vein filling, weight loss, low urine output, and increased specific gravity. Phipps and others (1987) and Ferrell (1986) provided the rationale for plans for implementation that were initiated regarding threatened intake of water (IV replacement, clear liquid diet). According to the data, C.L. does not exhibit symptoms of fluid volume deficit and is participating in the implementation of plans to prevent inadequate intake of water (drinking fluids and receiving IV fluids), and is, therefore, maintaining sufficient intake of water. This self-care requisite remains a potential health concern.

3. *Maintenance of sufficient intake of food:* Williams (1986) states that adequate protein intake is of prime importance postoperatively because of the loss of protein from tissue breakdown and loss of plasma proteins. Essential amino acids are necessary for wound healing. The goal is to reach 60 gm protein daily. One liter of 5% dextrose solution contains 50 g sugar and 200 calories. According to the above information, compared with the data, C.L. is not maintaining sufficient intake of food. Progressing from a clear liquid diet to a regular diet should be done as soon as C.L. can tolerate it. Overall eating habits remain a data gap.

4. *Adequate elimination processes and excrements:* Phipps and others (1987) state that intake of fluids exceeds output for about the first 48 hours after surgery. This is due to the loss of fluid in surgery, insensible fluid loss, vomiting, and increased secretion of antidiuretic hormone (ADH). The client should be expected to void within 6-8 hours after sugery. Data indicate that C.L. has voided within the recommended time and that her fluid intake does exceed her fluid output. According to the above data and norms for the postoperative client, C.L. is maintaining adequate urinary output (1/15/89: 7-3, 3-11: I, 2120; 0, 850). Phipps and others (1987) state that bowel patterns are altered after surgery because of the stress response, anesthesia, use of narcotics, and immobility. Even on a clear liquid diet and IV replacement, a client should have bowel movements if peristalis is present. C.L. has not had a bowel movement at this time. Bowel function remains a potential health concern. Further data need to be obtained in regard to bowel function, such as usual bowel function habits.

5. *Maintenance of balance between activity and rest:* Phipps and others (1987) and Ferrell (1986) indicate that early activity and ambulation are beneficial for increasing alertness, morale, ventilation, muscle tone, and peristalsis; facilitating voiding and wound healing; and decreasing venous stasis. Adequate rest is necessary for an accurate perception of pain and events surrounding recovery from surgery. Quadriceps-setting exercises began on the unaffected side. According to the data, C.L. has had minimum activity and interrupted rest periods related to pain. Therefore, an imbalance exists between activity and rest.

6. *Maintenance of balance between solitude and social interaction:* Data indicate minimum interactions with others at this time (except with C.L.'s mother), because of C.L.'s need for rest and her sedation from the anesthesia and analgesics. Data gaps remain concerning visitors and cards and phone calls from friends and other family members.

7. *Prevention of hazards to human life, functioning, and well-being:* Data indicate that C.L. is more aware of potential hazards (eg, CDB for adequate air exchange and importance of moving in bed to maintain skin integrity) and is participating with preventive measures coopera-

tively. Because of the surgery, this remains a health concern at this time.

8. *Promotion of human functioning and development within the individual's potential and desire to be normal:* Data obtained reflect biophysical health promotion at this time because of the recent surgery and actual and potential changes in biophysical health. C.L. needs assistance in promoting aspects of human functioning. C.L. responds to positive feedback of participating in self-care activities and her progress.

According to the previous review of universal self-care requisites, the following strengths and health concerns are identifed:

### Strengths

1. Adequate intake of air
2. Adequate intake of water

3. Adequate urinary excretion
4. Cooperative in actively participating in methods to decrease hazards to human functioning

### Health concerns

1. Potential alteration of intake of air and water
2. Inadequate intake of food
3. Potential alteration of bowel elimination
4. Inadequate activity
5. Hazards to human functioning

In view of the concerns listed, C.L. continues to have a therapeutic self-care demand and health-deviation self-care requisites. Because of her recent surgery and inability to maintain most universal self-care requisites and therapeutic self-care demands without assistance, C.L. is in a wholly compensatory nursing system.

No incongruencies in the data were identified.

## NURSING DIAGNOSES: Day 2

| Date | Diagnoses | Priority |
|---|---|---|
| 1/14/89 | 1. Hazards to human functioning related to surgery and lack of knowledge concerning surgery. | 3 |
| 1/14/89 | 2. Potential alteration of air, water, and food intake related to surgery (anesthesia, NPO/cl liq status). | 1 |
| 1/14/89 | 3. Decreased self-concept related to alteration in role of active sportsperson. | 5 |
| 1/14/89 | 4. Inadequate activity related to right knee injuries and upcoming surgery. | 2 |
| 1/15/89 | 5. Potential alteration in bowel elimination related to immobility. | 4 |

## DATA COLLECTION: Day 3—day after surgery 1/16/89

| Interactions | Observations | Measurements |
|---|---|---|
| **From 7-3 report from nurse:** She's had a good day today. C.L. is doing quad-setting exercises and straight leg raises on unaffected leg and she's done them every couple of hours. <br><br> She sleeps well with basal PCA. Started her on a soft diet this morning, and she's tolerating it well. I tried to get her out of bed this afternoon. She had pain and tensed up, so she couldn't get into the chair. PT was notified to come and fit her for crutches. She had quite a few visitors today, so she's pretty tired and has been sleeping off and on. | From chart: <br> New orders: Out of bed in chair at least tid <br> PT to fit for crutches <br> Tolerating soft diet well <br> Vital signs stable (see Measurements) <br><br><br><br><br><br><br><br><br><br> Washed self except for back in AM. <br> IV running at 75 cc/hr. | *1/16/86 Evening* <br> Circulation checks: <br> Warm rt foot; can move rt toes <br> Pedal pulses bilaterally 3+ <br> Capillary refill <5 sec on toes <br><br> **From chart:** <br> Vital signs: BP: 106/68-112/74; T: 98.4-99°; P: 68-76; R: 12-18 <br><br><br><br><br> PCA pump morphine 13 mg (11-7) <br> I and O (11-7): <br> I: 600 cc (IV)-400 cc (PO) <br> O: 400 cc urine |

## DATA COLLECTION: Day 3—day after surgery 1/16/89—cont'd

| Interactions | Observations | Measurements |
|---|---|---|
| | | PCA pump morphine 14 mg (7-3)<br>I and O:<br>  I:  600 cc (IV)-1005 cc (PO)<br>  O: 450 cc urine |
| **From client:**<br>I'm doing OK. I had a hard time trying to get out of bed, though. Guess I didn't do well. | **From client:**<br>Looks at nurse and smiles. | **From client:**<br>Vital signs at 1600:<br>  BP: 110/72<br>  TPR: 98.4°, 76, 16 |
| Yeah, I pressed pain button. Oh, OK (in response to waiting half an hour, then getting up into a chair).<br>Are these exercises to keep my good leg strong? That's what I thought.<br>Yeah, I remember some of the possible complications.<br>Well, bad circulation, pneumonia, funny feeling in my leg.<br>That's why you have me do all this—like breathing and coughing, and the exercises on my left leg, keeping my leg up, isn't it?<br>OK (in response to suggestion to rest now). | C.L. focuses eyes on rt leg.<br>Rt toes warm to touch.<br><br><br><br>Wriggles rt toes when requested.<br>Rt leg elevated on two pillows.<br>Ice bag to rt knee.<br>No drainage noted through cast.<br>No irritation around cast edges. | Capillary return <5 sec when rt toenails blanched<br>Pedal pulses 3+ bilaterally |
| *Later:*<br>Oh, boy, here we go!<br>OK (in response to instruction on how I will support her leg while turning her body and holding rt leg for her).<br><br>Yeah, I'm OK. | Environment:<br>  Two plants and one vase of flowers at bedside; several cards on bedside stand.<br>C.L. helped herself to move to rt side of bed by sliding her body across mattress with support of her arms.<br>Nurse supported rt leg.<br>Blank facial expression.<br>Looked at rt leg while standing.<br>Took a few deep breaths upon instruction.<br>Stood on lt leg and pivoted to chair at side of bed.<br>Sat in chair using arms to support herself as she sat. | |
| Well it's OK now. It felt bad for a second.<br>Thanks. | Rt leg elevated on pillow on second chair.<br>Bedside tray with supper placed in front of C.L. | |
| *Later:*<br>I need to use the commode. Then I'm ready to go back to bed.<br><br>It was easier this time.<br>My pain is better today.<br>It hurts less. | C.L. had eaten two thirds of food on tray.<br>Lifted herself up and pivoted to commode.<br>Assisted back to bed.<br>Nurse held rt leg while C.L. stood on lt leg and pivoted. CDB five times on request. | Oral intake: 450 cc (supper)<br>Voided 500 cc urine |

*Continued.*

## DATA COLLECTION: Day 3—day after surgery 1/16/89—cont'd

| Interactions | Observations | Measurements |
|---|---|---|
| The doctor told me today that I should be able to run again. | Smiled at nurse. | |
| Sure, that makes me happy. The track team means a lot to me. | | |
| At least I know it'll be OK sometime. | | |
| I can still be the timekeeper until I can run. That way I can still be with my friends. | | |
| Yeah, they gave me most of these—and those flowers. | Pointed with rt hand to flowers. | |
| The rest are from my relatives. | Rt leg elevated on two pillows. | Pedal pulses 3+ |
| Maybe if I work hard at exercising I'll be able to run sooner! | Rt foot warm to touch. | PCA pump: Morphine 15 mg (3-11) |
| See you later. | Hair groomed, wearing own nightgown. | I and O (3-11): |
| | Drank <240 cc 7-Up. | I: 690 cc (PO) |
| | | O: 500 cc urine |

## ANALYSIS/SYNTHESIS OF DATA: Day 3

Orem's concepts of universal self-care requisites are addressed individually.

### Analysis/Synthesis

1. *Maintenance of sufficient intake of air:* According to data and norms given in analysis/synthesis for day 2, C.L. is maintaining adequate air intake. VS stable. C.L. coughs on her own and produces nonproductive cough. Circulation checks of legs WNL. This still remains a potential health concern because of her decreased mobility and inactivity.

2. *Maintenance of sufficient intake of water:* According to the norms given in the last analysis/synthesis regarding intake of water, C.L. is meeting this health care requisite. This requisite also remains a potential health concern because of her surgery.

3. *Maintenance of sufficient intake of food:* Data show that C.L. has started eating a soft diet and is tolerating it. According to the projected ideal intake of food and calories given in analysis/synthesis day 2, C.L. has a greater chance to meet the requirements now that she is eating solid foods. Data gaps exist regarding the nutritional value of the food she is eating. This is a potential health concern.

4. *Adequate elimination processes and excrements:* C.L.'s intake still exceeds her output, which was stated as a norm for postoperative clients

in the last analysis/synthesis on 1/16/89 (11-7, 7-3, 3-11: I—2755, O—1350). Bowel function remains a potential health concern and a data gap.

5. *Maintenance of balance between activity and rest:* According to the data, C.L.'s activities are increasing. She is now up in the chair and transfers from bed to chair with help. She states she has more uninterrupted periods of sleep. The activities recommended in the discussion of analysis/synthesis day 2 have been implemented. This remains a health concern until C.L. is more mobile independently.

6. *Maintenance of balance between solitude and social interaction:* Data indicate that C.L. is having more contact with friends and family. A data gap still exists with respect to the quality of these relationships and how they satisfy C.L.'s needs and can be of assistance to her during her recovery.

7. *Prevention of hazards to human life, functioning, and well-being:* Data indicate that C.L. is aware of these hazards and is cooperating in preventive measures to decrease the potential of complications developing. C.L. coughs and deep breathes, eats more, exercises the unaffected leg with encouragement, and shows more interest in social interactions. Continued monitoring of these measures is needed until C.L. is more independently mobile and able to get up.

8. *Promotion of human functioning and development within the individual's potential and desire to be normal:* The norms given in analysis/synthesis day 1 regarding adolescent development compared with these data support C.L.'s concern with her self-concept and relation to peers. This remains a health concern, and will require greater focus, because C.L.'s role will be altered for an extended period.

The following list represent C.L.'s strengths and health concerns at this time:

### Strengths

1. Adequate intake of air
2. Adequate intake of water
3. Adequate urinary excretion
4. Social interaction with significant other people

### Health concerns

1. Potential alteration of air, food, and water
2. Potential alteration in bowel elimination
3. Inadequate activity
4. Hazards to human functioning
5. Altered self-concept

According to the concerns identified, C.L. still has a therapeutic self-care demand and health-deviation self-care requisites. Because C.L. remains somewhat dependent on others to maintain universal self-care requisites and therapeutic self-care demand, she is in a partly compensatory nursing system.

No incongruencies in the data were identified.

## NURSING DIAGNOSES: Day 3

| Date | Diagnoses | Priority |
|---|---|---|
| 1/14/89 | 1. Hazards to human functioning related to upcoming surgery and lack of knowledge regarding surgery (resolved 1/16/89). | 5 |
| 1/14/89 | 2. Potential alteration of air, water, and food intake related to surgery (anesthesia, NPO/cl liq status) | 2 |
| 1/14/89 | 3. Decreased self-concept related to alteration in role of active sportsperson | 3 |
| 1/14/89 | 4. Inadequate activity related to right knee injuries and upcoming surgery | 1 |
| 1/15/89 | 5. Potential alteration in bowel elimination related to immobility | 4 |

Plans for diagnoses 1, 2, 3, and 5 are given on the following pages. Initial plans for diagnosis 4 are included in plans for diagnosis 2. A more detailed plan is needed regarding increasing C.L.'s activity and discharge planning.

As of the second day postop, C.L. is not able to return to her previous level of functioning. Therapeutic self-care demands are still present, for example, C.L. needs to learn crutch walking. However, as C.L.'s recovery progresses and the nurse continues to assist her to increase self-care capabilities, it is anticipated that C.L. will begin to achieve more independence and a sense of well-being.

## PLANS FOR IMPLEMENTATION

**Nursing diagnosis 1:** *Hazards to human functioning related to upcoming surgery and lack of knowledge (1/14/89).*
**Goal:** *The client will decrease hazards to human functioning by increasing knowledge of upcoming surgery by 1/17/89.*

| Objectives | Nursing orders | Scientific rationale | Evaluation |
|---|---|---|---|
| 1. Client will name the sequence of events leading to surgery by 1/14/89. | 1a. Nurse and client will discuss previous experiences the client has had with surgery on 1/14/89. | 1a. Teaching/learning strategy by Pohl (1981). Principle of learning: new learning is based on previous knowledge experience. | **Criteria statement:** Client will cite sequence of four events leading to surgery as noted in 1c. Nurse implemented orders 1a–1d 1/14/89. |

*Continued.*

**PLANS FOR IMPLEMENTATION—cont'd**

| Objectives | Nursing orders | Scientific rationale | Evaluation |
|---|---|---|---|
| | 1b. On 1/14/89 the nurse will use open communication techniques, such as: Open-ended questions and statements Clarifying statements Summary statements. | 1b. Principles of teaching: Good nurse-learner rapport is important. Teaching requires effective communication. | Client responded that she understood the sequence of events on 1/14/89. Objective 1 met 1/14/89. |
| | 1c. Nurse will explain the events leading to surgery on 1/14/89: Injection in AM To holding area and then surgery Return to room about 4 hr later. | 1c. Increase C.L.'s sense of physical control and knowledge to promote powerfulness of client (Roberts, 1978). | |
| | 1d. Nurse will ask C.L. if she understands the sequence of events on 1/14/89. | 1d. Evaluation is an integral part of learning (Pohl, 1981). | |
| 2. Client will state changes in activity level surgery by 1/17/89. | 2a. Nurse will discuss with C.L. and C.L.'s mom their knowledge of the purpose of surgery by 1/16/89. | 2a. Principles of teaching and learning (Pohl, 1981): New learning is based on previous knowledge and experience. Planning time for teaching and learning requires special attention. Physical and mental readiness is necessary for learning. | **Criteria statement:** Client will name at least three changes in activity, as noted in 2b postop. 1/16/89: Orders 2a-2d implemented. C.L. and C.L.'s mom indicated general knowledge of surgery and need for crutches, limits on activity, and feelings about it. Objective met. |
| | 2b. Nurse will review the effects of surgery on human functioning: Bent long leg cast to immobilize rt knee. Use of crutches 3 days postop, non-weight–bearing. Walk with crutches 6-8 wk postop. Hospitalized for 4-5 days. Nurse will state that some differences may occur because of physician's individual practice. | 2b. Principles of medical-surgical (orthopedic) nursing practice strategy: Immobilization of the right knee joint allows for healing of traumatized tissue (Ferrell, 1986). Exercises facilitate strengthening of muscles around traumatized tissue (Ferrell, 1986). Knowledge of what to expect after surgery increases the client's sense of physical control and powerfulness (Roberts, 1978). | |

## PLANS FOR IMPLEMENTATION—cont'd

| Objectives | Nursing orders | Scientific rationale | Evaluation |
|---|---|---|---|
| | 2c. Nurse will ask C.L. and her mom to state changes in activity level on 1/17/89. | 2c. Effective learning requires active participation of the learner. Evaluation is an integral part of learning (Pohl, 1981). | **Summative evaluation:** Goal met 1/16/89. C.L. increased her knowledge regarding surgery and the main effects surgery will have on her. |
| | 2d. Nurse and client will discuss the client's feelings about altered functioning on 1/17/89. | 2d. A positive body image is particularly important to the adolescent (Roberts, 1978). | |

**Nursing diagnosis 2:** *Potential alteration of air, water, and food intake related to upcoming surgery (1/14/89).*
**Goal:** *The client will decrease the degree of alteration of air, water, and food intake by using preventive postoperative measures by 1/16/89.*

| Objectives | Nursing orders | Scientific rationale | Evaluation |
|---|---|---|---|
| 1. Client will state three possible postop problems on 1/14/89. | 1a. Nurse will ask C.L. what she knows about possible problems caused by surgery on 1/14/89. | 1a. Teaching-learning strategy by Pohl (1981). Principle of learning: new learning is based on previous knowledge and experience. | **Criteria statement:** Client will state three of the possible problems as noted in 1b. |
| | 1b. On 1/14/89 the nurse will use open communication techniques to discuss postop problems as: Decreased air intake and circulation. Decreased sensation. Discomfort. Decreased physical activity. Decreased food and water intake. | 1b. Principle of teaching: Teaching requires effective communication. Principles of medical-surgical (orthopedic) nursing practice strategy. These are considered possible problems after surgery due to the effect of anesthesia and immobility on general body systems. The possible decrease in circulation, sensation, and discomfort in the right leg is related to swelling of tissue as a response to surgical intervention (Phipps et al., 1987). | Order 1b was implemented on 1/14/89. C.L. acknowledged information given to her. Orders 1a and 1c were implemented on 1/14/89. C.L. able to state two problems on 1/14/89; objective not met 1/14/89. |

*Continued.*

## PLANS FOR IMPLEMENTATION—cont'd

| Objectives | Nursing orders | Scientific rationale | Evaluation |
|---|---|---|---|
| | 1c. Nurse will ask C.L. to state three of the possible occurrences mentioned above on 1/14/89. | 1c. Principles by Pohl: Effective learning requires active participation of the learner. Evaluation is an integral part of learning. | Objective met on 1/15/89 when C.L. was able to state three possible problems postop. |
| 2. Client will name three preventive measures for possible postop problems on 1/14/89. | 2a. Nurse will discuss preventive measures for possible postop problems on 1/14/89. | 2a. Principle of teaching: Teaching requires effective communication. Principles of nursing practice: | **Criteria statement:** Client will name four of the preventive measures as listed in 2a. |
| | CDB every 2 hours. | To increase ventilation of lungs and facilitate removal of secretions (Phipps et al, 1987). | Objective 2 not met. To be implemented on 1/15/89 and 1/16/89. |
| | Elevate rt knee on pillows. | To facilitate venous return and decrease swelling (Ferrell, 1986). | Order 2a partially implemented 1/15. C.L. acknowledged nurse's information. |
| | Ice bag to rt knee. | To decrease swelling and pain and facilitate circulation. | Order 2b not implemented 1/15 because of client's health status. |
| | Positioning for comfort and analgesics. | To decrease pain and increase comfort. | Order 2b implemented 1/16. C.L. identified four preventive measures. |
| | IVs and clear liquid diet as tolerated to regular diet as tolerated. | Fluid is lost during surgery and must be replaced. ADH is stimulated post trauma. GI function slowed (Phipps et al, 1987). | Objective met on 1/16/89. |
| | Out of bed within 2 days. | Increases morale, alertness, ventilation, muscle tone, and peristalsis. Facilitates healing and voiding. Decreases pain and venous stasis. | |
| | 2b. Nurse will ask C.L. to name four of the above preventive measures on 1/14/89. | 2b. Principles by Pohl: Effective learning requires active participation of the learner. Evaluation is an integral part of learning. | |
| 3. Client will participate in at least four postop preventive measures by 1/16/89. | 3a. Nurse will demonstrate CDB on 1/14/89. | 3a. Learning may occur through imitation (Pohl, 1981). | **Criteria statement:** Client will participate in at least four of the following preventive measures as noted in 3c. |
| | 3b. C.L. will demonstrate the above on 1/14/89. | 3b. Effective learning requires active participation of the learner. Repetition strengthens learning. | |
| | 3c. Nurse will provide necessary equipment and monitor their ef- | 3c. Nurse is responsible and accountable for the client's physical | Order 3b done 1/16/89. C.L. showed nurse how to CDB. |

## PLANS FOR IMPLEMENTATION — cont'd

| Objectives | Nursing orders | Scientific rationale | Evaluation |
|---|---|---|---|
| | fectiveness for the following preventive measures on 1/15/89: Elevate rt leg on pillows. Ice bag to rt knee. Position rt leg for comfort. Administer analgesics per physician order as needed via PCA. IVs and clear liquid diet as tolerated to regular diet. | safety and well-being postoperatively (Phipps et al, 1987). (See rationale for each preventive measure in objective 2.) | Order 3c done 1/15 and 1/16/89. Order 3d implemented 1/15 and 1/16/89. I and O maintained by nurse. Order 3e implemented 1/15 and 1/16/89. Objective met. |
| | 3d. Nurse will monitor intake and output postoperatively 1/15/89 and as needed. | 3d. Physiological changes due to surgical intervention and anesthesia interfere with usual intake and output (Phipps et al, 1987). | **Summative evaluation:** Goal met (needs monitoring until C.L. is more mobile) 1/16/89. C.L. is knowledgeable of possible postop occurrences and preventive measures and is actively participating with postop care. |
| | 3e. Nurse will initiate use of measures in 3c when appropriate. | 3e. Health restoration and maintenance are the responsibility of the nurse (Phipps et al, 1987). | |

**Nursing diagnosis 3:** *Decreased self-concept related to alteration in role of active sportsperson (1/14/89).*
**Goal:** *The client will accept a realistic self-concept considering her role change by 1/18/89.*

| Objectives | Nursing orders | Scientific rationale | Evaluation |
|---|---|---|---|
| 1. Client will verbalize at least two feelings regarding loss of function by 1/18/89. | 1a. Nurse and client will discuss C.L.'s perception of the loss of function from surgery on 1/17/89. | 1a. Strategies of therapeutic use of self, problem solving, and principles of medical-surgical nursing practice. Client reaction to a temporary or permanent loss depends on the client's perception of the loss (Pohl, 1981). | **Criteria statement:** Client will verbalize at least two feelings, such as sadness, anger, neutrality, frustration, pleasure, and joy on 1/17/89. Orders not implemented because of dates not yet occurring. C.L. is anxious to get back to sports. She feels frustrated by inactivity. Nurse supported C.L. in her feelings. |
| | 1b. Nurse will ask C.L. how and what she feels regarding the loss of function of her rt leg on 1/17 or 1/18. | 1b. Nurse needs to facilitate ventilation of feelings regarding loss (Phipps et al, 1987). In adolescence, the body acts as a source of acceptance or rejection by others (Murray and Zentner, 1988). | |

**PLANS FOR IMPLEMENTATION—cont'd**

| Objectives | Nursing orders | Scientific rationale | Evaluation |
|---|---|---|---|
| | | Problem identification step of problem-solving process (Ford et al, 1979). | |
| | 1c. Nurse will accept and support C.L.'s response in 1b on 1/17 and 1/18. | 1c. Nurse needs to support client in all phases of body image change (Roberts, 1978). | Objective met. |
| | 1d. Nurse will ask C.L. to think about coping methods on 1/17, to be discussed on 1/18. | 1d. Active participation by the learner promotes learning (Pohl, 1981). Generation of options of problem solving (Ford et al, 1979). | |
| 2. Client will state three ways she can cope with altered body function by 1/18/89. | 2a. Nurse and C.L. will discuss possible ways of coping with altered body function on 1/18/89 such as: Take care of own body. Participate in diversional activities. Learn to use crutches and increase mobility to the best of her ability within limits. Ask family to arrange home to allow C.L. increased mobility. Ask friends to carry books for her at school. Plan to continue being timekeeper for track team. Initiate social contact with friends (cognitive domain). | 2a. Identification of options in problem-solving process (Ford et al, 1979). Nurse is responsible for health promotion (Phipps, 1987). Nurse needs to participate in supporting the client with all aspects of changed body image (Roberts, 1978). | **Criteria statement:** Client will name three of the coping methods identified in 2a. Orders not implemented because of dates not yet occurring. Objective not met. |
| | 2b. Nurse and client will discuss the feasibility of each possible coping measure on 1/18/89. | 2b. Analyzing alternatives in problem-solving process (Ford et al, 1979). Increasing C.L.'s sense of physical, psychological, and environmental control and knowledge to promote powerfulness (Roberts, 1978). | |
| | 2c. C.L. will choose at least three ways she will cope with altered body function on 1/18/89. | 2c. Increasing sense of powerfulness Making the decision in the problem-solving process (Ford et al, 1979). | |

## PLANS FOR IMPLEMENTATION—cont'd

| Objectives | Nursing orders | Scientific rationale | Evaluation |
|---|---|---|---|
| | | A positive body image is built or reconstructed through encouragement of movement and activities (Roberts, 1978). | |
| 3. Client will exhibit at least two signs of acceptance of altered body function by 1/18/89. | 3a. Nurse will ask and encourage C.L. to initiate use of at least two coping measures by 1/18/89. | 3a. Increase C.L.'s sense of physical, psychological, and environmental control and powerfulness (Roberts, 1978). | **Criteria statement:** Client will participate in at least two of the coping measures listed in criteria statement for objective 2 by 1/18/89. |
| | 3b. Nurse will monitor and evaluate the use of coping measures by 1/18/89. | 3b. Nurse is responsible for promotion of health (Phipps et al, 1987). Evaluation is an integral part of teaching (Pohl, 1981). | Orders not implemented because of dates not yet occurring. Objective not met. |
| | 3c. Nurse will give positive reinforcement to C.L. for using coping measures by 1/18/89. | 3c. Nurse needs to participate in and support the client with all aspects of changed body image (Roberts, 1978). | **Summative evaluation:** Goal not met. |

**Nursing diagnosis 5:** *Potential alteration in bowel elimination related to immobility (1/15/89).*
**Goal:** *The client will resume normal pattern of bowel elimination by 1/18/89.*

| Objectives | Nursing orders | Scientific rationale | Evaluation |
|---|---|---|---|
| 1. Client will identify (state) decreased bowel function as a possible complication of surgery and immobility by 1/16/89. | 1a. Nurse will ask the client if she knows of any bowel changes that might occur as a result of surgery and immobility. | 1a. Teaching-learning strategy by Pohl (1981): new learning is based on previous learning and experience. | **Criteria statement:** Client verbally states or acknowledges with an affirmative word or gesture that bowel function is a possible complication by 1/16/89. |
| | 1b. According to C.L.'s response, the nurse will explain to C.L. the possible complication of altered bowel function on 1/16/89. | 1b. Principles of medical-surgical nursing practice strategy: anesthesia and immobility decrease peristalsis and therefore potentially alter bowel function (Phipps et al, 1987). | Orders not implemented because of dates not yet occurring. Objective not met. |
| | 1c. Nurse will ask C.L. to acknowledge information given above on 1/16/89. | 1c. Evaluation is an integral part of teaching. | |

*Continued.*

## PLANS FOR IMPLEMENTATION—cont'd

| Objectives | Nursing orders | Scientific rationale | Evaluation |
|---|---|---|---|
| 2. Client will participate in the assessment of bowel function by 1/16/89. | 2a. Nurse will ask C.L. if she has felt any need to defecate or any "rumbling" in lower abdomen or passed any flatus ("gas") since surgery on 1/16/89. | 2a. Subjective data are an important source regarding bowel function (Phipps et al, 1987). | **Criteria statement:** Client will answer questions and position body to facilitate data collection of bowel function upon request on 1/16/89. |
| | 2b. Nurse will use the following physical assessment techniques to collect data about bowel function on 1/16/89: Inspection Auscultation Palpation Percussion | 2b. Physical assessment techniques used to identify distention, bowel sounds, bowel segments, and fluid, gas, and solid elements in bowel (Malasanos et al, 1986). | Orders not implemented because of dates not yet occurring. Objective not met. |
| 3. Client will participate in three measures to stimulate bowel function by 1/16/89. | 3a. Nurse will ask C.L. to identify 2 ways to promote bowel function on 1/16/89. | 3a. Pohl's learning principle: new learning is based on previous learning and experience. Learning needs must be assessed. | **Criteria statement:** C.L. lists three ways to promote bowel movement. |
| | 3b. According to the above response, the nurse will identify measures to increase bowel activity on 1/16/89: Fluids to 2000-3000 cc per day. Maximum safe physical activity. Fruit juice intake. Mild laxative. Stool softeners. | 3b. Development of concepts is a part of learning. These measures increase fluid volume in bowel and stimulate peristalsis (Phipps et al, 1987). | Client will participate in three measures listed in order 3b on 1/18/89. Orders not implemented because of dates not yet occurring. Objective not met. |
| | 3c. Nurse will encourage C.L. to participate in the first three measures above if needed on 1/16/89. | 3c. Nurse is responsible for health promotion and maintenance (Phipps et al, 1987). | **Summative evaluation:** Goal not met. |

### REFERENCES AND READINGS

Edelman C and Mandle C: Health promotion throughout the life span, St Louis, 1986, The CV Mosby Co.

Erickson, EH: Identity, youth and crisis, New York, 1968, WW Norton & Co.

Ferrell J: Illustrated guide to orthopedic nursing, ed 3, Philadelphia, 1986, JB Lippincott Co.

Ford JG, Trygstad-Durland LN, and Nelms BC: Applied decision making for nurses, St Louis, 1979, The CV Mosby Co.

Long D, Lepley M, and Baker B: Health assessment across the life span, New York, 1984, McGraw-Hill Book Co.

Malasanos L, Barkauskas V, Moss, M, et al: Health assessment, ed 3, St Louis, 1986, The CV Mosby Co.

Murray RB and Zentner JP: Nursing assessment and health promotion through the life span, Englewood Cliffs, NJ, 1988, Prentice-Hall, Inc.

Orem DE: Nursing: concepts of practice, ed 3, New York, 1985, McGraw-Hill Book Co.

Phipps WJ, Long BC, and Woods NF: Medical-surgical nursing: concepts and clinical practice, ed 3, 1987, The CV Mosby Co.

Pohl ML: The teaching function of the nurse practitioner, ed 4, Dubuque, Ia, 1981, William C Brown Co.

Redman B: The process of patient education, ed 6, St Louis, 1988, The CV Mosby Co.

Roberts SL: Behavioral concepts and nursing throughout the life span, Englewood Cliffs, NJ, 1978, Prentice-Hall, Inc.

Stuart GW and Sundeen SJ: Principles and practice of psychiatric nursing, ed 3, St Louis, 1987, The CV Mosby Co.

Sundeen SJ, Stuart GW, Rankin ED et al: Nurse-client interaction: implementing the nursing process, ed 4, St Louis, 1989, The CV Mosby Co.

Whaley L and Wong D: Nursing care of infants and children, ed 3, St Louis, 1987, The CV Mosby Co.

Williams SR: Essentials of nutrition and diet therapy, ed 4, St Louis, 1986, The CV Mosby Co.

# CHAPTER 14

# Nursing Process of the Individual Client in the Community

ELIZABETH S. FAYRAM

## MODEL FOR ASSESSMENT

The client in this community-based case study is F.N., a 38-year-old black woman who has been coming to an urban clinic for control of hypertension. She has come to the clinic monthly for 4 months. Although she is taking antihypertension medications, her blood pressure remains elevated.

The Roy Adaptation Model (1984) is incorporated into the nursing process for this case study. This model is used for a variety of reasons: the nurse's philosophy and past experiences, the client situation, and the focus of the model. The goal of nursing according to Roy (1984) is to promote adaptation. The nurse has observed that many of the clients coming to the urban clinic, including F.N., require the nurse's assistance to promote adaptation. In addition, the model views clients holistically, with all dimensions addressed within the four adaptive modes. These adaptive modes are physiologic, self-concept, role function, and interdependence. The adaptation level is influenced by the focal, contextual, and residual stimuli present, and the response is either adaptive or ineffective (Roy, 1984).

Nursing activities as specified by Roy (1984) occur in six steps:

1. Assess behavior in each of the four adaptive modes.

2. Determine stimuli for ineffective behaviors.
3. Formulate nursing diagnoses.
4. Set goals.
5. Select interventions that will change the stimuli affecting adaptation.
6. Evaluate.

In this case study, data are collected and then analyzed according to the four adaptive modes. A judgment is made concerning the adaptive response. If responses are found to be ineffective, the stimuli affecting the behavior are identified and the nursing diagnoses are formulated. Plans, including goals, objectives, strategies, and nursing orders, are made. Evaluation completes the process.

The nursing process is organized into two sections. First, the assessment, analysis/synthesis, and nursing diagnoses are presented for each of two visits. This is followed by plans for each nursing diagnosis, consisting of goals, objectives, strategies, nursing orders, scientific rationale, and evaluation. Although the plans are placed last, they are initiated, implemented, and evaluated concurrently with the assessment visits. They are placed in the second section because they are ongoing and subject to revision, and demonstrate the continuity of the nursing process.

## DATA COLLECTION: Visit 1 2/4/89

| Interactions | Observations | Measurements |
|---|---|---|
| | **From chart:** | **From chart:** |
| | Client's initials: F.N. | Age: 38 yr. |
| | Reason for clinic appointment: hypertension. First seen at clinic 10/18/88. Chief complaint 10/18/88: headaches on awakening. Hypertension diagnosed. | Blood pressure:<br>10/18/88 (sitting):  210/124(right)  208/120(left)<br>11/15/88 (sitting):  186/112(right)  182/104(left)<br>12/13/88 (sitting):  184/102(right)  186/108(left)<br>1/10/89 (sitting):  168/96(right)  170/98(left) |
| | Separated from husband. Lives with four children in an apartment. Receives public assistance. Met with social worker on 11/15/88 and 1/10/89; marital difficulties discussed. | Height: 5'4"<br>Weight 10/18/88: 163 lb<br>Urinalysis 10/18/88:<br>Color: yellow<br>Opacity: clear<br>Specific gravity: 1.018<br>pH: 6.9 |
| | ECG 10/18/88: Left ventricular hypertrophy. | Glucose: neg<br>Protein: neg<br>RBC: neg<br>WBC: neg |
| | Eye exam 10/18/88: Arteriolar narrowing. | Serum electrolytes 10/18/88:<br>Sodium: 138<br>Potassium: 4.2<br>1/10/89: Potassium: 3.7 |
| | | Complete blood count 10/18/88:<br>WBC: 7.8<br>RBC: 4.6<br>Hgb: 13.4<br>Hct: 42.3 |
| | | Medications:<br>Prazosin (Minipress) 1 mg tid<br>Propranolol (Inderal) 120 mg bid<br>Hydrochlorothiazide (Hydrodiuril) 50 mg bid<br>Potassium chloride 10 mEq tid |
| **From client during clinic visit:** | | |
| Hi. Sure, I can answer some questions. | Eye contact with nurse, arms crossed, not smiling. Sitting on chair next to desk. | |
| I'm feeling better but my pressure's still up. | | BP (sitting):<br>162/96(right)<br>158/94(left)<br>Weight: 162 lb. |
| I'm still having problems with my husband. That's probably why it's up.<br>Too much water in me makes the pressure go up, I guess. | Looking out window, speaking softly. | |

*Continued.*

## DATA COLLECTION: Visit 1 2/4/89—cont'd

| Interactions | Observations | Measurements |
|---|---|---|
| My father had high blood pressure. My brother does too. | Eye contact. | |
| I guess I've had it since I was 25. | | |
| No, I was never given pills before. | | |
| I take my pills with my meals. Boy, I don't like the way the potassium tastes! | Smiles. | |
| I guess I shouldn't eat that chicken from the take-out restaurant. | Shakes head. | |
| I know I'm supposed to stay away from salty foods. | | |
| You mean I can't put salt on my food? Food doesn't taste good without it. | | |
| I know my weight isn't good for my pressure. What can I do to lose weight? | Shifting around in chair. | |
| I eat when I'm upset. | | |
| I've gained too much weight. Oh, about 20 pounds in the last year. | Abdomen obese; overall distribution of weight even. | |
| I'm not trying very hard to lose weight. | | |
| I eat snacks. Oh, cookies and cake, mostly. I can't remember everything I've eaten in the last 3 days. At work I eat chicken or hamburger and fries from the take-out place. | Black skin with reddish tone; clean, neat, tight clothes; small amount of make-up, perfume, and jewelry; nails short with polish. | |
| At home I have eggs, bacon, bread, cheese. I want to lose weight. Can you give me a diet? I think I look good at about 135 pounds. | | |
| Write down everything I eat for 3 days? Yeah, I can do that. Even all the snacks! | Nods head, smiling. | |
| No, I'm not having any more of those headaches. | | |
| I really don't exercise. I work 6 days a week as a sales clerk at a resale shop. | | |
| No, I've never smoked. | Sitting on exam table. | Pulse: 60/min<br>Respirations: 20/min |
| I do get short of breath when I climb a flight of stairs. | Breath sounds regular and quiet; no use of accessory muscles. Pulses strong; extremities warm. | |
| I drink a lot of pop. I'm always thirsty. | Moist mucous membranes; skin shiny; no dependent edema in lower extremities. | |
| I go to the bathroom a lot with this water pill. Oh, about 10 or 12 times a day. | | |

## DATA COLLECTION: Visit 1 2/4/89—cont'd

| Interactions | Observations | Measurements |
| --- | --- | --- |
| Sometimes my rings get tight when my fingers get puffy. | Holds out hands to show tightness of rings on fingers. | |
| I'm getting a divorce soon, in about 3 weeks. I'm hoping he'll finally be convinced it's over and leave me alone. | No eye contact, shifting around on table; voice tone louder. | |
| I've been married 21 years. | | |
| Yeah, I guess you could say I have a lot of stress. | Nods head. | |
| I have some friends at work and neighbors to talk to. I can't tell them everything. | | |
| Yes, I did talk to the social worker. It helped to talk to someone. I told her I'd come back when I needed to. | Nods head. | |
| Well, my weight and getting my pressure down. I think those are the most important things right now. | Eye contact. | |
| I used to get more exercise. Hard to find the time now. | | |
| Well, walking, I guess. My daughter would probably go with me. We could go before dinner. | | |
| Sure, I'll try it. If it'll help my pressure and my weight, it's worth a try. | Nods head. | |

## ANALYSIS/SYNTHESIS OF DATA: Visit 1

The four adaptive modes identified by Roy (1984) are addressed in this analysis with reference to appropriate data. Supporting theories, norms, and standards are also included. The adaptive or ineffective responses are identified. Stimuli influencing an ineffective adaptive response are also identified and classified as focal, contextual, and residual when possible.

### Analysis/Synthesis

A. Physiologic Mode
  1. *Oxygenation:* Data indicate an ineffective adaptive response in the oxygenation pattern. Blood pressure measurements ranging from 158/94 to 210/124 are elevated (Bates, 1987). According to Bullock and Rosendahl (1988), F.N.'s diastolic pressure of 120 and 124 is considered to be severely elevated. Diastolic BP between 102 and 112 is moderately elevated, and between 96 and 98 is mildly elevated. F.N. has previously experienced headaches on awakening, which can be a symptom of hypertension (Luckmann and Sorenson, 1987). Pulse (60) and respiratory rates (20) are within normal limits (Bates, 1987). F.N. describes symptoms of dyspnea on exertion, indicative of respiratory or cardiovascular difficulty (Luckmann and Sorenson, 1987). Other data include normal values in the complete blood count (Fischbach, 1988), quiet and regular breath sounds without the use of accessory muscles at rest, skin with reddish tones, strong pulses and warm extremities, and no dependent edema in the lower extremities. Edema is present in the fingers, indicating fluid retention or circulatory congestion (Bates, 1987). Contextual stimuli contributing to the ineffective response include many of the risk factors of

hypertension (Kochar and Woods, 1985): family history, black female, diet high in sodium and calories, limited exercise, and stress from relationship with husband.

Other stimuli include a history of hypertension since age 25, which was not treated with medications. There is a data gap in regard to other methods of blood pressure control used in the past. Positive stimuli include no history of smoking and taking medications prescribed to help control hypertension regularly. Elevated blood pressure over a period of about 13 years has contributed to changes within the cardiovascular/pulmonary systems: left ventricular hypertrophy, arteriolar narrowing in retina, dyspnea on exertion, and edema in upper extremities (Bullock and Rosendahl, 1988). The effect of propranolol on the cardiovascular system has affected the pulse rate, which is in the lower limits of normal (Bates, 1987). One effect of the beta-adrenergic blocking agents is slowing of the heart rate (Govoni and Hayes, 1988).

2. *Nutrition:* The nutritional pattern data indicate ineffective adaptation. F.N.'s weight of 163 lb is 20% over the ideal weight for her height (5 ft, 4 in.); therefore, she is considered to be obese (Williams, 1985). Appearance indicates an obese abdomen. Data regarding eating patterns are limited, but indicate that F.N. eats take-out food and snacks regularly, uses salt on food, and is not presently trying to lose weight. Contextual stimuli include F.N.'s inadequate knowledge of foods included in a low-sodium, low-calorie diet, eating when under stress, financial limitations, and limited exercise. Cultural influences on F.N.'s diet are unknown. Positive stimuli are indicated by F.N.'s request for a diet and assistance in losing weight.

3. *Elimination:* No data have been obtained about intestinal elimination. Data regarding urinary elimination include normal urinalysis (Fischbach, 1988) and frequent urination. The prescribed diuretic (hydrochlorothiazide) contributes to frequent urination (Luckmann and Sorenson, 1987). Effective adaptation is occurring in the urinary elimination pattern.

4. *Activity and rest:* Physical activity is limited. A data gap exists as to how much exercise F.N. gets at work. An exercise program should consist of 30 minutes of exercise three times per week (Luckmann and Sorenson, 1987). The focal stimulus contributing to the ineffective adaptation of activity is time for exercise. A factor that could affect F.N.'s ability to exercise involves her dyspnea on exertion. Data gaps include F.N.'s attitude toward exercise and environmental factors. F.N. indicated a willingness to try an exercise program. Data gaps regarding motor function and rest are present, and no inference about these items can be made at this time.

5. *Skin integrity:* Data on skin integrity indicate effective adaptation. The skin has reddish tones and is warm to the touch. Mucous membranes are moist. Data are limited regarding condition of skin (eg, lesions), hair, nails, perspiration, and sensation. A stimulus that may contribute to the development of ineffective skin integrity involves edema of the fingers and tight rings and is an area to continue to assess (Bates, 1987).

6. *The senses:* Minimal data have been obtained regarding the senses. An eye exam on 10/18/88 indicated arteriolar narrowing. No other data have been obtained regarding the senses. Data on pain also are limited. F.N. experienced headaches in the past. Headaches are a symptom of hypertension, and did occur while F.N.'s hypertension was considered to be severe (Bullock and Rosendahl, 1988). No inference regarding adaptation of the senses can be made at this time.

7. *Fluid and electrolytes:* Data regarding fluid and electrolytes include the measurements obtained in the urinalysis, such as specific gravity (1.018) and sodium (138) and potassium levels (4.2), which are within normal limits (Metheny, 1987). An abnormal finding, edema in the fingers, indicates ineffective adaptation regarding fluids. Focal stimuli include ingestion of foods high in sodium and the use of salt on food. The presence of left ventricular hypertrophy limits the pumping action of the left ventricle, causing fluid to back up into the lungs and eventually into the systemic circulation (Luckmann and Sorenson, 1987). Further assessment is necessary before determining whether this is a stimulus. A contextual stimulus is the use of a diuretic that can deplete sodium and potassium. The use of a potassium supplement (potassium chloride) has contributed to the effective adaptation of electrolyte levels. A

data gap exists on the type and volume of fluids the client drinks.

8. *Neurological function:* Minimum data have been collected for this pattern. F.N.'s ability to answer questions indicates that the client is alert and oriented (Bates, 1987). Data have not been obtained regarding the cranial nerves or sensory and motor evaluation. A tentative inference is made that neurological function is adaptive.

9. *Endocrine system:* The only data on endocrine functioning are the urinalysis (glucose: neg) and the presence of adipose tissue. More data are needed regarding temperature changes, menstrual cycle, and sexual development before an inference can be made.

B.  Self-Concept Mode
1. *Physical self:* Physical self includes body sensation and body image (Buck, 1984). Data are limited on body sensation but include statements that F.N. is "feeling better" and is not experiencing headaches at the present time. Data regarding body image center mainly around weight and include statements of a 20-pound weight gain within the past year, a desire to lose weight, and an ideal weight of 135 pounds. According to Williams (1985), F.N.'s perception of ideal weight is within normal limits for a woman of medium frame. Grooming is adaptive as observed by F.N.'s appearance in neat, clean clothes and the wearing of a small amount of make-up, perfume, jewelry, and nail polish. A temporary inference is made that F.N. is adapting in regard to physical self.

2. *Personal self:* Buck (1984) includes self-consistency, self-ideal, and the moral-ethical-spiritual self as components of the personal self. No data have been collected on the personal self. This is a data gap.

C.  Role Function Mode
F.N. is a 38-year-old woman, separated from her husband, who lives with her four children. F.N.'s developmental stage as defined by Erikson (1963) is generative adult, which involves generativity versus stagnation. Tasks included in this stage involve a satisfying marriage relationship, aiding the development of children, managing a home, meeting the needs of aging parents, and interdependence with others beyond the spouse (Nuwayhid, 1984). Data indicate that F.N. has the primary role of mother and provider for four children. She also has the role of sales clerk and is a recipient of public

aid. F.N. has been married 21 years but is in the process of a divorce. She expresses a desire to terminate the marriage relationship. Friends include those at work and neighbors.

Data gaps are present regarding the development of the children, responsibilities for aging parents, and the exact nature of the relationships with co-workers and neighbors. Successful adaptation within this stage results in productivity and accepting responsibility with affection (Sato, 1984). A data gap exists regarding stimuli such as social and cultural norms, role models, knowledge of expected roles, and rewards and cooperation F.N. receives from the roles she has assumed (Nuwayhid, 1984). Due to the data gaps, an inference is deferred.

D.  Interdependence Mode
The interdependence mode is divided into two components: significant others and support systems (Tedrow, 1984). Significant others are four children. A data gap exists regarding F.N.'s relationship with the children. F.N. is seeking a divorce from her husband of 21 years, who cannot be considered a significant other at this time. F.N. expresses difficulty with her husband. More specific data about the relationship with the husband are needed. Support systems include friends at work, neighbors, and the social worker at the clinic. F.N. does state that she cannot tell her friends everything. Another support system is the public assistance this family receives. A data gap exists about other family members.

According to Sato (1984), the black culture relies heavily on family as a support system. Another cultural factor affecting this mode is the underutilization of health care services by blacks. It is not clear whether F.N. and her children use the health care system on a regular basis or only when a crisis or illness occurs, such as the headaches F.N. experienced.

More data are needed to be obtained and considered when planning care with F.N. From the minimal data, a temporary inference of ineffective adaptation of this mode is made. The focal stimulus affecting this mode is the difficult relationship with F.N.'s husband. Data gaps regarding the stimuli include F.N.'s expectations of relationships, her nurturing abilities, and interactional skills (Tedrow, 1984).

Considering the previous review of the adaptive modes, the following strengths and concerns are identified:

### Strengths

1. Adaptive response in seeking assistance for weight loss
2. Adaptive response in urinary elimination pattern
3. Adaptive response in willingness to implement an exercise program
4. Adaptive neurological response
5. Adaptive response in the physical self pattern
6. Adaptive response in use of support systems in the interdependence mode

### Health concerns

1. Ineffective adaptive response in oxygenation pattern
2. Ineffective adaptive response in nutrition pattern
3. Ineffective adaptive response in activity pattern
4. Potential ineffective adaptive response in skin integrity pattern
5. Ineffective adaptive response in fluid pattern
6. Potential ineffective adaptive response in role function mode
7. Ineffective adaptive response in interdependence mode

## NURSING DIAGNOSES: Visit 1

| Date | Diagnoses | Priority |
|---|---|---|
| 2/4/89 | 1. Ineffective blood pressure control related to excessive intake of sodium and calories, lack of exercise, and stress. | 1 |
| 2/4/89 | 2. Alterations in nutrition, more than body requirements, related to knowledge deficit (low calorie, sodium), eating patterns, financial limitations, and limited exercise. | 2 |
| 2/4/89 | 3. Inadequate physical activity related to lack of providing time for exercise. | 3 |
| 2/4/89 | 4. Potential impairment of circulatory integrity of fingers related to fluid excess and tight rings. | 6 |
| 2/4/89 | 5. Fluid volume excess related to excessive sodium intake | 4 |
| 2/4/89 | 6. Potential ineffective role transition related to coping with change in marital status | 7 |
| 2/4/89 | 7. Ineffective interdependence related to stress from relationship with husband | 5 |

## DATA COLLECTION: Visit 2—2/18/89

| Interactions | Observations | Measurements |
|---|---|---|
| **From client during clinic visit:** | | |
| I'm doing much better, I think. | Sitting in waiting room: smiles when name called; erect posture, coordinated gait. | |
| | Sits on exam table. | Weight: 160 lb |
| | | BP (sitting):<br>152/94 (right)<br>156/98 (left)<br>Pulse: 60/min<br>Respirations: 20/min |
| I'm walking a lot. Yesterday we walked about 25 minutes. Usually three times a week for about 20 or 30 minutes. I like it. | | |
| I was tired after the first day. No, no trouble breathing. | Eye contact.<br>Extremities warm. No edema in lower extremities. | |
| I think it helps me relax.<br>I go to bed about 10:30 and get up at 6:30. I don't have trouble sleeping. | Quiet, regular respirations. | |
| Yeah, I wrote it all down for 3 days. I'm eating three meals a day, but I eat too | Looking away, swinging legs. | |

## DATA COLLECTION: Visit 2—2/18/89—cont'd

| Interactions | Observations | Measurements |
|---|---|---|
| many sweets. I usually eat with my kids or a friend at work. I snack at work when there's no customers. | | |
| I've been cutting back on my salt. I might have salt when I eat things I fix for my kids that I put salt in. | Able to remove rings from fingers. | Pitting edema (+1) in fingers. |
| Yeah, I had a list of foods high in salt. I think it got lost. | | |
| Yeah, I could use more information on that. Sure, I'll answer some more questions first. My BM's once a day. Soft, brown. No pain or bleeding. | | |
| No bad smell or urine infections. | | |
| No diabetes in my family. No, no thyroid changes. Heat and cold don't bother me. | | |
| I had my first period when I was 12 years old. Lasts about 5 days. No, no problem. | | |
| No, I don't check my breasts. Don't know how. | Shrugs shoulders. | |
| No, I don't wear glasses. I can see all right. | No squinting. | |
| I'm a Christian. The Lord has helped me get through this time with my husband. | Direct eye contact. | |
| It takes a lot to get me mad. I don't usually stay mad for long. | Looking down at hands in lap. | |
| It's hard for me to say something to someone. I guess I'm a kind-hearted, good person. At least, I try to be. | Looking up, smiling. | |
| My kids are great. I tell them they have to try hard. They do real well in school. They don't always understand they have to wait for things. You can only stretch a dollar so far. They have everything they need. I don't think kids should have everything they want. | Continues to smile. | Four children: Ages: 9, 12, 14, 17 |
| They don't want me to go out with friends. They want me to stay home. I need to get out, too. | Louder tone of voice. | |
| I don't know what it would be like to date again after 20 years of being married. | | |
| Sometimes I can't talk to others. I don't trust them with my feelings. I've been hurt too many times before. Some people just like to gossip. Most of the time I just keep my feelings inside. | Leans forward. | |
| I would like to better myself, but I do what I can and I'm all right for now. | Eye contact. | |
| My kids and my faith are the most important things in my life. We all help each other. | | |

*Continued.*

## DATA COLLECTION: Visit 2—2/18/89—cont'd

| Interactions | Observations | Measurements |
| --- | --- | --- |

I don't like taking money from public
aid. But I work, and it's too hard to
make the dollar stretch when you
have four kids.
My husband's hardly ever worked since
we've been married. I always worked.
I'm used to it.
The nurse and client then reviewed the
3-day food diary for foods high and
low in sodium and for factors influencing an increased caloric intake.

## ANALYSIS/SYNTHESIS OF DATA: Visit 2

Previous analysis is still applicable and is integrated for comparison when applicable. Roy's four
adaptive modes are addressed.

### Analysis/Synthesis

A. Physiologic Mode
   1. *Oxygenation:* F.N.'s blood pressure remains
      elevated (156/98) (Bates, 1987). Data within
      normal ranges include a pulse of 60/min,
      quiet and regular respirations 20/min, warm
      extremities, and no edema in the lower ex-
      tremities (Bates, 1987). Pitting edema (+1) is
      present in the fingers but has improved in
      that F.N. is able to remove her rings.
      Though progress has been made, the oxy-
      genation pattern remains in an ineffective
      adaptive response. Stimuli contributing to
      more effective adaptation are that F.N. is try-
      ing to reduce sodium intake and the imple-
      mentation of an exercise program. The exer-
      cise program has increased her relaxation
      level and is being tolerated (no shortness of
      breath). Stress from the marital relationship
      remains a data gap, as are the methods of
      stress management F.N. uses.
   2. *Nutrition:* F.N. has lost 3 pounds in 2 weeks.
      The food diary was reviewed for eating pat-
      terns: eating times, eating companions, and
      snacking habits; food quantity and quality;
      foods high and low in sodium; activity level;
      and food-related cues. F.N. states that she is
      attempting to reduce sodium intake but con-
      tinues to cook with it. She has received in-
      formation about high-sodium foods in the
      past, but has misplaced the written informa-
      tion. Her nutritional pattern remains an inef-

fective adaptive response. A positive stimulus is the establishment of an exercise program, which will influence caloric expenditure (Carpenito, 1987). Other positive stimuli
include F.N.'s attempt to reduce sodium intake, the recognition that she eats too many
sweets, and the interest in obtaining information about high-sodium foods.
   3. *Elimination:* Data obtained about intestinal
      elimination indicate effective adaptation
      (Servonsky, 1984). Minimal data on urinary
      elimination have been collected, such as nor-
      mal smell and no urinary infections. The uri-
      nary elimination pattern remains in adapta-
      tion.
   4. *Activity and rest:* F.N. has established a walk-
      ing program, which she does 3 times a week
      for 20 or 30 minutes. Data indicate that F.N.
      is tolerating the exercise program and has
      not developed shortness of breath or fatigue.
      Reasons for varying the length of time F.N.
      exercised were not explored. Data regarding
      motor function include F.N. walking with
      erect posture and coordinated gait and the
      ability to sit on the exam table, swing legs,
      and shrug shoulders. Motor function from
      the data is considered to be within normal
      limits (Bates, 1987). Data regarding rest indi-
      cate that F.N. does not have difficulty sleep-
      ing and sleeps for 8 hours, which is within
      normal limits (Potter and Perry, 1989). The
      activity and rest pattern is in adaptation but
      will need to be supported, especially in the
      area of activity.
   5. *Skin integrity:* Minimal data have been col-
      lected. Extremities remain warm, and no
      edema is present in the lower extremities.

Edema is still present in the fingers but has decreased. Effective adaptation of skin integrity has been maintained.

6. *The senses:* Again, a data gap remains. The only additional data are that F.N. is not squinting, does not wear glasses, and states she can see "all right." No additional data have been obtained about headaches or the other senses. No inference regarding adaptation of the senses is made at this time.

7. *Fluid and electrolytes:* Limited data have been collected for this pattern. Fluid volume excess continues to be present but to a lesser degree. The 3-day food diary was reviewed for foods high and low in sodium. Stimuli contributing to the reduction in fluid retention is F.N.'s attempt to reduce sodium intake (Luckmann and Sorenson, 1987). Further analysis of the 3-day recall will yield additional data in regard to sodium, fluid, and potassium intake.

8. *Neurological function:* F.N. continues to be alert and oriented, responding when her name is called and answering questions appropriately, demonstrating short- and long-term memory (Bates, 1987). Additional data regarding motor function is described in the activity and rest pattern. A data gap remains regarding cranial nerve and sensory evaluation. An inference is made that neurological function is adaptive.

9. *Endocrine system:* Additional data have been obtained regarding family history of diabetes, thyroid disorder, menstrual cycle, and breast self-exam. Specific data such as symptoms of diabetes were not explored. The endocrine pattern is adaptive (Luckmann and Sorenson, 1987). However, F.N. acknowledges a lack of knowledge to perform a breast self-exam.

B. Self-Concept Mode
1. *Physical self:* Data continue to be limited regarding body sensation and image. F.N. indicates that she is "doing much better" and is more relaxed since initiating an exercise program. Other relaxation techniques were not explored. Physical self is in adaptive response.

2. *Personal self:* Data have been obtained regarding self-consistency, self-ideal, and moral-ethical-spiritual components. Data regarding self-consistency include F.N.'s description of herself as a kind-hearted, good person who does not get mad easily. F.N. does not like

to receive public assistance but has accepted the need to do so. Nonverbal communication also adds data involving self-consistency: F.N. speaks freely about herself and uses direct eye contact, appropriate tone of voice, and facial expressions (Buck, 1984). Data regarding self-ideal are limited. Her statement that she would like to better herself is unclear and nonspecific. The statement, "I do what I can and I'm all right for now," indicates that F.N. accepts her self-concept at the present time. The third component, the moral-ethical-spiritual self, includes the client's belief system and morals (Buck, 1984). Data indicate a strong spiritual belief that gives F.N. strength to cope with difficult situations, such as the relationship with her husband. Other beliefs center around the children: valuing education and meeting children's needs but not necessarily all material desires. From the data obtained, an inference is made that F.N.'s personal self is adaptive.

C. Role Function Mode
Additional data have been obtained on F.N.'s role as parent. From statements such as "my kids are great," a tentative conclusion is made that F.N. is satisfied in her role as parent of four children. She identifies them as one of the most important things in her life. Another role is that of sales clerk. Little additional data have been provided. F.N. is in role transition at this point in time because of changes in marital status. She has begun to discuss dating, expressing some anxiety about dating after 20 years of marriage. There also is a concern between F.N. and the children about her visiting with friends. This may be an area of conflict. Further assessment is needed. Based on F.N.'s satisfaction with her roles, the role function mode is adaptive. However, there is a potential ineffective adaptation regarding role transition and role conflict.

D. Interdependence Mode
Significant others continue to be the four children. Main support systems are friends and religion. F.N. states that she has difficulty expressing feelings to others and keeps them inside. A factor influencing friends as a support system is the conflict between F.N. and the children regarding her visiting friends. Financial support is obtained through employment and public assistance. Financial support from F.N.'s husband is not provided. Health promo-

tion practices continue to be a data gap except for the data indicating that F.N. does not perform breast self-exam. The focal stimulus is lack of knowledge. No additional data have been obtained about the relationship with F.N.'s husband. It is difficult to conclude whether this continues to be a problem. Interdependence continues to be an area of concern with the possibility of inadequate support systems for dealing with stress and her relationship with her husband.

The following are F.N.'s strengths and health concerns at this time:

### Strengths

1. Adaptive response in nutrition pattern with a 3-lb weight loss in 2 weeks and attempt to reduce sodium intake
2. Adaptive response in elimination pattern
3. Adaptive response in activity and rest pattern

4. Adaptive response in skin integrity
5. Adaptive response in neurological function
6. Adaptive response in endocrine pattern
7. Adaptive response in self-concept mode
8. Adaptive response to roles as parent and employee
9. Adaptive response to interdependence with children, religion, and financial support

### Health concerns

1. Ineffective adaptive response in oxygenation pattern
2. Ineffective adaptive response in nutrition pattern
3. Ineffective response in fluid pattern
4. Potential ineffective adaptive response in role function (role transition and role conflict)
5. Potential ineffective adaptive response in interdependence mode (emotional support)
6. Ineffective adaptive response to health maintenance practices (breast self-exam)
7. Ineffective adaptive response in interdependence mode (relationship with husband)

## NURSING DIAGNOSES: Visit 2

| Date | Diagnoses | Priority | Resolved |
|---|---|---|---|
| 2/4/89 | 1. Ineffective blood pressure control related to lack of knowledge of high-sodium foods, excessive intake of calories, and stress. | 1 | |
| 2/4/89 | 2. Alteration in nutrition, more than body requirements, related to knowledge deficit, eating patterns, and financial limitations. | 2 | |
| 2/4/89 | 3. Inadequate physical activity related to lack of providing time for exercise. | | 2/18/89 |
| 2/4/89 | 4. Potential impairment of circulatory integrity of fingers related to fluid excess and tight rings. | 5 | |
| 2/4/89 | 5. Fluid volume excess related to excess sodium intake | 3 | |
| 2/4/89 | 6. Potential ineffective role transition related to coping with change in marital status. | 8 | |
| 2/4/89 | 7. Ineffective interdependence related to stress from relationship with husband. | 4 | |
| 2/18/89 | 8. Potential role conflict related to restricted time with friends. | 7 | |
| 2/18/89 | 9. Potential ineffective stress management related to inadequate emotional support system. | 6 | |
| 2/18/89 | 10. Alteration in health maintenance (breast self-exam) related to knowledge deficit. | 9 | |

Plans for diagnoses 1, 2, 3, and 7 are given on the following pages. Initial plans for diagnosis 5 are included in diagnosis 2. Potential diagnoses (4, 6, 8, and 9) and diagnosis 10 would be dealt with at a later time and are not included.

## PLANS FOR IMPLEMENTATION

**Nursing diagnosis 1:** *Ineffective blood pressure control related to lack of knowledge of high-sodium foods, excessive intake of calories, and stress (2/4/89).*
**Goal:** *Client will achieve blood pressure control by 4/1/89.*

| Objectives | Nursing orders | Scientific rationale | Evaluation |
|---|---|---|---|
| 1. Client will state four risk factors contributing to hypertension by 2/4/89. | 1a. Nurse will ask client to state what risk factors lead to development of hypertension on 2/4/89.<br><br>1b. Nurse and client will discuss additional risk factors unknown to client on 2/4/89.<br><br>1c. Client will state the risk factors applicable to her hypertension on 2/4/89. | *Content:* Control of hypertension<br>*Strategy:* Teaching/learning<br>1a. New learning is based on previous learning (Pohl, 1981).<br>1b. Teaching requires effective communication (Rorden, 1987). Risk factors include family history, racial predisposition, sodium intake, increased weight, stress and lack of exercise (Kochar and Woods, 1985).<br>1c. Active participation is part of effective learning (Pohl, 1981). Adult learners are motivated to learn when the information is applicable (Knowles, 1984). | **Criteria statement:**<br>Client will state four risk factors contributing to hypertension:<br>Family history<br>Racial predisposition<br>Sodium intake<br>Increased weight<br>Stress<br>Lack of exercise<br><br>Nurse implemented orders 1a-c on 2/4/89.<br>Client was able to state four risk factors: stress, sodium, weight, lack of exercise.<br>Objective met. |
| 2. Client will state two effects of hypertension on the body by 2/4/89. | 2a. Nurse and client will discuss the definition of hypertension on 2/4/89.<br>2b. Using audiovisual aids, nurse will explain how vasoconstriction influences pressure within the blood vessels on 2/4/89.<br>2c. Nurse will explain that:<br>(1) The higher the pressure, the greater the likelihood of organ damage.<br>(2) Hypertension is usually symptomless. | 2a. New learning is based on previous knowledge (Pohl, 1981).<br><br>2b. Audiovisual materials involve the learner actively, focus the learner's attention, and aid memory (Rorden, 1987).<br><br>2c. The possibility of organ damage increases as the pressure increases (Bullock and Rosendahl, 1988). Individuals with hypertension are usually without symptoms until the hypertension has progressed (Kochar and Woods 1985). | **Criteria statement:**<br>Client will state two effects of hypertension on the body:<br>Heart failure<br>Kidney failure<br>Stroke<br>Blood vessel changes in the eyes<br><br>Plan not implemented, due to other priorities and time constraints.<br>Objective not met. Nurse and client have agreed to implement this objective on 3/18/89. |

*Continued.*

## PLANS FOR IMPLEMENTATION—cont'd

| Objectives | Nursing orders | Scientific rationale | Evaluation |
|---|---|---|---|
| | (3) There are various consequences of hypertension on blood vessels and organs in the body on 2/4/89. | Complications of hypertension include heart and kidney failure, stroke, and blood vessle changes in the eye (Kochar and Woods, 1985). | |
| | 2d. Client will discuss concerns regarding the development of complications on 2/4/89. | 2d. An effective nurse-client relationship fosters expression of concern (Sundeen et al, 1989). | |
| 3. Client will name four measures used to control hypertension by 2/4/89. | 3a. Nurse and client will discuss reaching the blood pressure goal of 140/90 or less on 2/4/89. | 3a. Goals serve as guides to evaluate progress (Redman, 1988). | **Criteria statement:**<br>1. Client will name four measures used to control hypertension: Low-sodium diet Weight control Exercise program Medications Reduction in caffeine Stress management. |
| | 3b. Nurse will ask the client to state any control measures she is knowledgeable of on 2/4/89. | 3b. New learning is based on previous knowledge (Pohl, 1981). | 2. Client will state the individualized goal of BP less than 140/90, indicating a controlled blood pressure level. |
| | 3c. Nurse will explain control measures not stated by the client on 2/4/89. | 3c. Control measures include low-sodium diet, weight control, medications, exercise program, reduction in caffeine, and stress management (Luckmann and Sorenson, 1987). | 3. Client will state that blood pressure control is a life-long process.<br><br>Partial implementation of orders for objective 3. Client identified five control measures: medications, low-sodium diet, weight control, stress reduction, and exercise program. Further explanation and clarification is |
| | 3d. Nurse will explain that blood pressure control is a lifelong concern and that control measures should be continued on 2/4/89. | 3d. Hypertension is not curable but it is controllable (Kochar and Woods, 1985). | necessary (e.g., low-sodium diet). Objective not met. Nurse and client plan to continue with this objective on 3/18/89, emphasizing lifelong control and the difficulties client is experiencing with control measures. |
| | 3e. Using open-ended questions, nurse will encourage the client to express feelings about the difficulties following the control measures. | 3e. About 50% of clients with hypertension do not follow through with their prescribed regimens (McEntee and Peddicord, 1987). | **Summative evaluation:**<br>Client's blood pressure |

**PLANS FOR IMPLEMENTATION—cont'd**

| Objectives | Nursing orders | Scientific rationale | Evaluation |
|---|---|---|---|
| | | | level will be less than 140/90. |
| | | | Goal not achieved. F.N.'s blood pressure is decreasing but remains elevated. |
| | | | This plan, along with plans 2, 3, 5, and 7, should continue to be implemented to control hypertension. |

**Nursing diagnosis 2:** *Alteration in nutrition, more than body requirements, related to knowledge deficit, eating patterns, and financial limitations (2/4/89).*

**Goal:** *Client will improve nutritional status by decreasing caloric and sodium intake and achieving ideal weight by 6/15/89.*

| Objectives | Nursing orders | Scientific rationale | Evaluation |
|---|---|---|---|
| 1. Client will state three factors that lead to increased caloric intake by 2/18/89. | 1a. Nurse will explain factors that lead to increased caloric intake on 2/18/89: Eating patterns Food quantities Food quality Activity levels Food-related thoughts Food-related cues | *Content:* Nutrition *Strategy:* Teaching/learning 1a. Factors contributing to an increased caloric intake stem from emotions and eating habits. Refer to nursing order 1a (Snetselaar, 1983). | Orders 1a-d were implemented on 2/18/89. Food diary was reviewed. Factors contributing to increased caloric intake include eating patterns (snacking), food quality (high fat), previous sedentary activity level, and eating when under stress. Client was able to state four factors leading to increased caloric intake. Objective 1 met. |
| | 1b. Client will discuss with the nurse each factor in relation to own diet (time, place, financial considerations) on 2/18/89. | 1b. Active participation by the learner facilitates learning (Pohl, 1981). | |
| | 1c. Nurse and client will review the 3-day food diary on 2/18/89 in regard to factors listed in 1a. | 1c. Active participation by the learner facilitates learning (Pohl, 1981). | |
| | 1d. Client will state three factors that most likely lead her to increase caloric intake on 2/18/89. | 1d. Evaluation is a part of the teaching/learning process (Redman, 1988). | |

*Continued.*

## PLANS FOR IMPLEMENTATION—cont'd

| Objectives | Nursing orders | Scientific rationale | Evaluation |
|---|---|---|---|
| 2. Client will select three strategies to use to decrease caloric intake by 2/18/89. | 2a. Client will discuss with the nurse strategies used in the past to lose weight on 2/18/89.<br>2b. Nurse and client will discuss strategies to decrease caloric intake safely by 2/18/89:<br>Substituting non-food-related activities<br>Interposing time between eating episodes<br>Cue elimination (eating only in one room)<br>Reducing food quantity<br>Increasing activity while decreasing calories<br>Thinking positively about food intake<br>Including high-quality foods (e.g., protein, vitamin, minerals)<br>Using self-help groups<br>2c. Client will select at least three strategies to use to decrease caloric intake on 2/18/89. | 2a. New learning is based on previous knowledge and experience (Pohl, 1981).<br>2b. A variety of strategies is available to decrease caloric intake (Snetselaar, 1983).<br><br><br><br><br><br><br><br><br><br><br><br>2c. Active participation by the learner facilitates learning (Pohl, 1981). | Orders 2a-c not implemented because of time constraints. Nurse and client have agreed to implement this objective at the next visit on 3/18/89. |
| 3. Client will state five high-sodium foods consumed in her diet by 2/18/89. | 3a. Nurse and client will discuss factors that lead to high-sodium intake by 2/18/89:<br>Eating foods high in sodium<br>Salting food when cooking and at the table<br>Dislike of taste of foods without sodium<br>3b. Nurse and client will discuss ways to decrease sodium intake on 2/18/89.<br><br><br>3c. Nurse and client will review a written list of foods that have a high-sodium content on 2/18/89. | 3a. Factors contributing to a high-sodium intake are listed in 3a (Snetselaar, 1983).<br><br><br><br><br><br>3b. Factors leading to ingestion of a high-sodium diet can be modified by the choice of foods and the elimination of the use of sodium (Snetselaar, 1983).<br>3c. The use of written information and discussion reinforce learning (Rorden, 1987). | Orders 3a-d implemented by nurse and client out of sequence due to client's interest in high-sodium foods. All three factors contributed to the client's high-sodium intake. Client was given written list of foods high in sodium. The client was able with help to identify foods in the 3-day food diary that were high in sodium. She stated she was going to reduce her sodium intake by eliminating foods high in sodium and refraining from cooking with sodium and using it at the table. F.N. will try to use more spices and herbs in cooking instead of sodium, but she was unsure how her children would react. |

## PLANS FOR IMPLEMENTATION — cont'd

| Objectives | Nursing orders | Scientific rationale | Evaluation |
|---|---|---|---|
| | 3d. Client will identify foods from the high-sodium list that she eats regularly on 2/18/89. | 3d. Active participation by the learner facilitates learning (Pohl, 1981). | Objective met but needs further support and evaluation at future visits. |
| 4. Client will plan 3 days of menus, incorporating a 1450-calorie, low-sodium diet by 3/18/89. | 4a. Nurse and client will discuss the foods and daily requirements of the four basic food groups, using a handout from the American Dietetic Association on 3/18/89. | 4a. Basic knowledge of nutrition is necessary before the client can plan menus. | **Criteria statement:**<br>1. Client will plan 3 days of menus, incorporating a 1450-calorie, low-sodium diet.<br>2. Client will state financial considerations and palatability of the diet for the family. |
| | 4b. Nurse and client will discuss the reason to consume 1450 calories/day on 3/18/89. | 4b. Caloric requirement for a 1- to 2-lb weight loss per week is determined by the formula: Actual weight in pounds minus $15 \times 10$ ($160 - 15 \times 10 = 1450$) (Carpenito, 1987). | Orders 4a-d were not implemented at this point in time. Plan to be implemented at the next visit. |
| | 4c. Client will plan 3 days of menus using low-calorie and low-sodium handouts as a guide by 3/18/89. | 4c. Active participation by the learner is necessary for effective learning (Pohl, 1981). | |
| | 4d. Nurse and client will review menu plan for calorie and sodium content, financial considerations, and palatability by the client and family members on 3/18/89. | 4d. Evaluation is a part of the teaching/learning process (Redman, 1988). | |
| 5. Client will lose 1 to 2 lb per week until the ideal weight is reached. | 5a. Nurse and client will discuss proper weight loss of 1 to 2 lb per week on 3/18/89. | 5a. Safe weight loss is 1 to 2 lb per week (Carpenito, 1987). | **Criteria statement:**<br>1. Client will state that safe weight loss should be 1 to 2 lb per week.<br>2. Client will record weight on a weekly basis.<br>3. Client will lose 1 to 2 lb per week until ideal weight is reached. |
| | 5b. Nurse and client will discuss how new nutritional patterns are lifelong on 3/18/89. | 5b. Ability to maintain ideal weight, once achieved, requires continuation of new nutritional patterns (Williams, 1985). | |
| | 5c. Nurse and client will discuss the importance of continuing the exercise program while decreasing calories on 3/18/89. | 5c. Exercise aids in weight loss by increasing caloric requirements of the body (Carpenito, 1987). | Orders for objective 5 not implemented at the present time. After implementation of plans for objectives 2 and 4, this objective will be implemented. |
| | 5d. Client will weigh self weekly beginning 3/18/89. | 5d. Client will be able to note progress. | |

*Continued.*

## PLANS FOR IMPLEMENTATION—cont'd

| Objectives | Nursing orders | Scientific rationale | Evaluation |
|---|---|---|---|
| | 5e. Client will complete a 3-day food diary by 5/13/89. <br><br> 5f. Nurse and client will review progress with eating changes, problems, and acceptance on 5/13/89. | 5e. Evaluation is an integral part of the teaching/learning process (Redman, 1988). <br><br> 5f. Evaluation provides for review of progress and modifications necessary (Redman, 1988). | Weight between 2/4/89 and 2/18/89 did decrease by 3 pounds, which is an appropriate weight loss. Client attributed the weight loss to trying to reduce sodium intake and starting an activity program. She was encouraged by the weight loss and wanted to work on it in the future. <br><br> **Summative evaluation:** <br><br> Goal not met, but client's awareness of nutritional status has increased. Nurse and client agreed to continue to work on implementing the plan. |

**Nursing diagnosis 3:** *Inadequate physical activity related to lack of providing time for exercise (2/4/89).*
**Goal:** *The client will increase physical activity by 2/18/89.*

| Objective | Nursing orders | Scientific rationale | Evaluation |
|---|---|---|---|
| 1. Client will verbalize benefits of a regular exercise program by 2/4/89. | 1a. Nurse will ask the client to explain the benefits that occur from exercising regularly on 2/4/89. <br><br> 1b. On 2/4/89, the nurse and client will discuss benefits of a regular exercise program: Cardiovascular functioning Weight loss/control Relaxation <br><br> 1c. Client will state two benefits of a regular exercise program on 2/4/89. | *Content:* Activity *Strategies:* Teaching/ learning and problem solving. <br> 1a. New learning is based on previous knowledge (Pohl, 1981). <br> 1b. Regular exercise benefits cardiovascular functioning and will increase energy output, aiding in weight loss/control (Allan, 1985). When an enjoyable exercise program is initiated, relaxation may also be a benefit. <br> 1c. Active participation fosters learning (Pohl, 1981). | **Criteria statement:** <br> Client will state two benefits of a regular exercise program. Refer to 1b. <br><br> Nurse and client implemented orders 1a-c on 2/4/89. After implementation of the plan, the client stated that a regular exercise program would help reduce her blood pressure and weight. <br> Objective met. |

## PLANS FOR IMPLEMENTATION—cont'd

| Objectives | Nursing orders | Scientific rationale | Evaluation |
|---|---|---|---|
| 2. Client will select an exercise program based on interest and time constraints by 2/4/89. | 2a. On 2/4/89, the nurse and client will discuss different types of exercise programs: Swimming Walking Bicycling | 2a. A variety of exercise programs are available that provide moderate exercise (Luckmann and Sorenson, 1987). Programs mentioned by the nurse will be of low cost because of financial limitations of client. | Nurse and client implemented orders 2a-e. Client selected walking. Time for the exercise was before dinner. Enjoyment was enhanced by asking the client's daughter to accompany her. Objective met. |
| | 2b. Client will explain time constraints in present schedule on 2/4/89. | 2b. Active participation is a part of effective problem solving. The first step is accurate identification of the problem (Sullivan and Decker, 1988). | |
| | 2c. Nurse will discuss time commitments of an exercise program (3 times/week, 30 min duration) on 2/4/89. | 2c. Exercise, to be of benefit, should be performed at a frequency of 3 times/week for at least 30 min (Allan, 1985). | |
| | 2d. Client, with the nurse's assistance, will analyze possible exercise options according to enjoyment and scheduling on 2/4/89. | 2d. Problem solving includes determining possible solutions and analyzing the consequences. The nurse is the facilitator, guiding the client in the process (Sullivan and Decker, 1988). | |
| | 2e. Client will select one type of exercise program and the time to do it for the next 2 weeks on 2/4/89. | 2e. Next step of the problem-solving process is selection of a specific alternative by the client (Sullivan and Decker, 1988). | |
| 3. Client will implement the selected exercise program 3 times/week, increasing to 30 min by 2/18/89. | 3a. Client will select one type of exercise program to implement on 2/4/89. | 3a. Problem-solving includes selection of one alternative (Sullivan and Decker, 1988). | **Criteria statement:** 1. Client will implement the selected exercise program 3 times/week, increasing to 30-min duration. 2. Client will state the effects of the exercise program. Refer to 3d. 3. Client will state whether problems exist with the scheduling of the exercise program. |
| | 3b. Nurse and client will discuss precautions to take when implementing an exercise program on 2/4/89: Begin slowly. Include 5 min of warm-up and 5 min of cool-down exercises. | 3b. Activity intolerance can be prevented by beginning an exercise program slowly and including warm-up and cool-down exercises. Symptoms of activity intolerance should be assessed (Allan, 1985). | |

*Continued.*

## PLANS FOR IMPLEMENTATION — cont'd

| Objectives | Nursing orders | Scientific rationale | Evaluation |
|---|---|---|---|
| | Watch for activity intolerance: shortness of breath, lightheadedness, pain, fatigue. | | Client implemented the exercise program during the time frame of 2/4/89-2/18/89. |
| | 3c. Client will perform the exercise program 3 times/week, increasing to 30 min if tolerated by 2/18/89. | 3c. Implementation is the next step of the problem-solving process (Sullivan and Decker, 1988). | *Criteria 1:* Client states that she is walking, which is the exercise she selected. Frequency is usually 3 times/week with a duration of 20-30 min. Greater clarification should be obtained with F.N., such as the reason why the duration varies from 20-30 min. Client could write down the dates and times of exercising for a more accurate evaluation. |
| | 3d. Client will monitor the effects of the exercise program by 2/18/89: symptoms of activity intolerance, relaxation, and enjoyment. | 3d. Evaluation is an integral part of the problem-solving process (Sullivan and Decker, 1988). | *Criteria 2:* Client stated the effects of exercising were tiredness the first day, no shortness of breath, and greater relaxation. No specific mention is made regarding pain or lightheadedness. Client did state that she "likes it," indicating enjoyment. |
| | 3e. Nurse and client will evaluate the outcome of the implementation of the exercise program on 2/18/89: frequency, duration, enjoyment, time problems, and effects. | 3e. Evaluation is an integral part of the problem-solving process (Sullivan and Decker, 1988). | *Criteria 3:* No information was obtained regarding whether time difficulties occurred. This should be specifically addressed when evaluating this program. F.N. was able to "usually" find 3 days/week to implement the exercise program. Objective partially met. |
| | | | **Summative evaluation:** Client implemented an exercise program, so her physical activity has increased. Goal met. This pattern will need continued monitoring in terms of frequency and length of exercise as well as support. |

**Nursing diagnosis 7:** *Ineffective interdependence related to stress from relationship with husband (2/4/89).*
**Goal:** *Client will increase stress management techniques by 5/13/89.*

| Objectives | Nursing orders | Scientific rationale | Evaluation |
|---|---|---|---|
| 1. Client will list two personal reactions to stress from relationship with husband by 3/18/89. | 1a. Nurse will use open-ended statements and questions when discussing stressors and responses. | *Content:* Stress <br> *Strategies:* Stress management and teaching/learning <br> 1a. Open-ended statements and questions facilitate communication (Sundeen, and others, 1989). | Plan not implemented because of other priorities. Objective not met. |
| | 1b. Nurse will explain what stressors are and the body's response 3/18/89. | 1b. First stage in stress management according to Hamberger and Lohr (1984) involves education (e.g., nature of stress). | |
| | 1c. Client will identify two personal reactions to stress from relationship with husband by 3/18/89. | 1c. Stressors affect different people in different ways (Luckmann and Sorenson, 1987). | |
| 2. Client will choose two coping strategies to use to manage stress by 3/18/89. | 2a. Client will describe coping strategies she currently uses to deal with the stress from relationship with husband on 3/18/89. | 2a. Assessment of coping strategies currently used is a step in stress management (Hamberger and Lohr, 1984). | **Criteria statement:** <br> Client will select two coping strategies to use to manage stress. Refer to nursing order 2c. |
| | 2b. Nurse and client will discuss the effectiveness of methods client currently uses to manage stress on 3/18/89. | 2b. Learning needs of the client must be determined (Redman, 1988). | Plan not implemented because of other priorities. Objective not met. Plan to be implemented at next visit. |
| | 2c. Nurse will explain a variety of coping strategies available to manage the stress reaction on 3/18/89: <br> Relaxation techniques <br> Assertiveness training <br> Problem solving <br> Biofeedback | 2c. Stress management involves a variety of coping strategies that can be used by individuals (Hamberger and Lohr, 1984). Refer to nursing order 2c. | |
| | 2d. Client will react to each coping strategy on 3/18/89. | 2d. Client is an active participant. | |
| | 2e. Client will select two coping strategies to use for stress management on 3/18/89. | 2e. Client is an active participant in the selection of coping strategies, fostering motivation, and learning (Redman, 1988). | |
| 3. Client will use the selected coping strategies on a regular basis by 5/13/89. | 3a. Nurse will explain how each strategy is used correctly on 3/18/89. | 3a. Learning occurs through imitation (Rorden, 1987). | **Criteria statement:** <br> 1. Client will demonstrate the correct use of each coping strategy selected. |

*Continued.*

## PLANS FOR IMPLEMENTATION—cont'd

| Objectives | Nursing orders | Scientific rationale | Evaluation |
|---|---|---|---|
| | 3b. Client will practice with the nurse each technique selected on 3/18/89 and 4/15/89.<br><br>3c. Client will implement one strategy at a time on 3/18/89 and 4/15/89. | 3b. Effective learning requires active participation by the learner (Pohl, 1981).<br><br>3c. Learning is broken down into small steps to facilitate learning and achievement (Redman, 1988). | 2. Client will state the frequency each technique has been used to manage stress.<br>Plan not implemented.<br>Objective not met.<br>Plan to be implemented at a future date. |
| | 3d. Nurse and client will evaluate the technique according to use, ability to perform, and usefulness at managing the stress on 5/13/89. | 3d. Final stage of stress management is the application of coping strategies to an actual stressor and the evaluation of that application (Hamberger and Lohr, 1984). | **Summative evaluation:**<br>Goal not met. |

## REFERENCES AND READINGS

Allan JD: Exercise program. In Bulechek GM and McCloskey JC: Nursing interventions: treatments for nursing diagnoses, Philadelphia, 1985, WB Saunders Co.

Bates B: A guide to physical examination, Philadelphia, 1987, JB Lippincott Co.

Buck MH: Self-concept: theory and development. In Roy C Sr: Introduction to nursing: an adaptation model, Englewood Cliffs, NJ, 1984, Prentice-Hall, Inc.

Bullock BL and Rosendahl PP: Pathophysiology: adaptations and alterations in function, Glenview, Ill, 1988, Scott, Foresman & Co.

Carpenito LH: Nursing diagnosis: application to clinical practice, Philadelphia, 1987, JB Lippincott Co.

Erikson E: Childhood and society, New York, 1963, WW Norton Co, Inc.

Fink JW: The challenge of blood pressure control, Nurs Clin North Am 16:301, June 1981.

Fischbach TF: A manual of laboratory diagnostic tests, Philadelphia, 1988, JB Lippincott Co.

Foster SB and Kousch D: Adherence to therapy in hypertensive clients, Nurs Clin North Am 16:331, June 1981.

Govoni LE and Hayes JE: Drugs and nursing implications, Norwalk, Conn, 1988, Appleton & Lange.

Hamberger LK and Lohr JM: Stress and stress management: research and applications, New York, 1984, Springer Publishing Co, Inc.

Johnson MN et al: Psychological stress and blood pressure levels in Black women, J Nat Black Nurs Assoc 1:41, Fall 1986–Winter 1987.

Knowles M: The modern practice of adult education: from pedagogy to andragogy, Chicago, 1984, Follett Publishing Co.

Kochar MS and Woods KD: Hypertension control for nurses and other health professionals, New York, 1985, Springer Publishing Co.

Luckmann J and Sorenson KC: Medical-surgical nursing: a psychophysiologic approach, Philadelphia, 1987, WB Saunders Co.

MacDonald MB, Sawatzky JE, and Wilson TW: Lifestyle behaviors in treated hypertensives as prediction of blood pressure control, Rehab Nurs 13:82, March-April 1988.

McEntee MA and Peddicord K: Coping with hypertension, Nurs Clin North Am 22:583, September 1987.

Metheny NM: Fluid and electrolyte balance: nursing considerations, Philadelphia, 1987, JB Lippincott Co.

Nakagawa-Kogan H et al: Self-management of hypertension: predictors of success in diastolic blood pressure reduction, Res Nurs Health 11:105, April 1988.

Neighbors HW: Seeking professional help for personal problems: black Americans' use of health and mental health services, Community Ment Health J 21:156, Fall 1988.

Nuwayhid KA: Role function: theory and development. In Roy Sr C: Introduction to nursing: an adaptation model, Englewood Cliffs, NJ, 1984, Prentice-Hall, Inc.

Plawecki HM et al: Compliance and health beliefs in the black female hypertensive client, J Nat Black Nurs Assoc 2:38, Fall 1987–Winter 1988.

Pohl ML: The teaching function of the nursing practitioner, Dubuque, Ia, 1981, William C Brown Co.

Potter PA and Perry AG: Fundamentals of nursing: concepts, process, and practice, St Louis, 1989, The CV Mosby Co.

Powers MJ: Profile of the well-controlled, well-adjusted hypertensive patient, Nurs Res 36:106, March-April 1987.

Redman, BK: The process of patient education, St Louis, 1988, The CV Mosby Co.

Rorden JW: Nurses as health teachers: a practical guide, Philadelphia, 1987, WB Saunders Co.

Roy C Sr: Introduction to nursing: an adaptation model, Englewood Cliffs, NJ, 1984, Prentice-Hall, Inc.

Sato MK: Major factors influencing adaptation. In Roy Sr C: Introduction to nursing: an adaptation model, Englewood Cliffs, NJ, 1984, Prentice-Hall, Inc.

Servonsky J: Elimination. In Roy C Sr: Introduction to nursing: an adaptation model, Englewood Cliffs, NJ, 1984, Prentice-Hall, Inc.

Snetselaar LG: Nutrition counseling skills: assessment, treatment, and evaluation, Rockville, Md, 1983, Aspen Systems Corp.

Sullivan EJ and Decker PJ: Effective management in nursing, Menlo Park, Calif, 1988, Addison-Wesley Publishing Co.

Sundeen SJ et al: Nurse-client interaction: implementing the nursing process, St Louis, 1988, The CV Mosby Co.

Tedrow MP: Interdependence: theory and development. In Roy C Sr: Introduction to nursing: an adaptation model, Englewood Cliffs, NJ, 1984, Prentice-Hall, Inc.

Williams SR: Nutrition and diet therapy, St Louis, 1985, The CV Mosby Co.

# Nursing Process of the Family Client: Application of Neuman's Systems Model

## JOANNE R. CROSS

The community health nurse is working with the Ross family. This blended family consists of a married couple, Jim and Mary, both of whom have been formerly married, and their older children. Jim's 15-year-old son, Jim, Jr., and Mary's children, Danny, 23, and Mary, 20, reside in the home. The focus of this family nursing process is on Danny, who has Hodgkin's disease, and the stressors and family interactions related to his care.

The Neuman (1982) Systems Model, which is applicable with an individual, family, or community, was chosen as the framework to guide working with this family. In Neuman's model, the family is viewed as an open system in constant interaction with the environment. Successful transactions with the environment reflect adjustment to that environment by the family. Neuman's model was chosen because the major components of this model are stress and reaction to stress and this family is experiencing various stressors related to illness. Family stressors during illness and ways in which the family copes with stressors are also addressed by Neuman's model. Stressors are defined as follows:

*Intrafamily stressors* occur within the family unit—the individual interactions among family members. These interactions can be within the biological, psychological, sociological, developmental, and spiritual realms. They may include actual or potential stress problems, coping mechanisms, lifestyle changes, physical problems, strengths and weaknesses, general mood, and decision-making processes, among other factors.

*Interfamily stressors* occur between the family and the immediate or direct external environment. Examples include interaction with other families such as in-laws, neighbors, ex-spousal rela-

tionships, friends and community groups such as church and school groups, and work environments.

*Extrafamily stressors* occur between the family and the distal or indirect environment (political and social issues or support and other groups).

The process of interaction and adjustment within the family relies on the "lines of defense," which are biological, psychological, sociocultural, developmental, and spiritual in nature. The interaction and impact of each of these realms must continually be considered as they impinge on the family's stress points (Story and Ross, 1986). If a stressor breaks through the normal line of defense, the equilibrium is disturbed and a whole range of responses occurs. In addition, internal resistance factors (lines of resistance) are activated that attempt to stabilize and return the client or family to normal functioning.

Stressors not only create reactions within the client (individual or family), but also create strong emotional fields between the client and other extrapersonal forces. Nursing interventions can begin at any point at which a stressor is suspected or identified, and can be introduced at primary, secondary, or tertiary levels of prevention. Neuman's model facilitates attainment and maintenance of the highest possible level of function and addresses primary, secondary, and tertiary levels of care. This model guides the modes of nursing intervention for each level and focuses on returning the client to a previously healthy state. For a review of Neuman's major concepts, see Chapter 2.

In this nursing process of the family, the five nurse visits are presented sequentially, along with assessment data, analysis and synthesis of the data, and the list of nursing diagnoses for each visit. Then five nursing plans, which include goals, objectives, nursing orders, scientific rationale, and evaluation, are described. The plans are presented last because they are ongoing and subject to revision, and demonstrate the continuity of the entire nursing process. However, the nursing plans are initiated, implemented, and evaluated concurrently with the assessment visits.

## DATA COLLECTION: Preliminary information

Jim and Mary have been married for 3 ½ years. Jim's wife, Jill, died 5 years ago and his son, Jim, Jr., lives with Mary and him. Mary is divorced from her first husband, Bill. They had two children, Danny, 23, and Diane, 20, who are currently living with Jim and Mary. Danny is divorced and estranged from his ex-wife, Lois, who lives in Florida with their 2-year-old son. Danny has Hodgkin's disease and is currently undergoing a course of chemotherapy treatment.

*Source of referral:*
Oncology clinic at hospital where Danny is a client

*Collaborating agencies:*
John Shell, MD
Medical Oncology Unit
Cancer Society
United Way

*Communication with collaborating agency:*
Oncology unit at Sycamore Hospital

October 14, 1988: Information received from Dr. Shell, Danny's oncologist, in a phone conversation:
1. Diagnosed in February 1988. Stage IIIB Hodgkin's disease. Initial symptoms were night sweats, inguinal lymph node enlargement, severe lower back pain, and hematuria.
2. No response to MOPP,* first line therapy.
3. Has had 4 courses of ABVD therapy (Adriamycin, bleomycin, vinblastine, and DTIC).
4. Is in remission (not sure yet if complete remission). Lymph nodes and bone lesions have resolved.
5. If present therapy eventually fails, several other courses of therapy can be tried.
6. Not concerned about back pain; bone scan was negative.
   a. Received radiation therapy to this area in February 1988.
   b. Discontinued Dilaudid because he felt Danny was becoming too dependent on it.
7. Physician feels that right now Danny is coping with his disease well psychologically.
8. Since Danny has been feeling better, Dr. Shell has had no contact with the family (stepfather called him often during early phase of illness).

*MOPP = acronym for combination of nitrogen mustard, vincristine (Oncovin) procarbazine, and prednisone (Porth, 1986).

**Genogram**

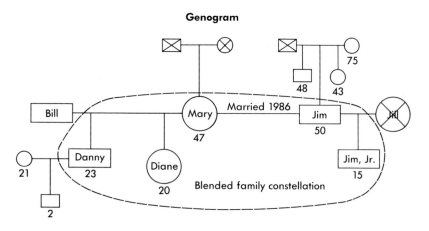

Ross family genogram.

## Biographical Data and Initial Contact

| Name | Age | Sex | Education | Occupation | Introductory data |
|------|-----|-----|-----------|------------|-------------------|
| Danny | 23 | M | Dropped out of high school in senior year | Unemployed | Impaired member—has Hodgkin's disease, is recently divorced, and has 2-yr-old son who lives with his ex-wife |
| Jim | 50 | M | Working toward master's degree in business | Salesman for large insurance company | Stepfather of Danny and Diane; father of Jim, Jr. |
| Mary | 42 | F | Did not finish high school | Housewife; grooms, breeds, and shows poodles | Mother of Danny and Diane; stepmother of Jim, Jr. |
| Jim, Jr. | 15 | M | Freshman in high school | N/A | Stepbrother of Danny and Diane |
| Diane | 20 | F | High school graduate | Unemployed; assists mother with grooming of poodles | Sister of Danny; stepsister of Jim, Jr. |

## DATA COLLECTION: Visit 1—October 22, 1988

*Setting:* Nurse talked with client in hospital room at Sycamore Medical Center where he had been since October 18 to receive chemotherapy. No other clients were present in the three-bed room. Data were received verbally from client, by observation of nurse, and from the chart.

| Interactions | Observations/Measurements (M)* |
|--------------|-------------------------------|
| **Biological data (from client)** | |
| Hi, Joan. I'm doing a little better today. My doctor says I will probably be getting these drugs for 6-8 more months. He says he thinks I am starting remission, and if I can live for 5 years, I will probably not get the cancer back. If this drug stops working, there is one other drug they can try, and if that doesn't work, I've had it. | Client lying in bed. Head of bed slightly raised. Bedcovers covering him up to waist. Danny appeared well nourished and of normal weight. Skin was pale. No alopecia was noted. Hair was shiny and neatly combed. Eyes alert. Wearing a clean pair of striped pajamas. |
| I get sick with this drug but not as bad. They give me THC† (like "joints"), and they let me smoke "joints" while I'm getting therapy. It makes me feel like I'm in a different place, and I don't mind the nausea as much. I still get the shakes, but if I can get my mind on something else, that helps, even if it's just tapping my fingers. I'm usually sick for 3-5 hr after getting the drug. | Client takes THC 7.5 mg every 4 hr when receiving chemotherapy (chart) **(M)**. Client demonstrated by tapping fingers on bedside stand. Smiled and rolled his eyes. |
| I ate supper last night after getting therapy in the late afternoon and kept it down. I just eat light foods. | |
| They've really messed up my veins. It's hard to find a good one any more. My doctor says they might have to start putting it in my neck or legs. I don't want them to do that. I'm afraid that will really hurt. | Both arms appeared "black and blue" at injection sites. |
| I still get tired rather easily. | Smoked filtered cigarettes continuously throughout interview. |
| My doctor says I should not get a job yet. I can feel fine for a while and then get sick again and would have to quit a job. | |

*(M) = measurement data.
†THC = Delta-9-tetrahydrocannabinol.

## DATA COLLECTION: Visit 1—October 22, 1988—cont'd

| Interactions | Observations/Measurements (M) |
|---|---|
| Still gets sweats but no bleeding from UT‡ now.<br>Denies any itching of skin.<br><br>Started having symptoms in January 1988—sweats, bleeding from kidney, lower back pain. "I was very sick. I couldn't stand or sit without severe pain."<br>They did a lot of tests and finally diagnosed it as cancer. At first they thought I would only live about 5 months.<br>For the past 2 months I have been receiving one drug as an outpatient 1 day every month, and then 2 weeks later, 5 days of DTIC‖ in the hospital. | Smoked 4 cigarettes/hr **(M)**.<br>Sat up, showed part of back that was affected (midlumbar).<br><br>**From chart (also from physician):**<br>Feb-Aug: received MOPP§ chemotherapy, which caused severe nausea and vomiting. This therapy was then found to be ineffective.<br>Received radiation therapy to coccygeal area in Feb 88 which helped to relieve pain. |
| **Sociological data**<br>I quit high school 3 weeks before graduation in 1983. That was really a mistake. I would like to get my high school diploma.<br>I was married for 2 years and got divorced in February '86. I have a 2-yr-old son who lives with my ex-wife in Florida.<br>I worked as a machinist in a brush company repairing $5,000 machines. It was a very responsible job, and I learned a lot. I also had a job laying pipes for a construction company.<br>I would really like to get a job now, but I would have to give up my Social Security. Then I might get really sick again and have to quit.<br>I'm just now starting to receive Social Security and Medicaid. I have not been able to work since December. I have been receiving General Relief funds.<br>I have friends who really help. One friend in particular I see about every day. He sort of inspires me to do things that I didn't think I could still do. We play pool or ping-pong, ride cycles, or just go drink beer.<br>My mother and stepfather have been married for 3½ years. I didn't approve of him, but since I have been sick I feel differently. He has really shown that he cares about me and has helped me financially.<br>My real dad lives in Florida. We're pretty close; I talk with him on the phone every 2 weeks. I'm going to visit him for 3 weeks in Feb. I haven't had a vacation in the past year, and my mom and stepdad think I should go for my birthday. | Looked wistfully out the window but sounded hopeful.<br><br><br>Sat up, looked alert, and gestured with hands.<br><br><br>Smiled and looked contented. |
| **Psychological data**<br>I felt really bad when Mike and Larry, my roommates on the oncology unit, died. It really makes you think about your life.<br>I started with the GED program at Montgomery County Vocational School twice to get my high school diploma but had to quit both times. I need a more structured | Sad expression on face while looking out window. |

‡UT = urinary tract.
§MOPP = acronym for combination of nitrogen mustard, vincristine (Oncovin), procarbazine hydrochloride, and prednisone (Porth, 1986).
‖DTIC = dacarbazine

*Continued.*

## DATA COLLECTION: Visit 1—October 22, 1988—cont'd

| Interactions | Observations/Measurements (M) |
| --- | --- |
| classroom setting and help. I have difficulty doing everything on my own. | |
| My goal is to become an electrical engineer. | |
| I wouldn't mind working as an orderly at a hospital or as a pharmacy aide. | |
| I like my physician very much and I think he is very competent. | |
| My marriage seemed to be a disaster from the beginning, but we had a beautiful child. My son looks just like me, a really nice-looking kid. I still love my wife. That really messes up my head. During my marriage I drank a lot, wrecked my new car 3 times, quit a good job, and didn't do what I should have for my family. I guess I still had wildness in me. | Smiled broadly.<br><br>Voice sounded regretful. |
| I cope by trying to have a cheerful attitude. I pretend in my mind that I don't have cancer. I usually manage to have a good mental attitude. | He spoke cheerfully and appeared "high spirited." |
| It is difficult for me to have a close relationship with a woman. When I tell them about my condition they back away. I know it's because they don't want to get hurt. | His outward appearance throughout the interview was cheerful and friendly. |

**Spiritual data**

| | |
| --- | --- |
| I've been going to the Church of the Nazarene on Main Street. I really like that church. I used to be Catholic, but I didn't believe in everything the Catholic Church teaches. Now I just say I'm a Christian. | |
| I have never believed in divorce. My mom and dad were divorced after being married 22 years, and I didn't think that was right. It was really hard for me when my wife wanted a divorce. | Sad expression on face; hands folded behind neck, cradling his head. |

## ANALYSIS/SYNTHESIS: Visit 1—October 22, 1988

The central focus of the Neuman model is on the family's relationship during stress and their reaction to stressors and factors of reconstitution. In assessing the client, the various types of stressors—intrapersonal/family, interpersonal/family, and extrapersonal/family—are considered. The illness has not only penetrated the normal line of defense, but also threatens the very core of Danny himself as well as the family structure.

### Intrapersonal/Intrafamily Stressors

According to Neuman, the balance and harmony within this family have been disrupted due to Danny's life-threatening illness, Hodgkin's disease, Stage IIIB. Initially, biological stressors and the lines of defense are analyzed. In this disease, the malignant proliferation of abnormal histiocytes replaces the normal cellular elements within the lymph nodes. The disease causes painless enlargement of the lymph nodes in one site and then spreads to other nodes throughout the body. This neoplastic process may spread to other organs such as spleen, liver, ureters, bowel, bone marrow, and the bones themselves (Brunner and Suddarth, 1986). Pain occurs if a nerve or nearby structure is infiltrated or compressed.

Hodgkin's disease is often classified in four stages according to the extent of the spread of the disease in the body. In Stage III, groups of nodes are involved, both above and below the diaphragm. The stages are subdivided into groups: A, no general symptoms, and B, presence of symptoms such as weight loss, fever, and night sweats (Brunner and Suddarth, 1986; LeBlanc, 1978).

*Normal line of defense invaded; physical integrity compromised.* Danny's initial symptoms were night sweats, inguinal lymph node enlargement, severe lower back pain, and hematuria. His back pain and hematuria could have been due to infiltration of the neoplasm into bone and urinary tract structures. After radiation therapy to his lower back and chemotherapy, the pain was relieved and the hematuria subsided. He still suffers from night sweats and fatigue. His energy integrity is compromised. The fatigue is probably due to anemia caused by decreased erythrocytes. Both Hodgkin's disease itself and chemotherapy can cause abnormal erythrocyte destruction and production (Brunner and Suddarth, 1986).

An additional factor that could be affecting Danny's energy level is inadequate nutrition. He seems to be coping fairly well with the nausea and vomiting associated with chemotherapy by using THC and marijuana and diverting his thoughts elsewhere. (THC is the major psychoactive compound in cannabis sativa, the hemp plant that is the source of marijuana. Cannabis is a psychotropic agent that causes altered consciousness and a dreamlike state.) A nutritional assessment should be done because one of the symptoms of Hodgkin's disease is anorexia (Brunner and Suddarth, 1986). Data are also needed about other symptoms Danny may be having associated with his disease process or the effects of chemotherapy.

Another stressor involving the physical line of defense is the apparent collapse of Danny's arm veins due to frequent IV infusions. In summation, there are two nursing concerns in relation to Danny's energy and resistance level: he is at high risk for nutritional deficiencies, and he has reduced venous access due to repeated IV infusions.

There is a data gap in information about Danny's prognosis. He may be experiencing an objective remission in response to his current chemotherapy. LeBlanc (1978) defines objective remission as regression of the disease and complete remission as the return to normal function with no physical, biochemical, or roentgenographic evidence of disease. According to Brunner and Suddarth (1986), late-stage patients treated with combined chemotherapy had an arrest rate greater than 70% in 1980.

Other intrapersonal stressors affecting Danny's well-being, as well as that of the family, are in the developmental and psychosocial realms. Danny seems to be working through the developmental tasks in two of Erikson's stages, identity versus role confusion and intimacy versus isolation (Eshleman, 1988). A major event in the ego identity stage is emancipation from parents. When a young adult develops a chronic illness he often has to resume dependence on parents for financial support and care (Valentine, 1978). This aptly describes Danny's situation. Because he had no medical insurance and could not work, he chooses to live with his mother and stepfather and be dependent on them. Part of forming a healthy adult self-concept is finding a satisfying occupation. Danny seems to want to pursue this goal but has several obstacles in his path—the limitations imposed by his illness and inability to complete high school. These have curtailed his occupational desires.

In the intimacy versus isolation stage, a person develops the ability to form a close, loving interpersonal relationship with another person, without losing his or her own identity (Valentine, 1978). Danny mentioned that it is difficult for him to develop a close relationship with a woman because of his illness. Even before his illness, he was having some difficulty in mastering the tasks in both of Erikson's stages just mentioned. He regrets now that he did not assume his full responsibilities in being a husband and father. He still seems to be experiencing conflict and remorse about his divorce. This analysis leads to the following nursing diagnosis for Danny: alterations in self-concept and disruption of interpersonal relationships related to illness.

Danny is aware that his disease may be fatal and apparently does have anxiety about his treatment and prognosis. He mentioned two ways in which he copes with his illness. He makes an effort to be cheerful and he pretends in his mind that he doesn't have cancer. This seems to be a conscious denial of the reality of the situation. Denial is a normal protective means of adapting to the diagnosis of cancer, and some patients continue to use it throughout their entire cancer experience (Watson, 1978). Danny apparently receives acceptance and support from his family, physician, and friends. He may be coping adequately with his condition; however, the nursing diagnosis—anxiety related to life-threatening illness—is appropriate.

### Interpersonal/Interfamily Stressors

From this first visit, little data support the perceived threat to family relationships, status, and goals. The only role change apparent at this time is Danny's change from husband and father to dependent son, which has a major impact on both Danny and the entire family. There is a data gap concerning the family's past experience with the same or similar situations and their response to the present situation.

### Extrapersonal/Extrafamily Stressors

There are many data gaps regarding resources that are available to the family. How are the medical bills being paid? Is there financial strain on the family? Danny seems to receive spiritual support from the church that he attends. The spiritual resources of the other family members represent a data gap. Danny and his stepfather seem to have a closer relationship as a result of this illness, and Danny expresses a close relationship with his biological father.

## NURSING DIAGNOSES FOLLOWING FIRST VISIT

| Date | Diagnosis | Priority |
|------|-----------|----------|
| 10/22/88 | 1. Potential alterations in nutrition related to chemotherapy treatments | 5 |
| 10/22/88 | 2. Alterations in comfort related to nausea and vomiting | 1 |
| 10/22/88 | 3. Alterations in self-concept (body image) related to illness and treatment | 2 |
| 10/22/88 | 4. Anxiety related to life-threatening illness | 3 |
| 10/22/88 | 5. Potential alteration in family coping related to life-threatening illness of family member | 6 |
| 10/22/88 | 6. Inadequate venous access related to repeated chemotherapy treatments | 7 |
| 10/22/88 | 7. Alterations in interpersonal relationships related to life-threatening illness | 4 |

## DATA COLLECTION: Visit 2—November 1, 1988

*Setting:* Talked with Danny in living room of his family's home in a middle-class, suburban neighborhood. House is brick, three-bedroom, split-level with wood siding, 10 years old, and well kept. Client's house and lawn were neat, with motorboat and two cars in driveway. City bus line is one block away. Inside, home is orderly, clean, carpeted. Furniture appears new with two TV sets and a stereo system. Danny sleeps at the end of family room in an area set apart by room dividers. He has two posters and album covers decorating the wall, and his other personal items, bed, dresser, and shelves. Danny has a large collection of records and tapes. Mother keeps four poodles in the one-car garage.

When nurse arrived for visit, Danny had just gotten home and said he forgot she was coming.

| Interactions | Observations/Measurements (M)* |
|--------------|-------------------------------|
| **Biological data** | |
| I see my doctor Thursday. I may get more chemotherapy then, but my white blood count may still be too low. | |
| My pain medication was reduced to 1 mg every 4 hr from 4 mg every 4 hr. Now it does not relieve the pain in my back. It is a dull ache. I know my doctor is afraid I will become addicted to drugs, but I usually only need it in the evening when I am tired. | Indicated midlumbar back area as where pain was. Now takes Dilaudid 1 mg every 4 hr (previously 4 mg every 4 hr) **(M)**. |
| Mom gets *Prevention* magazine and has been trying to get me to eat green, leafy vegetables. She gets after me for eating junk food. | Pointed to end table where 3 or 4 *Prevention* magazines lay neatly stacked. |
| The doctor says it is okay for me to drink beer. It has helped me gain weight. | Talked with Danny in living room of home. |

*(M) = measurement data.

## DATA COLLECTION: Visit 2—November 1, 1988—cont'd

| Interactions | Observations/Measurements (M) |
|---|---|
| When I eat out with friends, I eat fast food. It's more convenient. | Danny sitting up in chair. Wearing plaid flannel shirt, corduroy pants, and slippers with heavy socks. Hair combed neatly. Alert and eyes bright. |
| What should I eat to increase my white blood count more rapidly? | |
| Mother and Jim both see a doctor in Englewood when they need medication; neither take any medication now except Ornade. | |
| Jim is a disabled vet—no physical disabilities now. | Danny smoked 9 cigarettes throughout this interview **(M)**. |
| The doctor says I am either in remission or entering remission. | |
| I have been exercising my arms with weights. | Danny extended arms and displayed his arm muscles. |

### Sociological data

Our family shops at the commissary once a month for food. We spend about $350. We have a freezer.

Usually our family eats together in the evening. Mother fixes meals. One night a week everyone fixes their own dinner.

Jim provides for the family. Mom contributes a little with money earned by grooming dogs or prize money from dog shows. I help buy food the last week of the month when food begins to run out.

Mom cleans the house but everyone chips in a little. I keep my bedroom and family room straightened up. My sisters helps with the dogs.

I went to Bowling Green Lanes last night with a friend. We drank beer, played pool, Tron, and other games.

I lived with another family for 9 months while my mom and dad got their divorce. This family told me if I get my GED,* I would have a painting job with them. I don't know if I could physically handle the job yet.

Jim told me that if I don't get my GED, I could stay in Florida with my real father.

My mother and stepfather make the decisions in the family, but we do have family discussions.

Jim, Jr., my stepbrother, is bussed to high school.

With five people living together in the house, sometimes things just blow up.

    (He mentioned disagreements between mom and stepfather, himself and stepfather, sister and stepfather. During one altercation, sister took mother's side against stepfather, became angry, threw coffee table, hit ceiling in family room; they had to have it repaired.)

    *Danny sat forward with an intense look in his eyes. He gestured with his hands as he described this incident. Then he frowned and shook his head from side to side.*

I almost hit my stepfather with my crutch one time. He was angry because I wouldn't eat. We usually explode, then cool down, next day apologize, and forget all about it.

I always lose in an argument with Jim.

Every once in a while, when everyone is on edge, we all sit down together and just talk about things.

    *Sat back in his chair in a relaxed position with his arms at rest on the sides of chair and legs crossed.*

My stepfather and mother have been involved in a group trying to get permission for a Vietnam veteran

---

*GED = Graduate equivalency diploma.

*Continued.*

## DATA COLLECTION: Visit 2—November 1, 1988—cont'd

| Interactions | Observations/Measurements (M) |
|---|---|
| who is walking to Washington DC to walk through Ohio. They finally took him to KY, so he could walk from there. | Danny frowned, grimaced, and shook his head. |
| Jim is still talking about his Vietnam venture. When he does something, he wants to be sure everyone knows about it. I don't mean to belittle the man, but that is one thing I get tired of. | |
| I had a long talk with my girlfriend and we ironed out our differences. | Smiled. |
| I have been getting General Relief ($67 a month). Now I will get $250 a month from Social Security. | |
| (Extended family) Jim's mom lives in Versailles. She sent cards when I was ill in the hospital. | |
| I keep in touch with aunts, uncles, cousins on my real father's side; none live close. My mother is an only child and all of her family are dead. She has one really close friend in Boston. | He sat back in chair and placed his hands behind his neck and cradled head in hands. |
| (When Danny was really sick, Jim handled things within the immediate family; the only outside help came from Cancer Control to help pay for medication.) | |
| My sister and I go places together. She has a car and I pay for the gas. | |
| Our family plays cards and watches TV together— programs like *Nova* and *Cosmos*. Jim insists that we watch these kinds of shows. I like the stereo especially. | Smiled. Got up and walked over to his stereo system. |

**Psychological data**

| | |
|---|---|
| My real father is always on the run and likes to keep busy. | |
| I started going to vocational school to take classes for GED—2 evenings a week for 2 hr each evening. | |
| After I get my GED, I would like to learn to play a synthesizer. I can take classes at the vocational school in reading music. | Eyes alert, bright; spoke animatedly. |
| I really enjoy music. I sang in the school choir for 6 yr. I could have made the best singing group in high school, but my grades weren't good enough. I was thought of as a "trouble maker." | |
| (Talked again about wife.) I called her parents to get her address, so I could have Social Security sent to my son. They told me their daughter was getting along fine without my money. | |
| When I was married I never saw my friends; now my friends are very important to me. | Thoughtful expression on face. |
| I really appreciate being able to stay at home and not have to pay for room and board. | |
| My mom is very particular about the house. I often have to wait for her when we're ready to go somewhere while she empties the ashtrays. If there is one piece of silverware in the sink, she washes it. | Rolled his eyes, then smiled. |

## ANALYSIS/SYNTHESIS: Visit 2—November 1, 1988

### Intrapersonal/Intrafamily Stressors

Most of the previous analysis of October 22 continues to be appropriate. Using Neuman's model and considering the intrusion of this life-threatening illness on the basic lines of defense, the lines of resistance, and on the intrinsic core of energy, Danny continues to demonstrate acute symptoms. He is still experiencing back pain and also has pain in his left leg, especially in the evening when he is tired. The pain medication he is now receiving does not relieve the pain. He has some degree of leukopenia with his chemotherapy, which could put him at risk for infection (Brunner and Suddarth, 1989). He expressed an interest in what to do about this. A positive aspect of his illness is that his physician has told him that he is going into remission.

In considering energy conservation, a nutritional analysis is planned. On the positive side, his mother prepares meals for the family on most days and is apparently aware that good nutrition is important, but there is a data gap about what she prepares (tertiary and primary levels of prevention). Danny eats junk food and eats at fast food places when he is with friends, but it is not known how often this occurs. Danny seems to smoke regularly, which is detrimental to his energy level (Ardell, 1986). It might, however, be very difficult for him to quit smoking while having to cope with his illness. In conclusion, the nursing diagnoses are (1) alterations in comfort related to lower back pain and (2) potential for infection related to leukopenia.

The basic core of the family appears intact, albeit somewhat stressed. It is normal that life-threatening illness challenges family stability, adaptability, resources, and, most intensely, beliefs and assumptions.

### Interpersonal/Interfamily Stressors

Regarding Danny's personal response to shifting roles, new data support the diagnosis of alterations in self-concept. He is undecided about what kind of occupation he might like to pursue, but he has started working toward a high school diploma. It is unknown whether he is sufficiently motivated to do the required work or whether he has enrolled in the program only because other people have encouraged him to do so. Because of his wife's and in-laws' attitudes, he is unable to fulfill his financial obligation to his son. Although he feels affection for his son, he is unable to be in touch with him. He does try to contribute what he can to his own immediate family.

In considering the perceived threat to family relationships, status, and goals, a data gap still exists because Danny is the only member of the family who has talked with me. The roles in the family seem to be mostly traditional, with the wife taking care of the home and cooking and the husband providing most of the income. Their communication patterns seem somewhat dysfunctional, especially between the father and his stepchildren, and some members of the family have difficulty dealing with their anger in a functional manner. Some of the anger seems to be related to family tensions due to Danny's illness. Danny still seems to feel animosity toward his stepfather, and one gets the feeling from talking with Danny that he has little power in the family. The stepfather seems to be authoritarian in his approach to his grown children. Possible diagnoses could be family tensions related to Danny's illness and dysfunctional family communication.

### Extrapersonal/Extrafamily Stressors

Some of the resources available to the family were identified in this visit. They live in a clean, well-kept home in a residential neighborhood, with adequate transportation available. Each member of the family has adequate money for food and other necessities. There is affection between Danny and his sister, and in spite of their difficulties, Danny's stepfather is concerned about him. The family spends time together at meals and watching TV or playing cards. Danny gets some support from his friends and the family he lived with while his parents were getting a divorce. The extended family has not responded to this crisis. According to Danny, his immediate family handled his hospitalization and initial illness, except for some help from the cancer control agency.

The next family visit will include Danny and his mother, to gather data about the effect of Danny's illness on the family, about communication and decision-making patterns, and about coping strategies used by the family. A review of Danny's systems will be done to see whether he is experiencing any other symptoms of Hodgkin's disease or any effects of chemotherapy. Also, the family support and communication patterns will be examined, which seems to have a great impact on the family functioning.

## NURSING DIAGNOSIS FOLLOWING SECOND VISIT

| Date | Diagnosis | Priority |
|------|-----------|----------|
| 10/22/88 | 1. Potential alterations in nutrition related to chemotherapy treatment | 6 |
| 10/22/88 | 2. Alterations in comfort related to nausea and vomiting | 1 |
| 10/22/88 | 3. Alterations in self-concept related to life-threatening illness | 7 |
| 10/22/88 | 4. Anxiety related to life-threatening illness | 3 |
| 10/22/88 | 5. Potential alterations in family coping related to life-threatening illness of family member | 8 |
| 10/22/88 | 6. Inadequate venous access related to repeated chemotherapy treatment | 10 |
| 10/22/88 | 7. Alterations in intrapersonal relationships related to illness | 4 |
| 11/1/88 | 8. Alterations in comfort related to lower back pain | 2 |
| 11/1/88 | 9. Potential for infection related to leukopenia | 5 |
| 11/1/88 | 10. Potential for dysfunctional family communication related to blending of two families | 9 |

## DATA COLLECTION: Visit 3—November 15, 1988

*Setting:* Meeting took place in living room of home. Mother wore new jeans, a bulky pink sweater, and loafers. Her hair is dark brown, shiny, and combed neatly off her shoulders. Eyes alert and facial expressions attentive. Danny wore a red T-shirt and jeans with Reebok running shoes. Danny and mother sat on opposite ends of couch, and nurse sat in chair facing them. The room is neat and orderly as in previous visit. (Jim came in later.)

| Interactions | Observations/Measurements (M)* |
|--------------|-------------------------------|
| **Biological data (from client):** | |
| I weighed 140 lb before my illness, then lost and gained about 30 lb. Now I weigh 139 lb, and I'm 5'7" tall. | Good eye contact with nurse while talking. |
| I had shingles on my left leg about 3 months ago. I wasn't able to walk on the leg for 6 weeks. That leg is still weak. Sometimes it buckles under me. | |
| I still have pain in the coccygeal region of my back. It aches worse when I lie down. | |
| My doctor has taken me off Dilaudid, now I can take Zomax but haven't tried this medication yet. | |
| My doctor is concerned about the back pain. I was to have a bone scan Friday, November 12. | Jim, Sr., walked into the room wearing blue plaid shirt and corduroy trousers. Hair is shiny and combed back. He greets us, smiles, and sits next to Mary on the sofa. |
| I received chemotherapy as an outpatient about a week ago (Adriamycin, bleomycin, and one other drug). I was very nauseated about 6 hr after treatment. The nausea lasted about 24 hr. I used THC and smoked marijuana at home to relieve nausea and vomiting. | |
| (Review of systems revealed no other symptoms of Hodgkin's disease or side effects of chemotherapy at this time). | |
| Here is my 3-day diet diary. I was careful to keep track of almost everything I ate. I took 3 days that I wasn't nauseated. | |

*(M) = measurement data.

## DATA COLLECTION: Visit 3—November 15, 1988—cont'd

| Interactions | Observations/Measurements (M) |
|---|---|

**Biological data from other members of family:**

*Mary:* My husband Jim has back and leg pain. He cannot sit or stand still for very long periods of time. Uses TNS unit for pain relief. It goes back to Vietnam days.

I have no medical problems, except that my allergies kick up once in a while.

We all smoke except Jim, Jr. My husband and I each smoke about 3 packs a day. We seem to smoke more since Danny's been so sick.

Jim, Jr., is picky in his food habits, too. It's difficult to get him to eat his vegetables and salad greens.

Jim and I eat fairly healthy foods. Diane goes out a lot and eats at fast food places with Danny.

**3-day diet diary (M)**

*Day 1*

| | |
|---|---|
| 1 egg | 9 AM alone at home |
| 1 pc toast w/butter | |
| 1 glass milk | |
| | |
| 1 quarter pounder | 1 PM w/sister |
| 1 reg french fry | |
| 1 milk | |
| | |
| 6-8 oz liver | 5:30 PM at home w/ family |
| 1 cup mashed potatoes (w/blue cheese, sour cream, garlic, onion, and butter) | |
| 1 pc bread & butter | |
| 2 glasses milk | |
| 1 cup each of broccoli & brussel sprouts | |
| 2 cookies | |
| | |
| 6 beers | 8-11 PM w/friends |

*Day 2*

| | |
|---|---|
| 2 eggs | morning, alone |
| 2 pc toast w/butter | |
| 3 cup coffee | |
| | |
| 2 big slices Godfather Pizza | 6 PM at home w/family |
| 1/2 gal milk | |
| | |
| single lg bag potato chips (4 oz) | in PM |

*Day 3*

| | |
|---|---|
| 3 cups coffee | morning, alone |
| | |
| 2 Big Macs | 2 PM w/friends |
| Small coke (8 oz) | |
| | |
| 2 TV dinners w/shrimp, fish, scallops, potato, peas | 6 PM at home |
| 2 glasses (8 oz) milk | |
| | |
| single bag potato chips (½ oz) | evening |

**Sociological data:**

*Mary:* When Danny first became so ill, we all got together and helped each other out in our chores and helped Danny, too. Even Jim, Jr., helped out.

*Continued.*

**DATA COLLECTION: Visit 3—November 15, 1988—cont'd**

| Interactions | Observations/Measurements (M) |
|---|---|
| Outside of our immediate family the only person to help out was Jim's mother, especially when Danny was hospitalized. She lives in Versailles. She prepared and brought food and provided emotional support to the entire family. | |
| When Danny is feeling well, as he has been lately, he forgets how important a good diet is for him and stops eating well. This causes friction, because Jim and I are concerned about him and realize how important diet is. | Mary leaned forward and gestured with her hands—eyes intense and focused on nurse. |
| *Jim:* During the first part of Danny's illness, he was very weak and dependent (he couldn't walk 6 ft without becoming short of breath). Mary tried to let him do as much for himself as possible, but this was very difficult for her to do, I mean, stand by and watch heroic effort. | Jim shifted position on couch and crossed legs to get more comfortable. |
| Roles in any family change during a crisis period. Diane, Jim, Jr., and I took over some of Mary's chores at home, because she spent so much time at the hospital. I got up at 3:00 AM to study before going to school. That helps, but is exhausting after a while. | |
| **Psychological data:** | |
| *Mary:* During the crisis period, Jim, Jr., did things to irritate me (left messes in the kitchen, etc). I knew this was for attention but I just could not deal with it at that time. I tried to ignore his behavior—not easy. | |
| Jim, Jr., is a loner, he has only one friend. He can talk with his father, but he really doesn't have much to do with other members of the family. | |
| I get along well with Jim, Diane, and Danny. With Jim, Jr., our positive relationship is sporadic. | |
| It was such a shock when Danny was so ill. We have always been very health-conscious and wanted to know why this was happening. Jim and I read Jim's psychology and sociology books and got books from the library. We read about diseases being caused by stress. | Look of concern on Mary's face. Jim's face also concerned as he looked at Mary. |
| I had feelings of helplessness. We wanted to help Danny as much as we could, but there didn't seem to be much we could do. | |
| I read the book *Focusing* by Gendlin and encouraged Danny to use this technique to combat N&V with chemotherapy. | |
| I am not assertive (always afraid of hurting someone's feelings), so when I get upset with Danny, Jim, Jr., or Diane, I just keep it inside until I finally blow up and tell Jim about it. When he sees that I am upset, he lays down the law to the others. | Jim nodded his head in affirmation. Somber expression on his face. |
| My husband and I have the final say with most of the decisions in the family. My decisions mostly concern the running of the house and those concerning the children. | |
| *Danny:* I am worried that I will never again be as muscular and strong as I was before this illness. | Sad expression in Danny's eyes. He leaned forward and extended his right arm, which is very thin. |
| I missed my appointment last Friday for the bone scan because I forgot. I feel that Dr. Shelly was put out with me. | |
| *Jim:* The father of one of Danny's friends told Danny that he was worthless, because he wasn't working—some friend! | |

## DATA COLLECTION: Visit 3—November 15, 1988—cont'd

| Interactions | Observations/Measurements (M) |
|---|---|
| *Danny:* I was upset and angry because of this remark. Then I realized he just doesn't understand. | Danny's eyes alert at first; some expression of anger in voice and eyes. Then he settled back in chair and looked resigned. |
| **Spiritual data:** | |
| *Mary:* Danny is the only one in the family who attends church right now. It's difficult for me to go to church and pray. Why would a good God let something like this happen to us? What have we done? | Eyes sad, intense. Jim reached over and took Mary's hand. |

## ANALYSIS/SYNTHESIS: Visit 3—November 15, 1988

### Intrapersonal/Intrafamily Stressors

Previous analyses remain appropriate. Considering Danny's physical stamina and defense system, he still experiences back pain (lumbosacral area). His physician may suspect bone metastasis because he has ordered a bone scan. The left leg weakness that he is experiencing could be related to an episode of shingles, which he had about 3 months ago. Shingles or herpes zoster is an acute viral infection of the nervous system, characterized by a vesicular skin eruption, pain, and sometimes segmental motor and sensory loss along the course of a nerve or group of nerves, usually on only one side of the body (Patrick et al, 1986).

Considering energy and basic core structure, Danny is back to his pre-illness weight, which is normal for his height (Williams, 1989). A comparison of Danny's 3-day diet diary with RDA standards reveals deficiencies in fruits, vegetables, and vitamin C. Vitamin A was adequate only because of one large serving of liver. Protein and calcium are adequate. He is eating more than twice as much meat and milk products as are recommended for an adult. He eats more than enough carbohydrates and fats and consumes adequate amounts of grains (Williams, 1989). An environmental condition that may be a family stressor is that four members of the family smoke, which is a potential for a multitude of problems. Smoking may be a coping mechanism used by individual family members to relieve stress in the family environment.

### Interpersonal/Interfamily Stressors

Regarding Danny's other intrapersonal stressors, this interview revealed other ways in which his illness threatens his self-concept. It bothers him that others may think he is lazy because he doesn't have a job. He is also concerned about his physical appearance and stamina. New data from this interview support the previous cue that the mother and stepfather are concerned about his welfare and want to help him as much as they can.

New data were gathered about past experience with stressful situations. During the period when Danny was very ill and hospitalized, the family coped by doing some role changing and by learning more about the causes of his illness and how they might be able to help. Mary mentioned difficulty coping with Jim, Jr., at this time. This may be related to the fact that he seems to be an "outsider" in the family.

Mary seems to act as hub for most of the communication in the family. Everyone except Jim, Jr., seems to communicate well with her. New data support previous diagnosis of dysfunctional family communication. Jim, Jr., has difficulty talking with anyone but his father. Mary does not express her feelings until she really becomes upset and then she tells her husband, who speaks to the others. As other data indicate, Jim seems to use an authoritarian manner, which may be the reason that Danny and his sister have difficulty communicating with him.

### Extrapersonal/Extrafamily Stressors

The family has expressed in many different ways that they get very little support from outside sources in times of crisis or stress.

### Summary

Data gaps still exist concerning the spiritual resources of the family, their coping behaviors, and communication patterns. Information on these gaps will be completed in later interviews, with as many family members as possible.

## NURSING DIAGNOSIS FOLLOWING THIRD VISIT

| Date | Diagnosis | Priority |
|---|---|---|
| 10/22/88 | 1. Alterations in nutrition related to chemotherapy treatment and lifestyle | 2 |
| 10/22/88 | 2. Alterations in comfort related to nausea and vomiting | 9 |
| 10/22/88 | 3. Alterations in self-concept (body image) related to life-threatening illness | 5 |
| 10/22/88 | 4. Anxiety related to life-threatening illness | 3 |
| 10/22/88 | 5. Dysfunctional communication related to blending of two families and illness in family | 4 |
| 10/22/88 | 6. Potential inadequate venous access related to repeated chemotherapy treatment | 10 |
| 10/22/88 | 7. Alterations in family coping related to illness of family member | 6 |
| 11/1/88 | 8. Alterations in comfort related to low back pain | 1 |
| 11/1/88 | 9. Potential for infection related to leukopenia | 7 |
| 11/15/88 | 10. Social isolation related to life-threatening illness | 8 |

## DATA COLLECTION: Visit 4—December 1, 1988

*Setting:* Mary sat on couch dressed in jeans and yellow blouse. Hair shiny and arranged neatly off shoulders. Danny is dressed in plaid flannel shirt and faded blue jeans wearing house slippers. He is sitting in a recliner chair tilted back.

| Interactions | Observations/Measurements (M) |
|---|---|
| **Biological data:**<br><br>*Danny:* I still have back pain. Zomax does not relieve it.<br>I haven't had the bone scan yet, because I had the flu on the day of my appointment.<br>I go to the hospital tomorrow for chemotherapy. I hope they find veins for the treatment.<br>I had flu last week. I vomited for about 8 hours, then I developed chest pain, could not breathe, and was very frightened. I went to emergency room at Sycamore Hospital. They took an x-ray and said maybe I had pulled a chest muscle, that it was an anxiety attack. They gave me Vistaril and sent me home. I felt better the next day.<br>I have a lot of numbness and weakness in my left leg.<br>I have been urinating a lot and have needed more sleep lately, 10-11 hours per night.<br>I drink about 12 beers a week.<br>We have a lot of vegetables and greens but not much fruit. I don't like vegetables that much.<br>*Mary:* Yes, Danny seems to be having some trouble with his leg—numbness and weakness too. Sometimes it buckles under him.<br>I buy both fruits and vegetables, but the fruit gets eaten more quickly, especially by Diane and Jim Jr. Fruit in the winter is also more expensive, so we run out of it faster. | Has redness and dryness at corner of right eye and corner of mouth. No sore areas or lesions within mouth.<br>Worried look on Danny's face.<br><br>Danny's face appeared more pale than usual.<br><br>Continued to sit contentedly in chair without much movement. |

## DATA COLLECTION: Visit 4—December 1, 1988—cont'd

| Interactions | Observations/Measurements (M) |
|---|---|

**Sociological data:**

*Danny:* I am doing well in school. I plan to help mom with her math. She is considering getting her GED and starting her own business.

*Mary:* Yes, we've been talking about my getting my high school diploma. Jim thinks it's a good idea too. Danny has promised to help me with the math. He is good at that! I really can't go further, career-wise, if I don't have the basic diploma. I would like to operate my own business in dog grooming on a full-time scale. It's exciting!

Danny smiled and looked at his mom.

Mary's eyes lit up with enthusiasm and her body posture became more alert and focused.

**Psychological data:**

*Danny:* I dread going to the hospital tomorrow, because the chemotherapy makes me feel so bad.

I am also concerned about the effects of the chemotherapy on my future children. I have one son who is perfect, but I will probably never see him again.

I am concerned about weakness in my left leg, because this is the foot I used to support myself when riding my cycle.

You can call Dr. Shell. I told him you would be calling. Otherwise he probably won't tell you anything.

I am not interested in learning any other relaxation techniques to help me cope with nausea and pain.

I am also worried about whether they will have difficulty finding veins for my treatment.

*Mary:* I am aware that I need to be more assertive in some situations, especially within the family. (Mary expressed interest in reading *Stand Up, Speak Out, Talk Back.*)

Danny stared into space with a concerned look on his face.

Danny pointed to his left leg.

**Spiritual data:**

*Danny:* Yes, I still go to church when I feel well enough to go. I always pray though, whether I go to church or not. It gives me a lot of strength especially now when I have to deal with this illness and pain.

*Mary:* Jim and I used to go to church. None of us goes at this point. We've just gotten away from it.

Sometimes I wonder if there is a God when I see people with these terrible diseases and the suffering with it.

It doesn't make sense.

Looking thoughtful. Staring out of the window, speaking in a low voice almost to herself.

## ANALYSIS/SYNTHESIS: Visit 4—December 1, 1988

### Intrapersonal/Intrafamily Stressors

The previous analyses are still relevant. Considering Danny's diminished physical stamina and penetration of lines of resistance, new symptoms are present that may be related to side effects of his chemotherapy treatment.

Numbness and weakness of his left leg could be from neurotoxicity. Redness and dryness at corners of eye and mouth are symptoms of skin and mucosal effects of bleomycin and adriamycin. Drug effects are on the basal layers of mucosa preventing replication and replacement of most superficial cell structures (Fredetta and Glorian, 1981). He has no lesions or sore areas within his mouth, however. Frequency of urination and increased need for sleep could be signs of a urinary tract infection. This and Danny's harsh bout of intestinal flu could be associated with leukopenia. Adriamycin suppresses bone marrow functions, especially granulocytes and neutrophils (Fredetta and Glorian, 1981). He seems to be having an increased problem with nausea during chemotherapy, so the diagnosis of discomfort related to nausea due to chemotherapy seems appropriate.

In considering diet and nutrition, there seem to be incongruencies about Mary's knowledge of good nutrition and concern about Danny's diet. In earlier interviews, Danny mentioned his parents' concern for his diet and his mother's knowledge in this area. But his food diary showing the meals eaten at home and the fact that Danny says there is not much fruit available there indicate the possibility that Mary does not actually have much knowledge about what is necessary for good nutrition. Although it is true that Mary spoke about greens, vegetables, and the family eating the fruits (and not liking vegetables), there is still a possible deficit in this area.

### Interpersonal/Interfamily Stressors

Regarding interpersonal stressors, Danny is doing well in his school work and also has offered to help his mother with her math classes when she goes back to school for a high school diploma. The bonding relationship between mother and son is being enhanced by their sharing of interests, talents, and time. This is definitely helping his self-concept. On the other hand, Danny's self-image is compromised because of the weakness in his legs and its effect on his ability and mobility in the future as well as now.

The diagnosis of anxiety related to diagnosis, treatment, and prognosis is still relevant. He dreads his chemotherapy because of the discomfort associated with the treatments and is concerned about iatrogenic effects of the drugs he is being given.

Few events in life provide deeper and more poignant emotions than a life-threatening illness of a young family member. It frequently shakes the very foundation, organization, and equilibrium of family life. Feelings of injustice, anger, hopelessness, and spiritual confusion are engendered among family members as they care for the endangered child (McFarland and Wasli, 1986). From the spiritual data obtained in this most recent visit, it seems that despite all of Danny's emotional fears, he is coming to peace with himself and with his God, for in this relationship he feels secure and loved. This assists him in coping with the illness. Conversely, it would seem that his parents are facing a sense of helplessness, powerlessness, and an overall anger directed toward God because of this illness, which has threatened the family's equilibrium. A diagnosis of the family's spiritual distress related to life-threatening illness seems appropriate at this time.

*data gap wrt this issue* [handwritten annotation]

In summation, although Danny is exhibiting more symptoms and side effects from chemotherapy, he also is integrating his spiritual needs into his life in a wholesome manner. The family members continue to meet their physical needs, but are having problems dealing with the group's spiritual integrity. Data gaps are in the areas of specific nutritional knowledge and knowledge of and planning for the eventuality of Danny's prognosis.

## NURSING DIAGNOSIS FOLLOWING FOURTH VISIT

| Date | Diagnosis | Priority |
|------|-----------|----------|
| 10/22/88 | 1. Alterations in nutrition related to chemotherapy treatments and possible lack of knowledge | 2 |
| 10/22/88 | 2. Alterations in comfort related to effects of treatments | 1 |
| 10/22/88 | 3. Alterations in self-concept (body image) related to effects of chemotherapy | 3 |
| 10/22/88 | 4. Anxiety related to life-threatening illness | 6 |
| 10/22/88 | 5. Dysfunctional family communication related to family member's illness | 5 |
| 10/22/88 | 6. Inadequate venous access related to repeated chemotherapy treatment | 8 |
| 11/1/88 | 7. Potential for infection related to leukopenia | 4 |
| 12/1/88 | 8. Spiritual distress of family related to severe illness in family member | 7 |

## INTERIM—December 1 to January 25

Two appointments to visit with the family were canceled due to the fact that one or more family members could not be there. Finally, on January 25 the nurse visited with Danny and his mother again; Diane was working and could not be there, and Jim declined to participate in any more visits.

## DATA COLLECTION: Visit 5—January 25, 1989, 2:00 PM

*Setting:* Living room of home with Danny and his mother, Mary. Danny is dressed in corduroy pants, plaid shirt, socks, and slippers. He is sitting in a recliner. His hair is dry and lusterless. Mary is dressed in a green shirtdress with hose and black flat shoes. She had just returned from shopping. She is sitting on the couch. She looks tired (rings under eyes).

| Interactions | Observations/Measurements (M) |
|---|---|
| **Biological data:** | |
| *Physician interview:* Dan has recently been in the hospital for chemotherapy and various tests (EKG, chest x-ray, body scan). He is still in remission and I am quite pleased with Danny's progress. | EKG, chest x-ray, body scan carried out. Results: he's still in remission. Physical exam revealed inguinal hernia. |
| *Danny:* I still have periods when all my muscles ache, and I feel very tired. | |
| I have been having less pain in my back. | |
| I have a right inguinal hernia but my physician does not want me to have surgery at this time. | Danny pointed to his lower abdomen and rubbed that area gently. |
| I want to have my hernia repaired as soon as possible, because it causes me some discomfort. | |
| The doctor says my leukocyte count is very good at this time. | |
| *Mary:* Danny will have just two more rounds of chemotherapy and then he will be examined periodically. | |
| When receiving chemotherapy treatments, Danny eats very little—a light diet. He is usually able to eat more the day after the treatment. | |
| He has been out with his friends a lot and when not home for meals, he doesn't eat as well. I always check on this. | Mary's face showed concern—eyes intent, alert, and focused on both nurse and Danny. |
| He tends to forget that he is ill and that a good diet is important for him. | Mary's diet assessment shows she eats a well-balanced nutritious diet. |
| *Danny:* I am bothered that my hair is becoming dry and unruly. | |
| I try to prevent tension on my hair. I wash it only when necessary and let it air dry. I very seldom use a hair dryer. | |
| I realize that this is a side effect of my chemotherapy treatment. | |
| **Psychological data/sociological data:** | |
| *Danny:* My doctor has told me that I need to have another lymphography. I am really dreading the procedure, because it was so painful when I had one last January. | Frowned—concerned look on face. |
| I will be relieved when chemotherapy is over. I am able to cope fairly well with nausea by sleeping or directing my thoughts on something else (focusing). | |
| I have been feeling bored and fed up with not being able to work and be as active as I would like. If I stay out late, I am tired for several days. | Voice indicated an irritable tone. He gestured widely with hands. |
| No, I don't think I would be interested in attending a support group. | Voice had an emphatic tone. |
| I cope well by having a positive attitude and not dwelling on the thought that I have cancer. | |

*Continued.*

**DATA COLLECTION: Visit 5—January 25, 1989, 2:00 PM—cont'd**

| Interactions | Observations/Measurements (M) |
|---|---|
| It depresses me when I become acquainted with other cancer patients in the hospital who seem to be getting along fine, and then I find out later that they have died! | Voice sounded somewhat upset, almost an angry tone. |
| In a support group I wouldn't be able to tell people that because they hadn't experienced it. They couldn't understand what I've been through. | |
| I am still attending evening school, working toward GED. | |
| *Mary:* Dan is looking forward to visiting his real father in Florida for a few weeks, whenever it is possible. | Mary looked hopefully at Danny. |
| Although we had some difficulty coping with Danny's illness when he was first diagnosed we have been able to cope well by maintaining a positive attitude, trying to accept things as they are, and doing what we can to help. We try to treat Danny as normally as possible—not like an invalid. | Mary smiled and glanced at Danny. |
| I have read most of *Stand Up, Speak Out, Talk Back* and find it helpful. | |
| I have decided I do not want to role play assertive behavior. I would rather just practice in specific situations where I want to be more assertive. Like with my own family at home, especially with Jim and the children. We have started to discuss things openly. It's a start but sometimes painful. | Facial expression alert, pleased with herself. |
| Yes, I know about the daily food guide and what should be eaten every day. | Mary repeated the four basic food groups. |
| **Spiritual data:** | |
| *Danny:* I don't worry much about dying. I feel I can accept death if it happens. Just so they let me listen to my music. | Mary's eyes filled with tears. Danny appeared calm and assured. |

**ANALYSIS/SYNTHESIS: Visit 5—January 25, 1989**

Most of the previous analysis is still appropriate, with the following additional considerations. The reactions to the interpersonal/interfamily stressors during this visit indicate that Danny's energy integrity is still not in proper balance. Although he is having less back pain, he still complains of fatigue. Even though he understands what he should eat, Danny is apparently not motivated to eat fruits and vegetables, so his diet is still deficient in this area. His basic core structure and lines of resistance are penetrated by Hodgkin's disease. Now, however, he is in remission. His physician is evidently still assessing the extent of this remission, because he feels it is necessary for Danny to have another lymphography. Danny also has recently developed a hernia, which is causing him concern. Although the family's values and belief systems have been challenged, role adjustments and interdependence have been maintained throughout. The basic core of the family is felt to be intact.

Intrapersonal/intrafamily stressors are those that impinge upon a client's sense of identity and self-worth. Danny is still having problems working through the developmental tasks in the state defined by Erikson as identity versus role confusion (Eshleman, 1988). He says he is bored and "fed up" with not being able to work and be as active as he would like.

Danny still has anxieties about his treatment, especially in relation to the lymphography. Although he will be relieved when his chemotherapy is over, he is coping fairly well with the nausea. There are some incongruencies in what he says concerning the possibility that Hodgkin's disease may be fatal. He states he will be able to accept death if it happens and he doesn't worry much about dying. It does bother him that other cancer patients seem to be getting along fine and then die. However, he is coming to terms with the possibility of his own death through a strong personal commitment to God. The family members, on the other hand, may be in spiritual distress, because they have not dealt with this problem and still express anger and powerlessness toward God.

The response of significant others in the family toward Danny's disease is still one of concern and support while, as Mary says, they try not to treat Danny as if he were an invalid. At this time, there still are a few perceived threats to family relationships, status, and goals due to Danny's illness, and his role change from independence to being again dependent on his parents. This role change began a year ago when he first became ill. Mary feels that learning some assertiveness skills may be helpful to their family communication, especially in some situations.

In regard to other interpersonal/interfamily stressors, the family is coping fairly well with Danny's illness at this time. Coping strategies include maintaining a positive attitude, trying to accept things they cannot change and being as supportive of Danny as possible. Danny apparently still copes by denying his illness to a certain extent and does not think he would be interested in attending a support group. He feels that he is coping well at this time, and he thought that the people in a support group would not understand what he has been through.

No further information was obtained about the family's past experience with similar illness situations, so there is still a data gap in this area. All the previous diagnoses are still essentially correct.

## SUMMARY

In using Neuman's systems model to assess the stressors that impinge on Danny and his family, it is felt that although Danny's inner structure of defense is not in proper balance yet, the disease is in remission and Danny is on a trajectory toward reconstitution. Other intrapersonal stressors that re-

## FINAL NURSING DIAGNOSIS LIST

| Date | Diagnosis | Priority |
|------|-----------|----------|
| | **Intrafamily (Intrapersonal)** | |
| 10/22/88 | 1. Alteration in nutrition—less than body requirements related to anorexia, nausea/vomiting, and malabsorption | 2 |
| 12/1/88 | 2. Activity intolerance, fatigue | 3 |
| 10/22/88 | *3. Alteration in comfort: pain and discomfort related to illness and treatment | 1 |
| 12/1/88 | 4. Alteration in tissue integrity (alopecia) related to chemotherapy treatments | 6 |
| 10/22/88 | *5. Altered body image and self-esteem related to changes in appearance, functions, and roles | 5 |
| 10/22/88 | 6. Anxiety related to life-threatening illness | 4 |
| | **Interfamily (Interpersonal)** | |
| 11/1/88 | *1. Alterations in family process related to dysfunctional communication | 9 |
| 10/22/88 | 2. Disrupted interpersonal relations related to illness | 7 |
| 11/15/88 | 3. Difficulty with role changes related to family member's illness | 8 |
| 12/15/88 | *4. Grieving related to anticipatory loss | 10 |
| 12/1/88 | 5. Spiritual distress related to search for meaning in family member's illness | 11 |
| | **Extrafamily (Extrapersonal)** | |
| 12/1/88 | 1. Inadequate resources related to impact of catastrophic illness in family | 13 |
| 11/15/88 | 2. Inadequate support group related to Danny's diminished self-concept and life-threatening illness | 12 |
| 12/1/88 | 3. Potential for financial crises related to illness and required therapy | 14 |

*Plans for nursing implementation for these diagnoses are shown on pp. 296-303.

late to Danny's inability to work and anxieties about his treatment are still present. Although he is not interested in a support group, information about such a group was given to him in the event he would reconsider this option.

Whereas the family in general is coping, it is felt that some education in assertiveness skills may assist them in improving family communication, thereby helping them to reach a higher level of functioning.

## PLANS FOR IMPLEMENTATION

**Nursing diagnosis 1:** *Alteration in comfort: Pain and discomfort related to illness and treatment (10/22/88).*
**Goal:** *The client will use various methods to relieve pain and discomfort by 12/15/88.*

| Objectives | Nursing orders | Scientific rationale | Evaluation |
|---|---|---|---|
| 1. Danny will have a decreased level of pain and discomfort by 12/15/88. | 1a. Nurse will assess pain and discomfort characteristics: location, quality, frequency, duration, timing, disruption of activities, etc. <br> 1b. Danny will verbalize the specific characteristics of his discomfort (same as above). | *Content:* Pain. <br> *Strategy:* Principles of nursing practice. <br> 1a. Baseline data provides information for assessing changes in pain level and evaluation of intervention (Brunner and Suddarth, 1989). | **Formative:** <br> Danny reported that the level of pain and discomfort has decreased with the use of measures such as humor, music, analgesics, relaxation, and rest. |
| | 1c. Nurse will assure Danny that she knows pain and discomfort is real and will facilitate some measures to reduce it: <br> • Pain medication to be taken before pain peaks <br> • Use of humor and distraction <br> • Adequate rest periods | 1c. A client's fear that pain will not be considered real increases anxiety and reduces pain tolerance (Brunner and Suddarth, 1989). | Analgesic therapy was modified to adjust to the level of pain and to prevent narcotic addiction. |
| 2. Danny will verbalize awareness of those factors that contribute to pain in order to prevent them by 12/1/88. | 2a. Nurse will explain and list the many factors that can contribute to pain, such as fear, fatigue, anger, etc. <br> 2b. Client will identify those factors in his life that contribute to his pain (ie, lack of rest) | 2a. Holistic assessment provides a basis for dealing with other factors that decrease a client's ability to tolerate pain and increase pain level (Brunner and Suddarth, 1989). | Danny reported less disruption from pain and discomfort. <br> He verbalized that fatigue and fear contributed to the severity of pain and discomfort. <br> He used pain medication as prescribed and reports an increased level of relief after adjustment. |
| 3. Danny will use 3-4 new strategies to deal with pain by 12/15/88. | 3a. Client will verbalize how he responds and deals with pain (ie, tenses up muscles, goes to bed, takes too many analgesics, tires easily, etc.) | 3a. To fully relieve pain, a total assessment is necessary, and all additional information provides basis for appropriate intervention. | Danny verbalized the ways he responded to pain: weary, tired, fatigued, irritable, and grimacing. |
| | 3b. Nurse will explain and teach new and different strategies in dealing with pain: <br> • Use of humor <br> • Relaxation techniques | 3b. The use of humor in relieving pain and discomfort has a therapeutic effect in relieving the accompanying depression and | He identified additional effective pain relief strategies. |

## PLANS FOR IMPLEMENTATION—cont'd

| Objectives | Nursing orders | Scientific rationale | Evaluation |
|---|---|---|---|
| | • Imagery, distraction<br>• Cutaneous stimulation<br>• Use of analgesics before peak pain in cycle<br>• Music | one overpowering aspect of stress (Prerost, 1988). | |
| | 3c. Client will select and use appropriate measure to deal with pain and discomfort:<br>• Analgesics within prescribed regimen<br>• Relaxation techniques<br>• Diversion, humor, and music | 3c. Analgesics tend to be more effective when administered early in pain cycle (Brunner and Suddarth, 1989; McCaffery, 1972). Client's participation in his own self-care improves self-esteem and gives more control over his illness (Pohl, 1978). | He reported the effective use of new pain relief strategies and the decrease in pain intensity:<br>• Imagery, music<br>• Humor<br>• Diversion |
| 4. Danny will identify measures that maintain a pain management regimen by 12/15/88. | 4a. Danny will cooperate and collaborate with nurses, physician, other health care team members, as well as family, when changes in pain management are necessary (ie, when medication does not appear to relieve pain, the dosage is too small, side effects are present, relief of stress is needed, etc). | 4a. New methods of administration of analgesics must be acceptable to patient, physician, health care team members, and family in order to be effective: the patient's participation decreases his sense of powerlessness (Brunner and Suddarth, 1989). | Danny exhibits decreased physical and behavioral responses to pain:<br>• Interest in surroundings<br>• Interest in school<br>Danny takes responsibility for taking analgesics at appropriate times.<br><br>**Summative:**<br>Danny achieved more relief from pain and discomfort through use of new coping strategies and adjustment in medications. |

**Nursing diagnosis 2:** *Altered body image and self-esteem related to changes in appearance, function, and roles (10/22/88).*

**Goal:** *The client will develop an improved body image and self-esteem by 12/15/88.*

| Objectives | Nursing orders | Scientific rationale | Evaluation |
|---|---|---|---|
| 1. Danny will identify concerns related to body image and self-esteem by 11/5/88. | 1a. Nurse will assess client's feelings about body image and level of self-esteem:<br>• Dependence on family<br>• Inability to provide for his son (infant)<br>• Changes in appearance | *Content:* Body image.<br>*Strategy:* Principles of nursing practice; therapeutic use of self; and stress management.<br>1a. Provides baseline assessment for evaluation of changes and assessing effectiveness of interventions (Brunner and Suddarth, 1989). | **Formative:**<br>Danny identified areas of importance:<br>• Loss of strength<br>• Loss of hair<br>• Loss of role as father<br>• Dependence on family by not being able to work |

*Continued.*

**PLANS FOR IMPLEMENTATION—cont'd**

| Objectives | Nursing orders | Scientific rationale | Evaluation |
|---|---|---|---|
| | 1b. Nurse will identify potential threats to self-esteem (altered appearance, decreased sexual function, hair loss, energy, role changes). Danny will validate with nurse his specific concerns. | 1b. Anticipation of changes permits client to identify the importance of these areas to self. Effective learning requires active participation (Pohl, 1978). | |
| 2. Danny will continue an active role in activities and decision-making by 11/15/88. | 2a. Nurse will encourage continued participation and decision-making in personal and family life. | 2a. Active participation of client in his own self-care is critical to reconstruction and upward trajectory (Neuman, 1982; Pohl, 1978). | He continued to take an active role in both personal and family decision-making. |
| | 2b. Danny will be active in choices of social life, family decision-making, and responsibilities in household. | 2b. Active role in family living reduces depersonalization and emphasizes patient's self-worth (McFarland and Wasli, 1986). | He verbalized his feelings and reactions to impending losses (fatherhood, sexuality, loss of muscle tone and activity, loss of body image: hair, muscles). |
| | 2c. Nurse will encourage Danny to voice concerns regarding self-care. | 2c. Identifying concerns is an important step in coping with them (Brunner and Suddarth, 1989). | |
| | 2d. Danny will voice concerns to himself, family, and nurse. | | |
| 3. Danny will participate in self-care when side effects compromise his independence by 12/1/88. | 3a. Family (or other caregivers) will assist Danny when fatigue, lethargy, nausea, vomiting, and other symptoms alter his independence (appropriate foods for a nutritious diet; adequate rest periods provided, etc). | 3a. Physical well being improves self-esteem (Brunner and Suddarth, 1989). | Danny allowed nurses and family to assist him when in distress from chemotherapy (diet; passive exercise [ROM], walking, etc). |
| | 3b. Client will maintain self-care and, yet, accept assistance in times of severe distress (choosing eating times and types of food that are less aggravating to his system; taking appropriate rest periods). | 3b. Accepting of assistance with appropriate self-care measures when possible assists in maintaining self-esteem and helps with upward trajectory in rehabilitation (reconstruction) (Neuman, 1983; Hill and Smith, 1985). | |
| 4. Danny will select activities that will increase his general well-being in dealing with his illness by 12/1/88. | 4a. Nurse will provide information about methods of problem solving with hair loss, loss of muscle tone, general body image, and self-esteem (use of hairpiece; care of hair and skin; preservation of muscle tone). | 4a. Providing current information to client regarding prostheses, and activities that maintain an improved body image are necessary and preliminary to self-care measures (Hill and Smith, 1985). | Danny exhibited interest in appearance and was anxious to participate in self-care. He does not use a hairpiece yet but is very cautious in taking care of his hair (washes with gentle shampoo; uses no hair dryer). |

| Objectives | Nursing orders | Scientific rationale | Evaluation |
|---|---|---|---|
| | 4b. Danny will choose alternatives and ways to work with these impending losses:<br>• Hair care<br>• Weight lifting<br>• Extended rest periods | 4b. Client participation in improving body image will increase self-esteem (Brunner and Suddarth, 1989). Alternating rest periods with passive exercise will maintain and improve physical well-being (Brunner and Suddarth, 1989). | |
| 5. Danny will share concerns about possible altered sexual functions and social relationships with partner by 12/15/88. | 5a. Nurse and client will explore and verbalize concerns about socializing with girlfriend (sexual relationships; effects of illness on time commitment; knowledge about illness).<br>5b. Danny will share these concerns with girlfriend.<br>5c. Danny and girlfriend will explore alternatives and various ways to express affection.<br>5d. Nurse and Danny will provide knowledge and encourage girlfriend to verbalize her concerns regarding his illness. | 5a. The client's participation in selecting options and in decision-making regarding the socialization process is paramount to preserving self-esteem (Hill and Smith, 1985).<br>5b. The provision of both knowledge and opportunity for expression of concern, affection, and acceptance is basic to maintenance of self-esteem (Stuart and Sundeen, 1987; Brunner and Suddarth, 1989). | Danny participated with others in conversations, social events, and activities (he and his sister go to parties, or go "cruising").<br>He verbalized concern about his girlfriend's reluctance to get involved after he told her of his illness.<br>Danny is willing to explore better ways to communicate with girlfriend and to explore alternate ways of expressing concern and affection.<br><br>**Summative:**<br>Danny fulfilled the objectives and verbalized that he was coping and feeling good about himself. |

**Nursing diagnosis 3:** *Grieving related to anticipatory loss (altered role functioning) (11/15/88).*
**Goal:** *The client and family will progress within the grieving process by 1/22/89.*

| Objectives | Nursing orders | Scientific rationale | Evaluation |
|---|---|---|---|
| 1. The family and ill client will verbalize expressions of grief by 12/1/88. | 1a. Nurse will encourage and explore verbalization of fears, concerns, and questions regarding disease, treatment, and future implications:<br>• Chemotherapy and side effects<br>• Role changes<br>• Prognosis/remission | *Content:* Grief/loss.<br>*Strategy:* Therapeutic use of self and stress management.<br>1a. An increased and accurate knowledge base will decrease family anxiety and dispel misconception. | **Formative:**<br>• Partially met<br>• Mother just beginning to express grief (crying), and also expressed spiritual distress |

*Continued.*

**PLANS FOR IMPLEMENTATION—cont'd**

| Objectives | Nursing orders | Scientific rationale | Evaluation |
|---|---|---|---|
| 2. The family will identify internal and external resources available to aid coping strategies during grieving by 12/15/88. | 2a. The nurse will encourage active participation of both ill patient and family in care and treatment decisions:<br>• Medications<br>• Pain relief<br>• Decisions about work<br>2b. Nurse will visit family frequently to maintain interpersonal relationship and physical closeness.<br>2c. Nurse will inform Danny of support groups for those with cancer.<br><br>2d. Danny and family will speak with clergy or counselors as needed.<br>2e. The nurse will offer other aids such as the book *When Bad Things Happen to Good People* by Rabbi Harold Kushner (nurse and family can read and discuss this book together). | 2a. Active participation from ill client along with family helps with client independence and control.<br><br>2b. Frequent contacts promote trust and security and reduce feelings of fear and isolation.<br><br>2c. Support from others who are experiencing the same problems reduces isolation and the added knowledge releases anxiety.<br><br>2d. Professional support can aid the grieving process. | The family included Danny in household chores and in the financial support and management of the home.<br><br>A schedule was set up for visits from the nurse as needed.<br><br>Danny refused to go to support groups because of fear of members dying. This was a way to preserve his own use of denial.<br><br><br>Mary expressed an interest in this resource (book). |
| 3. The family will openly express grief as they need to by 1/10/89. | 3a. The nurse will encourage the ventilation of negative feelings including projected anger and hostility within acceptable limits:<br>• Oppositional behavior<br>• Verbalize anger at nurse<br>• Verbalize anger at God<br>3b. The nurse will support and give permission for periods of crying and expression of sadness:<br>• Support client through touch<br>• Verbal affirmation<br>• Cry with client<br>• Offer spiritual support and reinforcement | 3a. Ventilation of feelings allows for emotional expression without destruction of self-esteem. It also reverses the denial mechanism when the use of this defense technique becomes destructive and dysfunctional (Rawlins and Heacock, 1988).<br><br>3b. The expression of emotional grief (crying and sadness) are necessary in order to progress through the grief process (McFarland and Wasli, 1986). The meeting of spiritual needs is basic to integrating the human spirit (Carson, 1989). | *Objectives not met:* Anger was expressed somewhat openly in Danny's refusal to use a support group. Jim, Sr., not coming to these meetings was an expression of negative behavior. Anger was expressed indirectly.<br><br>Only mother directly expressed sadness and crying (other members still in denial?). |
| 4. The family will relieve their spiritual distress by 1/22/89. | 4a. The nurse will assess the spiritual needs of ill client and family as | 4a-b. Providing spiritual care is a requirement of holistic nursing. | Danny seemed to be at peace with himself and his God. The family con- |

| Objectives | Nursing orders | Scientific rationale | Evaluation |
|---|---|---|---|
| | they relate to grieving in life-threatening illness:<br>• Search for meaning<br>• Sense of forgiveness<br>• Hope<br>• Love<br>4b. Danny and family will become aware of these needs as nurse explores these concepts with them. | (1) As people approach finitude, they want to view their lives as having *purpose and meaning*. They need to integrate dying with personal goals and values.<br>(2) When people review their lives, guilt is experienced if their self-expectations are unfulfilled. They must have a sense of *forgiveness.*<br>(3) *Hope* is a feature of human existence critically ill patients need with concrete and abstract hope to carry them through the dying process.<br>(4) One of the spiritual needs of the dying is to experience love. This can be demonstrated through words and acts of kindness (Conrad, 1985). | tinues to struggle and is displacing their anger at God. |
| | 4c. The nurse will provide spiritual care support for this family.<br>(1) Use of communication skills:<br>  a. Openness<br>  b. Listen for cues; respond appropriately<br>  c. Willing to be involved with family<br>(2) Other intervention such as<br>  a. Prayer<br>  b. Meditation<br>  c. Guided meditation or Imagery<br>  d. Reading<br>  e. Music and art | 4c. Prayer is powerful and effective when used cautiously. Music has tremendous power for meeting the emotional and spiritual needs of a dying person. It can produce laughter and tears. It can sedate or stimulate (Conrad, 1985). | Danny verbalized his peace with God. The family has not yet done this.<br>Danny used music as his own support system.<br><br>**Summative:**<br>Goal partially met. |

**Nursing diagnosis 4:** *Alteration in family process related to dysfunctional communication (11/1/88).*
**Goal:** *Family will improve communication among its members by 1/15/89.*

| Objectives | Nursing orders | Scientific rationale | Evaluation |
|---|---|---|---|
| 1. Mary (mother) will verbalize her knowledge of assertiveness skills by 12/15/88. | 1a. The nurse will assess Mary's knowledge and "feelings" concerning assertiveness, that is:<br>• Meaning of word *assertive*<br>• When she is or isn't assertive<br>• When she would like to be assertive<br>• How she feels about it (guilt, etc) | *Content:* Communication.<br>*Strategy:* Teaching and learning.<br>1a. Assertiveness training is a type of behavior therapy in which the client learns to communicate both positive and negative feelings in an open, honest, direct, and appropriate way (McFarland and Wasli, 1986). | **Formative (primary prevention):**<br>Mary and nurse explored what her concept of assertiveness was:<br>• How she felt about it<br>• The discomfort<br>• Fear of antagonism<br>• Fear of confrontation<br>Mary read *Stand Up, Speak Out, Talk Back.* She felt she understood it and had no particular problems with it. She gave examples in her own family situations where it applied (ie, with children and husband; taking care of the situation when it occurs). |
|  | 1b. Nurse will explain:<br>• The difference between *passive, assertive,* and *aggressive* behavior<br>• That the key concept in learning assertiveness is choice | 1b. It is important to differentiate passive, assertive, and aggressive behavior so that the client can make an informed choice about the appropriate action to take (McFarland and Wasli, 1986). |  |
|  | 1c. Mary will read the book *Stand Up, Speak Out, Talk Back* by Alberti and Emmons (1975) before next visit and relate this to her own situation, giving specific examples.<br>1d. The nurse and client will discuss important points in the above book and clarify together any parts of the book about which the client has questions. | 1c. A client cannot change others, but he can change his own behaviors so that self-esteem and self-respect are enhanced (Rawlins and Heacock, 1988). |  |
| 2. Client (Mary) will use assertive techniques to improve family communication by 12/30/88. | 2a. Nurse will teach client the techniques and steps in assertiveness training using Alberti and Emmon's book as a guide.<br>2b. Client will practice these steps using "I" messages and role playing with nurse in practice situations.<br>2c. The *nurse* will *serve* as a *role model* in seeking clarification, showing | 2a. Each person should choose for himself how he or she will act (Alberti and Emmons, 1975).<br><br>2b. Effective learning requires active participation of the learner (Pohl, 1978).<br><br>2c. Teaching requires effective communication (Pohl, 1978). | Mary practiced the steps and techniques of assertiveness as outlined in book. She felt the book was helpful to her.<br>She only role played one situation and then decided against this method of learning.<br>She said she would rather practice on her own. |

## PLANS FOR IMPLEMENTATION—cont'd

| Objectives | Nursing orders | Scientific rationale | Evaluation |
|---|---|---|---|
| | respect, listening to expression of feelings, giving suggestions, expressing opinions, setting limits, and making clear statements. | | |
| | 2d. The nurse will give support by:<br>• Clarifying "I" and "we" messages<br>• Supporting trials of new behaviors<br>• Listening to expressions of fear of change<br>• Giving feedback after role play<br>• Helping client learn positive self-reinforcement | 2d. Changed behavior leads to changed attitudes about oneself and one's impact upon people and situations (Alberti and Emmons, 1975).<br><br>Positive reinforcement of behavior increases its occurrence (Bower and Bevis, 1984). | Mary practiced new behaviors with her family, and she felt rather awkward the first week. The family gave positive feedback at the end of the first week. Mary states that she still feels uncomfortable in being assertive. |
| | 2e. Client will try out new behaviors with the family asking for feedback for 1 week and then discuss these interactions with the nurse.<br>2f. Client will continue for 3 more weeks and meet with nurse to discuss progress. | 2e. Client has the right to make a request, and others have a right to refuse the request. Rights have accompanying responsibilities (Rawlins and Heacock, 1988). | **Summative:**<br>Goal partially met. |

## REFERENCES AND READINGS

Alberti R and Emmons M: Stand up, speak out, talk back, New York, 1975, Pocket Books.

Ardell D: High level wellness, New York, 1986, Bantam Books.

Backanan BF: Human environment interaction: a modification of the Neuman systems model for aggregates, families, and the community, Public Health Nurs 4:1, 1987.

Bower F and Bevis E: Fundamentals of nursing practice, St Louis, 1984, The CV Mosby Co.

Brunner LS and Suddarth DS: The Lippincott manual of nursing practice, Philadelphia, 1986, ed 4, JB Lippincott Co.

Brunner LS and Suddarth DS: Textbook of medical surgical nursing, Philadelphia, 1989, JB Lippincott Co.

Carson VB: Spiritual dimensions of nursing practice, Philadelphia, 1989, WB Saunders Co.

Conrad NL: Spiritual support for the dying, Nurs Clin North Am 20(2):415, 1985.

Cross J: Betty Neuman. In George J: Nursing theories: the base for professional nursing practice, ed 2, Englewood Cliffs, NJ, 1985, Prentice-Hall, Inc.

Eshleman JR: The family: an introduction, Boston 1988, ed 5, Allyn Bacon, Inc.

Fredette S and Gloriant F: Nursing diagnoses in cancer chemotherapy, Am J Nurs 11:2013, November 1981.

Gerald MC: Pharmacology: An introduction to drugs, Englewood Cliffs, NJ, 1981, Prentice-Hall, Inc.

Hill L and Smith N: Self-care nursing, Norwalk, Conn, 1985, Appleton-Century-Crofts.

Krause M and Mahan K: Food, nutrition and diet therapy, Philadelphia, 1979, WB Saunders Co.

Kushner H: When bad things happen to good people, New York, 1983, Avon Books.

Lauer P et al: Learning needs of cancer patients: a comparison of nurse and patient perceptions, Nurs Res 31(1):11, 1982.

Leahey M and Wright LM: Families and life threatening illness, Springhouse, Pa, 1987, Springhouse Corp.

LeBlanc D: People with Hodgkin disease: the nursing challenge, Nurs Clin North Am, 13(2):281, 1978.

Levitt DZ: Cancer chemotherapy, RN December:33, 1980.

Mayer MG and Watson AB: Nursing care plans and the Neuman systems model: I. In Neuman B: The Neuman systems model, East Norwalk, Conn, 1982, Appleton-Century-Crofts.

McCaffery M: Nursing management of the patient with pain, Philadelphia, 1979, JB Lippincott Co.

McFarland G and Wasli E: Nursing diagnosis and process in psychiatric mental health nursing, Philadelphia, 1986, JB Lippincott Co.

Miller S and Winstead-Fry P: Family systems theory in nursing practice, Englewood Cliffs, NJ, 1982, Reston Publishing Co.

Neuman B: The Neuman systems model: application to nursing education and practice, East Norwalk, Conn, 1982, Appleton-Century-Crofts.

Neuman B: Family interventions using the Betty Neuman Health Care Systems Model. In Clements I and Roberts B: Family health: a theoretical approach to nursing care, New York, 1983, John Wiley & Sons, Inc.

Patrick ML et al: Medical surgical nursing: pathophysiological concepts, Philadelphia, 1986, JB Lippincott Co.

Pohl M: The teaching function of the nursing practitioner, Dubuque, Iowa, 1978, Wm C Brown Co.

Porth CM: Pathophysiology: concepts of altered health states, ed 2, Philadelphia, 1986, JB Lippincott Co.

Prerost FJ: Use of human and guided imagery in therapy to alleviate stress, Ment Health Counsel 10(1):16, 1988.

Rawlins RP and Heacock PE: Clinical manual of psychiatric nursing, 1988, The CV Mosby Co.

Spiegel D et al: Group support for patients with metastatic cancer, Arch Gen Psychiatry 38:527, May 1981.

Story EL and Ross MM: Family centered community health nursing and the Betty Neuman systems model, Nursing Papers: Perspectives in Nursing, 18:2, Summer 1986.

Stuart GW, and Sundeen SJ: Principles and practice of psychiatric nursing, ed 3, St Louis, 1987, The CV Mosby Co.

Valentine AS: Caring for the young adult with cancer, Cancer Nurs 12:385, 1978.

Veninga K: An easy recipe for assessing your patient's nutrition, Nursing 82 12(11):57, 1982.

Watson P: Psychosocial aspects of the cancer experience, Canad Nurse 14:45, 1978.

Williams SR: Nutrition and diet therapy, St Louis, 1989, The CV Mosby Co.

Wright LM and Leahey M: Nurses and families: a guide to family assessment and intervention, 1984, FA Davis Co.

# Nursing Process of the Family Client: Application of Friedman's and Roy's Models

CYNTHIA MAKIELSKI MARTZ

The client in this chapter is a young family: husband, wife, and 2-year-old son, who are facing the birth of a new baby in the next 6 weeks. The community health nurse received a routine referral from the clinic physician for a home visit. No specific health concerns were identified in the referral other than the pregnancy and the changing family unit.

During the initial home visit, the nurse chose Friedman's (1986) Structural-Functional Model as the guide for the family nursing process. This model was chosen because it facilitates analysis of the interactions among family members and the family's interactions with the community, such as the educational and health care systems. Roy's (1984) Adaptation Model is also applied in this chapter for an appropriate focus on individual family members. Roy's model is congruent with Friedman's model in examining role function and interdependence. However, Roy's model also addresses the physiological and self-concept areas that the nurse believes are very important aspects of individual health.

The Structural-Functional Model by Marilyn Friedman (1986) describes the structure of the family as the manner in which it is organized. Four basic dimensions or subconcepts are considered: (1) role structure, (2) value systems, (3) communication patterns, and (4) power structure. Family functions, according to Friedman, are those outcomes of the family structure that meet the needs of the family members. Six family functions are consid-

ered: (1) affective functioning, (2) socialization and social placement, (3) reproduction, (4) family coping, (5) economic function, and (6) provision of physical necessities. Both structure and function need to be addressed in a family nursing process.

In Roy's Adaptation Model, the individual is viewed as a whole being in interaction with the environment, who adapts to changes through four adaptive modes: physiological needs, self-concept, role function, and interdependence. Friedman's Structural-Functional model and Roy's Adaptation Model are more fully described in Chapter 2.

In this chapter, the nursing process begins with an overview of the demographic data. Assessment data follow and are presented in three columns. The left-hand column shows interaction data; the middle column is the observations; and the right-hand column indicates the measurements. The nursing process is organized as follows: first, the assessment and analysis/synthesis for the first visit are presented, followed by the list of nursing diagnoses. Next, the second and third assessment visits and analysis/synthesis are included, along with an updated list of nursing diagnoses. The nursing plans, which include goals, objectives, strategies, nursing orders, scientific rationale, and evaluation, are presented last. The plans are last because they are ongoing and subject to revision, and because they demonstrate the continuity of the entire nursing process. However, they are initiated, implemented, and evaluated concurrently with the assessment visits.

## DATA COLLECTION: Preliminary Information

### Biographical data and initial contact

### Biographical data

| | | | |
|---|---|---|---|
| Father | David Smith | Age 24 | Full-time student, first-semester college senior |
| Mother | Carla (Jones) Smith | Age 23 | High school graduate |
| Son | Gabe | Age 2 years, 4 months | |

Race: Caucasian

Ethnicity: Mother, German and English; father, English and Swiss

Religion: Mother, Methodist; father does not attend religious services

Occupation: Father, full-time sales clerk, Guaranteed Auto Store; mother not employed outside the home

Language spoken: English

Marital status: Parents married to each other; neither married previously.

Carla and Dave have been married 4½ years. They both grew up in Kokomo, Indiana, but did not meet until they were out of high school. They dated 6 months before getting married. They moved to Bloomington 3½ years ago so Dave could go to Indiana University and pursue a degree in political science.

Carla's mother, father, and sister (4 years younger) still live in Kokomo. Dave's mother, stepfather, brother (3 years younger), and sister (4 years younger) also live in Kokomo. Dave's mother and father were divorced when Dave was 5 years old. Dave does not know where his father lives and has not seen him since the divorce.

### Source of referral

Physician at clinic where Carla was seeking prenatal care

### Initial contact

Initial contact was with Carla by telephone on Tuesday, October 24, 1989. At that time the nurse explained that all clinic patients received a home visit by the community health nurse to discuss concerns of pregnancy or any other health concerns of the family. Carla was very pleasant and seemed eager to cooperate. After discussion with Dave, a date was set for the first visit.

## DATA COLLECTION: Visit 1

*Time:* Monday, November 6, 1989, 2 PM

*Place:* The Smith home. Carla and 2-year-old Gabe were present. Dave had planned to be present but was called to work to cover for someone who was sick. Carla had been watching television, but turned it off. Gabe had just awakened from a nap. Carla offered the nurse something to drink. The visit lasted 1½ hours.

*Nursing goals:* (1) to establish rapport with the family members, (2) collect a health history on each family member, (3) begin to assess family life patterns, and (4) initiate at least one plan of intervention based on nursing diagnosis made during this visit.

| Interactions | Observations | Measurements |
|---|---|---|
| **Carla provided Gabe's health history** | | |
| Gabe was born July 7, 1987, after 18 hours of labor. Low forceps were used. I had pudendal anesthesia, and I received two pain shots during labor. I don't know what kind of medicine it was. | | |
| No allergies that I know of. | | |
| No childhood diseases. | | |

## DATA COLLECTION: Visit 1—cont'd

| Interactions | Observations | Measurements |
| --- | --- | --- |
| Immunizations are up-to-date; at least that's what the pediatricians have told me. | Carla went to desk and immediately found Gabe's immunization record booklet with the pediatricians' names on front of booklet. | |
| Not on any medications.<br>No chronic illnesses, only two or three colds, and he had a really bad ear infection about a year ago.<br>No surgeries or hospitalizations. | | Diptheria, pertussis and tetanus (DPT) given: 9-4-87; 10-9-87; 11-6-87; 1-13-89<br>Oral polio vaccine (OPV) given: 9-4-87; 11-6-87; 1-15-88; 1-13-89<br>Measles, mumps, and rubella (MMR) given: 10-14-88 |
| **Gabe's current health status provided by Carla** | | |
| I give Gabe a bath every night before bedtime, and I usually wash his hair about twice a week. We're in the process of potty training, and he does pretty well, but he usually has one or two accidents a day. Of course, that means my laundry builds up quickly. Thank God I have that washer and dryer. They were gifts from my mom and dad. | Gabe is dressed in shirt and over-alls that fit neatly, navy blue tennis shoes with white shoe laces. Hair is straight, brown, combed, and cut neatly. | |
| Well, I guess you could call me a health food nut when it comes to diet. I never bought any baby food that had salt or sugar in it. And Gabe never gets candy. He doesn't eat much, but I always make him eat a little bit of protein and some fruits and vegetables. He loves milk, and I make my own cookies with whole wheat flour and honey, which he loves. He usually has two or three snacks a day besides his three small meals. | Carla helped Gabe wash hands before snacktime and washed his face and hands after snack. Carla also helped Gabe wash hands after urinating in the potty chair. Carla washed her own hands before giving Gabe his snack and after emptying the potty chair receptacle. Washer and dryer are in the small bathroom off the kitchen. | Gabe had a snack of about 4 oz 2% milk and 25 raisins. |
| Gabe weighs 27 lb and is 35″ tall. | Gabe is a 2-year-old with dark-brown eyes and fair complexion. Skin soft, well hydrated. | Gabe has 16 teeth, missing only his second molars. |
| Gabe is such an active boy. We go for a walk every day, and I have to walk fast to keep up with him. He loves to do puzzles, and he loves it when Dave roughhouses with him. | Gabe half runs whenever he goes somewhere. Gabe did a four-piece puzzle quickly and easily. When Carla turned the TV on to "Sesame Street," Gabe became very excited and then settled in front of TV, sucking his thumb and holding a blanket. There are a few toys scattered over the living room floor: a small round ball, two puzzles, a large plastic truck, three books, and a See 'n Say talking toy about farm animals. Gabe played with all the toys during the | Gabe was on and off Carla's lap 7 times in 5 minutes. Gabe sat still for 10 minutes while watching TV show (the only quiet period of any length during the 1½-hour visit). |

*Continued.*

## DATA COLLECTION: Visit 1—cont'd

| Interactions | Observations | Measurements |
|---|---|---|
| | visit, but seemed to prefer the puzzles. He smiled, clapped his hands, and looked at Carla at the completion of the puzzles. | |
| I usually put Gabe to bed at 8 or 9 o'clock, and he sleeps till 6 or 7 in the morning. But sometimes I do keep him up later if he hasn't seen Dave. You know, with classes and work, some days Dave isn't home at all. Anyway, then Gabe usually takes a 2- or 3-hour nap during the day. | | |
| I get awfully tired being the only one here with Gabe all day. But I understand that Dave doesn't have a choice right now. Besides, if Dave didn't work full time, I'd have to work. And with the new baby coming, that isn't very feasible. I guess it won't last forever. | | |
| Gabe really is a mama's boy. And I know I let him get away with more than he should. But it takes so much more energy to fight with him than to let him have his way. I'm a little concerned how he will react when we bring the new baby home. | Gabe speaks several words clearly: Mommy, milk, no, potty, ball, Ernie, Bert, blanky, go, baby, tummy, and a few others. He speaks in three- to four-word sentences. Gabe said no to many of Carla's requests and demands, and Carla did not insist that he comply. Most of the time Carla would ignore Gabe's no's and let him do as he pleased. However, besides the negative behavior, Gabe was also openly affectionate with Carla, hugging and kissing her many times during the visit. Carla was also physically and verbally affectionate with Gabe, stroking his head and back, hugging and kissing, and saying, "Mommy loves you." At one point, Gabe said, "Gabe a good boy." | |
| Well, we've talked about the new baby. He knows the baby is in my belly, and we encourage him to love the baby. | Gabe pats Carla's abdomen and says, "baby." | |
| We're going to move Gabe into a youth bed that my mother has in her attic, and then the new baby will sleep in Gabe's crib. | | |
| My mother said she could come to take care of Gabe while I'm in the hospital, but we haven't made anything definite yet. I know Dave | | |

## DATA COLLECTION: Visit 1—cont'd

| Interactions | Observations | Measurements |
|---|---|---|

won't be able to stay home; he'll be getting ready for final exams.

I'm willing to do anything that will make this easier for Gabe and for Dave and me. The little girl next door started wetting her pants all the time after her baby sister was born. How can I deal with that if it happens with Gabe?

So should I have a special time with Gabe every day while the baby's sleeping and have Gabe help care for the baby in simple ways?

Well, it will be easy to keep telling Gabe how good and special he is and how much we love him. Dave and I have always been very demonstrative with Gabe.

Getting Gabe in the youth bed as soon as possible makes sense, too. I'm sure my mother would bring the bed this weekend if I asked her. I'd kind of enjoy a visit with her anyway. And then we could finalize the plans for her coming when the baby is born. I know, that's when we could talk to Gabe about grandma staying with him when mommy is gone. Don't you think that's a good idea?

I have another good idea! Since you say Gabe won't understand 2 or 3 days, do you suppose it will help if Dave and I go out for awhile when my mom is here? Gabe really does love my mom.

You know, all of this seems vaguely familiar. When Dave and I took prenatal classes before Gabe was born, it seems the instructor talked a little bit about preparing the older children for the new baby. But of course, Dave and I didn't pay much attention, since Gabe was our first. We didn't take the classes this time because of Dave's hectic schedule.

I'm going to call my mom tonight and try to set it up for her to come and bring the bed this weekend. I can let you know how it all goes the next time you come. At least this way, if Gabe reacts badly to the new baby, I'll know we did everything we could to prepare him.

Carla becomes more animated. She speaks faster and the pitch of her voice gets higher.

*Continued.*

## DATA COLLECTION: Visit 1—cont'd

| Interactions | Observations | Measurements |
|---|---|---|

**Carla's health history**

No allergies

I know I had the chickenpox and mumps. And I must have had rubella, because my obstetrician took a test for that and he said I don't have to worry about getting it because my titre is high.

No chronic illnesses, and no medications. I really am very healthy. Oh, I do take prenatal vitamins.

Carla smiled and said this is a very prideful tone of voice.

My mother's father died of a heart attack, but everyone else in my family is okay.

I had a tonsillectomy when I was 10, and I had a D and C last summer after I had my miscarriage.

Started my period at age 12, had a period every month, and had no problems with periods except occasional bad cramps.

I've been pregnant a total of three times. A year ago August when I had my miscarriage, I was only about 2 months along.

No problems with Gabe's pregnancy, except I had a lot of problems holding water near the end of my pregnancy. The doctor kept a close watch on my blood pressure. He said it was okay.

**Carla's current health status**

No problems with this pregnancy either, but I do get awfully tired chasing after Gabe all day.

Carla has a gravid uterus, apparently near term. She appears to have edema of the hands and feet and has dark circles around her eyes.

Carla is wearing an attractive maternity top and blue jeans. Her hair is shiny brown, curly, and neatly styled. She is wearing makeup. Her fingernails are nicely shaped, medium length, and painted with a light pink polish. Carla's loafers are polished.

The drinks Carla offered the nurse were orange juice and herbal tea.

LMP: 2-24-89; EDC: 12-1-89
Blood type A, Rh pos.
Uterus measures 35 cm from symphysis pubis to fundus.

As I said, I'm a health food nut. I loved home ec in high school then I worked in a nursing home in the kitchen after Dave and I were married. So I understand about the basic four and vitamins and all. Luckily, Dave will eat anything I fix. I like to try new recipes, and I

## DATA COLLECTION: Visit 1—cont'd

| Interactions | Observations | Measurements |
|---|---|---|

make great salads. It's a good thing, too. I lost all my baby weight after Gabe was born by eating mostly salads.

No, I don't smoke or drink coffee or pop. Dave and I have an occasional glass of wine, but I haven't had any while I've been pregnant.

My recreation consists mostly of socializing with the other mothers in the apartment complex. A lot of them have husbands in school, too, and we sort of get together and bolster one another. About once a week this one girl and I trade babysitting, so I get out during the day to run errands or go shopping. I really enjoy that. Dave and I try to get out about once a month to one of the free things on campus. We trade babysitting for that, too. Oh, I almost forgot: I love to take care of my plants. And I do a little needlepoint while I'm watching TV.

*(Observations)* There are many lovely and exotic-looking plants throughout the living room and kitchen. There are also two or three needle-point pictures hanging on the wall. A large stack of women's and home decorating magazines sits by the living room couch.

I'm tired all the time. I'm sure it's the pregnancy and running after Gabe. I wasn't this tired before I got pregnant. Anyway, I try to sleep whenever Gabe takes a nap, and I always get at least 8 hours at night.

Like I said, I take a walk every day. That's nice. And I do a few of the exercises that I remember from prenatal classes. The pelvic rock really helps the low back pain.

I certainly intend when Dave is through school to take my turn. I've heard too many stories about wives who put their husbands through school and end up divorced. I know I'll have to go part-time because of the kids, but I think it would be a lot more fun taking only one class at a time. Not so much pressure, like Dave has. I'd like to study interior decorating or home design.

*(Observations)* Carla is an articulate woman who uses grammar correctly.

I feel pretty good about myself. I truly enjoy being a mother, even though someday I want to be an interior decorator. I feel sorry for some of the other mothers in the complex. They're always complain-

*(Observations)* Carla walks with head and shoulders erect and speaks with confidence when talking about her role as a mother and about her plans to go to school and become an interior decorator.

*Continued.*

## DATA COLLECTION: Visit 1—cont'd

| Interactions | Observations | Measurements |
|---|---|---|

ing about their boring lives. Well, sure, some days are rough, but Gabe and this new baby won't be little forever. I'm not going to be one of those mothers who complains when they're around and then complains when they're gone.

I come from an emotional family. We love family get-togethers, and we're always hugging and kissing one another. Dave's family isn't that way, and I think it really took some getting used to on his part. But now I think he really enjoys all the affection.

I weigh 142 lb, and I'm 5'4" tall. I've gained 22 lb so far in the pregnancy. I guess you've noticed the water in my hands and feet. It's the same problem I had before. The doctor says my blood pressure is okay, though.

**Family life patterns**

Boy, making ends meet is tough, especially with only a sales clerk's income and a full-time college student. Luckily, our parents have been great. I don't know what we'd do without them. Dave's folks pay for all his tuition. They're just so happy he's finally getting a degree. And every time my mom and dad come down for a visit, they're always bringing several sacks of groceries and clothes for Gabe and me. Then, of course, we have our student loans, which we'll probably be paying back 50 years from now. And Dave's employee health benefits plus the student health insurance policy we took out cover most of the medical bills.

We've been in this apartment about 3 years. We had a one-bedroom apartment down by the College Mall when we first moved here. Then when I got pregnant with Gabe, we needed a bigger place. It's not a bad place. As I said, a lot of the families in the complex are going to school. I think most of

Carla laughs and smiles appropriately. She also frowns and shows concern appropriately. No evidence of anger during this visit.

Smiths live in a two-bedroom townhouse apartment in a large complex on Bloomington's west side. Several large factories are located on the west side, and the Smiths are within a mile of several grocery stores (supermarkets), fast-food places, and discount stores (eg, K-Mart). The apartment has

## DATA COLLECTION: Visit 1—cont'd

| Interactions | Observations | Measurements |
|---|---|---|

the others work at Otis or Cook's or RCA. This place is sort of like college: we know we won't have to be here forever, and it's okay for now.

Upstairs there are two bedrooms, a bathroom, and a linen closet.

an 11' × 15' living room furnished with a couch and chair, a Boston-type rocking chair, a bookshelf made of bricks and planks, a stereo record player with two small speakers, and an antique-looking desk. The dining room is an area between the living room and kitchen. It has a card table with two placemats, napkins and napkin rings, and a small vase with a few silk flowers in it. There is also Gabe's high chair sitting next to the card table. The kitchen has a window over the sink, overlooking an approximately 6' × 8' fenced-in patio area. Off the kitchen is a half-bath, where the washer and dryer and Gabe's potty chair are located. The nurse did not go upstairs. Everything looked orderly except the few toys scattered on the floor. The furnishings were few, but the plants made the apartment look very unique and well decorated. A small TV rests on the bookshelves. There is also a coat closet inside the front door and a closet under the stairway that is used for storing Gabe's toys. (See floor plan on this page.)

I belong to the First Methodist Church. You know, the one downtown. But I don't go very often. Sunday morning is one of the few times Dave and Gabe and I all have together, and frankly, I don't want to give up our time together to go to church. Does that sound awful?

I don't belong to any other organizations, and neither does Dave. We do have friends, though. I still see some of the girls I used to work with at Sears and, of course, the girls here in the complex. Dave has his college friends and some friends from Guaranteed Auto. I guess our best friends are the Gibsons. They live almost directly across the parking lot from us. They have a 6-month-old girl, and Gary goes to IU, too. Sharon and I probably talk on the phone or in

Continued.

## DATA COLLECTION: Visit 1—cont'd

| Interactions | Observations | Measurements |
|---|---|---|
| person almost every day. The four of us sometimes get together on weekends and play Trivial Pursuit or cards and eat popcorn. They're the ones we trade babysitting with so Dave and I can get out alone. They really are fun. | | |
| Well, I've already said our folks have been great. My mom and dad are terrific, and even though Laura [sister] is 4 years younger, we're good friends besides being sisters. I love Dave's dad. We get along great. Dave's mom is okay. I guess we are typical mother-in-law and daughter-in-law. Luckily, Dave usually agrees with me that his mom is being a little too nosy and pushy. But she has her good side, too. She sure loves Gabe. I'd say either my folks or Dave's come down or we go to Kokomo at least once every 2 months. It's easier for us to go there because we don't really have any room for them to stay here. We'll go up for Thanksgiving. The nice thing about Kokomo is that it's only 2 hours away, so if we want to go up for just a day's visit, it's not too bad a trip. I hope my mother can come this weekend. It's been awhile since we visited. | On the top of the desk are Carla and Dave's wedding pictures taken with each of their separate families (along with several pictures of Gabe). | |
| Sure, we can set up a time for you to come again. How about next week on Dave's day off? That's next Wednesday. Same time? | Carla goes to the desk and looks at a calendar. | |
| I'll check with Dave and call you at the clinic, if it's not okay. | | |
| I enjoyed your visit. Thanks for the information. We'll work on the bed thing, hopefully this weekend. Bye. | Gabe waves bye-bye at Carla's suggestion. | |

## ANALYSIS/SYNTHESIS OF DATA: Visit 1

### Analysis/Synthesis

I. An analysis/synthesis of the individuals according to Roy's (1984) adaptation model is presented first.
  A. Physiological Mode
     Gabe is very active most of the time and takes a walk with his mom nearly every day. He gets 12 to 13 hours of sleep in a 24-hour period, which according to Matt, Fazekas, and James (1985) is normal. Gabe eats small amounts of food, but Carla claims he eats from all four food groups. Gabe is in the process of being toilet trained, but no information was obtained on elimination patterns, which is a data gap. Gabe's skin is soft and well hydrated, which indicates ade-

quate fluids and electrolytes. Gabe's height of 35 inches and weight of 27 pounds put him in the 25th percentile for his age, according to Matt and co-authors. A total of 16 teeth is normal for his age. All this information, plus the fact that Gabe's health history reflects current immunizations and no disease, indicates that Gabe is adapting physiologically. Data gaps exist in the areas of oxygenation, elimination, the senses, and neurological and endocrine functions.

Carla gets adequate amounts of exercise and rest. Her diet includes the basic four food groups, and weight gain of 22 lb in 8 months of this pregnancy is adequate (Jensen and Bobak, 1989). No elimination information was obtained. Although edema of the hands and feet is a common phenomenon of pregnancy and Carla's blood pressure is "okay" according to her doctor, further assessment of Carla's edema is needed before ruling it out as a physiological threat. Carla's complaint of constant fatigue may also be only a phenomenon of pregnancy; however, other causes, such as anemia, have not been ruled out. Therefore, a data gap exists. Carla's health history is negative for disease, and Carla considers herself a healthy person. From the evidence gathered, physiologically she is adapting, which is a strength.

B. Self-Concept Mode

Gabe appears to be adapting in the self-concept mode, as evidenced by his stating, "Gabe a good boy" and by his obvious pleasure and pride after completing a puzzle.

Carla's self-concept can also be described as adaptive. She is attractively dressed and wears makeup. She states, "I feel pretty good about myself." She has a plan to get further education when Dave is through college.

Strengths are good self-concepts for both Gabe and Carla.

C. Role Function Mode

Data relating to Gabe's role as a 2-year-old firstborn son show that he is complying with toilet training, eating, and hygienic habits expected of him. He appears to be in Erikson's (1963) stage of development: autonomy vs. shame and doubt, which is appropriate for his age. He is developing autonomy as he learns to control himself and his environment.

Regarding Carla's role as mother, she states, "I truly enjoy being a mother," and feels it is important for her to be home with the children. She is conscientious in her mothering role, as evidenced by her attention to eating and hygienic habits as well as her concern for Gabe's emotional well-being. Data gap: Carla's role as wife. It can be concluded that Gabe and Carla are both adapting to their respective roles identified during this visit.

D. Interdependence Mode

Gabe appears to be still in the working stages of achieving independence from his mother. Getting on and off her lap so frequently may represent his working through needing her in close proximity and exploring the environment. He gives and gets verbal and nonverbal affection openly. Data gaps: separation anxiety/behaviors when Carla leaves the house without him, behaviors at bedtime, interdependence with Dave.

Carla obviously enjoys giving to and getting from Gabe verbal and nonverbal affection. She recognizes Gabe's dependence on her (calls him a mama's boy), yet recognizes the need to, and actually does, get out of the house without Gabe. Carla's interdependence with her family and Dave's shows that she can depend on them and is grateful for their help and support. Yet, independence also exists in that a family visit every 2 months seems reasonable. Data gap: Carla's interdependence with Dave.

Strengths from the evidence gathered: Gabe is at an appropriate level of interdependence adaptation for his age. Carla is adapting in the interdependence mode with Gabe and the extended families.

II. An analysis/synthesis of family data is presented according to the structural-functional approach. The four concepts of structure are addressed first, followed by the six concepts of family functions.

A. Family Structure

1. *Role:* The roles of Gabe as a 2-year-old firstborn son and Carla as mother have been addressed under Roy's model. However, the coming birth of the new baby will bring new roles for Gabe and Carla. Gabe will become a brother and for the first time have to share his parents' attention on an everyday basis. Carla is concerned about Gabe's adjustment to the new role, which is a strength. However, she has done very little (only talks

about the new baby to Gabe and has him pat her belly as a way of loving the baby) to prepare Gabe or help him accept the new role. This is a potential concern.

Carla's role as mother of one 2-year-old will change to mother of two children, including a newborn baby. More information is needed regarding Carla's new role. Another data gap is Dave's roles in the family.

2. *Values:* Carla's apparent values are: health (good nutrition, good hygiene, exercise, prenatal care), education, time together as a nuclear family, and extended family. The data gap is values that Dave and Carla hold together as a nuclear family.

3. *Communication:* Communication patterns between Carla and Gabe reflect much use of touch, stroking, sitting on the lap. When Gabe and Carla speak they look at one another, and Carla encourages the expression of feelings, which Satir (1972) says is a characteristic of a healthy family. Data gap: Dave's communication with the rest of the family, and theirs with him.

4. *Power:* Carla makes the decisions about nutrition and food on the table, but that is the only definite piece of data collected related to power structure. It is possible that Gabe's many "no" responses have become manipulative, and in that way Gabe may exert some power over Carla. However, more assessment is necessary, because the "no" could simply be a result of his age and stage of development. Data gaps: who makes what decisions and how; power hierarchy.

B. Family Functions

1. *Affective:* The open affection between Carla and Gabe has been mentioned and can be considered a strength. Data gaps: Dave's part in the family's affective function; his psychological response to members' needs.

2. *Socialization:* Initial assessment shows that childrearing practices in the Smith family are permissive, inasmuch as Carla does not insist that Gabe do what she ask. But a data gap exists, because Dave's input on child-rearing practices is not known and child-rearing practices were not actually discussed. Also, the environment was somewhat artificial because of the nurse's presence. Carla may have let

Gabe go to avoid any hassles during the visit. According to Piaget, Gabe should be in the preconceptual period of the preoperational phase of cognitive development. In this period the emergence of the symbolic function is shown in the rapid development of language (Hetherington and Parke, 1979). Data related to cognitive development show that Gabe is at the proper period, which is a strength.

Dave is in college, and Carla intends to get further education in the future. This will influence Gabe's attitude toward education.

In the area of community contacts, Dave is involved with an educational organization and with his work organization. Carla belongs to church but goes infrequently. So their contacts with actual organizations are somewhat limited. However, they do have contact with the community in terms of their friends and family, which is a strength.

3. *Reproduction:* Carla and Dave are participating in the reproductive function of the family. Data gaps: Were any of the three pregnancies planned? Are more children wanted? Sexual history; family planning.

4. *Coping:* More than once Carla said, "it's not forever," particularly in relation to Dave's being gone all the time because of school and work and in relation to their financial situation and their apartment. This telling herself, in effect, that the stress will end some day seems to be a coping pattern of Carla's. Also, she has made a plan to take her turn at higher education, and she talks of chatting with the other "college wives" and bolstering one another. These are also effective coping methods and can be considered strengths. Data gaps: Dave's coping patterns; past and current stressors and past coping patterns.

5. *Economics:* The family income is apparently meager, but the Smith's are able to provide for their food, clothing, shelter, and health care by using a variety of resources, such as help from family, loans, medical insurance, and even trading babysitting and attending free functions at the university for entertainment. The apartment is modest but satisfactory to Carla until something nicer can be afforded. The Smith's economic function,

according to Carla, is a strength. Data gaps: provision of transportation; Dave's attitude toward economic function.

The Smith family strengths are:

1. Adequate activity and rest, nutrition, fluids and regulation for Gabe
2. Adequate activity and rest, nutrition, fluids and regulation for Carla
3. Gabe and Carla have good self-concepts
4. Role adaptation of Gabe, and of Carla in her mothering role
5. Appropriate level of interdependence adaptation of Gabe for his age
6. Adaptation in the interdependence mode of Carla with Gabe and with the extended families
7. Carla's concern for Gabe's adjustment to his future new role as brother
8. Open expression of feelings between Carla and Gabe, with much verbal and nonverbal affection shown
9. Good contact with friends in the community and family for Carla
10. Effective coping mechanisms by Carla
11. Adequate economic provisions

## NURSING DIAGNOSES: Visit 1

| Date | Diagnoses | Priority |
|---|---|---|
| 11/6/89 | 1. Potential role conflict for Gabe related to inadequate preparation for new baby | 1 |
| 11/6/89 | 2. Incomplete data base, especially in areas related to Dave | 2 |

## DATA COLLECTION: Visit 2

*Time*: Wednesday, November 15, 1989 2:00 PM

*Place*: The Smith home. Dave opened the door, introduced himself, and immediately apologized for not having been present at the last visit. Carla greeted the nurse and told her that Gabe was still napping. The visit lasted 1 hour.

*Nursing goals*: To (1) establish rapport with Dave, (2) fill in the identified data gaps related to Dave and family life patterns, (3) evaluate previous nursing interventions, and (4) initiate at least one plan of intervention based on nursing diagnosis made during the visit.

| Interactions | Observations | Measurements |
|---|---|---|

**Dave's health history (provided by Dave)**

I'm not really sure about my childhood diseases. I think I had the mumps—that's the one men have to watch out for—my mom would know. She kept records just like Carla does for Gabe.

I don't have any chronic illnesses and I don't take any medications. I do take Alka-Seltzer Plus when I have a cold.

I couldn't really tell you whether or not my dad has any illnesses. I guess Carla told you I haven't seen him or talked to him in almost 20 years. I hardly remember

Dave is dressed in a flannel shirt and blue jeans. He is clean-shaven with shiny, dark-brown straight hair that is cut just covering the top of the ears. His nails are clean, and his oral hygiene is good.

Dave is a trim-looking man with muscular physique who does not have dark circles around his eyes.

*Continued.*

## DATA COLLECTION: Visit 2—cont'd

| Interactions | Observations | Measurements |
| --- | --- | --- |

what he looks like. But my family is all healthy.

No surgeries, but I did have to go to the hospital in high school when I broke my arm playing touch football, of all things.

**Dave's current health status (provided by Dave)**

Carla's a great cook. I'll eat anything she fixes. No, I don't smoke. But I do drink wine and an occasional beer.

My greatest recreation right now is sleeping. I know that sounds terrible, but with my schedule and all the studying I have to do, it's such a luxury to get a good night's sleep. When I'm not in the midst of a semester, I like sports of all kinds, to watch and play. I used to run 3 miles every day, but I've even given that up, too. Now my only real exercise is walking on campus between classes.

School is going great, in spite of the pressure it creates. My grades are good, and if everything goes according to schedule, I'll graduate next May. We'll both be glad.
— Carla is smiling.

You know, I feel good about myself, but I also feel a little selfish and guilty. I know my being gone all the time is hard for Carla. It will be worse when the new baby comes. I also know how much Carla wants to go to college. I guess I am grateful that I get to be the first one to go. I'll support her all the way when it's her turn.
— Dave is an articulate man, uses correct grammar.

Well, having Gabe has been great, although as I've said, I don't get to spend as much time with the family as I'd like. I think because my own father ran out, I want to do a good job as a father. Speaking of Gabe, there's the little guy now.
— Dave shows emotions appropriately.
Gabe comes walking down the stairs carrying a blanket in one hand and a stuffed Snoopy dog in the other hand. He goes immediately to Carla and climbs on her lap.

Dave: Carla told me that Gabe may wet his pants more and throw more temper tantrums and maybe even hit the new baby. I guess it's gonna be rough on him, huh?

## DATA COLLECTION: Visit 2—cont'd

| Interactions | Observations | Measurements |
|---|---|---|
| Carla: Well, maybe not. We did all the things to prepare him, and I'm sure I can spend a little time with just him every day, and I know I'll be careful about him getting rough with the baby. So maybe it won't be so bad.<br><br>My mom did come this past weekend and brought the youth bed. Gabe is really proud of his new bed now, but the first couple nights were pretty hairy. I think he was out of bed 50 times at least.<br>Dave: Gabe, come to daddy.<br>What's going to happen when mommy goes to the hospital to have our new baby?<br>Gabe: Mommy go bye-bye. Gabe stay with Gram.<br>Dave: Good boy, Gabe. Mommy and Daddy love you.<br>Carla, if you tell me what you want Gabe to have for a snack, I'll get it. | Carla and Dave are now sitting on the couch about a foot apart. They look at each other when they talk.<br><br><br><br><br><br><br><br><br><br>Gabe crawls into his dad's lap.<br><br><br><br><br>Dave looks at Carla, smiles, and then gives Gabe a hug.<br><br><br>Dave helps Gabe use his potty chair and washes his hands; then Dave washes his own hands and gets Gabe's snack. |  <br><br><br><br><br><br><br><br><br><br><br><br><br><br><br><br><br><br><br><br>Gabe ate half a banana and 4 oz 2% milk. |
| Carla: You know, something has been on my mind. I know it would be best if I nursed this baby, and I want to, but I'm afraid to try. I breast-fed Gabe for about 2 weeks and had to quit. I don't want to feel like such a failure again.<br>I think I received bad advice and conflicting advice from the nurses in the hospital and the clinic.<br>Gabe was really sleepy at first, and my nipples are kind of flat. So a nurse gave me a nipple shield to use. Things were going fine until another nurse told me to get rid of the shield. Then came the sore nipples! After we went home, I used the bottles of formula they sent home with us to give my sore nipples an occasional break. Well, by the end of a week it seemed like I didn't have enough milk. Poor Gabe wanted to eat every hour. And of all things, the nurse at the clinic told me to let him cry and not to nurse that often. I couldn't just let him cry, so I'd give him a bottle. By the end of 2 weeks I hardly had any milk at all, so I gave up and switched completely to formula. | After Gabe's snack and during the discussion on breast-feeding, Dave and Gabe are on the floor stacking and knocking down building blocks. Gabe is giggling loudly. |  |

*Continued.*

## DATA COLLECTION: Visit 2—cont'd

| Interactions | Observations | Measurements |
|---|---|---|

Carla: I didn't decide for sure to breastfeed until about 3 weeks before Gabe was born. I don't think I really listened to the prenatal instructor when she was talking about breastfeeding because I didn't think I would be doing it. My mom didn't breastfeed either of us, and Dave didn't really care one way or the other. So I didn't make that much effort to learn about it. I figured if I decided to do it, it was just a natural thing.

I just wasn't prepared for those awful sore nipples. They said in prenatal classes to rub the nipples with a towel in the last months of pregnancy to prepare them. And I did that. But my nipples got sore anyway.

My neighbor always looks so at ease breastfeeding. I think I need to know more about it. It was never easy for me.

Oh, I love to read, and I'm certainly interested in the subject. I read the little booklet the obstetrician gave me in the clinic, but I didn't get that much information from it.

*Carla goes to the bookshelf and pulls out the booklet. It is a 10-page booklet on feeding your baby published by a formula company.*

I've heard of LaLèche League, and I know its a bunch of breastfeeding mothers getting together, but that's about all I know.

I could go to at least one meeting and see what it's like. It's good to know they allow toddlers to come along. I'll be happy to have you bring the books about breastfeeding over, too. As for the nipples, I'll try to start preparing them. But if they're going to get sore anyway, I'm not sure it's worth the bother.

Dave: I'll sure support Carla if she decides to breastfeed. But I really feel the decision is up to her.

*Dave resumes his position next to Carla on the couch. Gabe promptly squeezes between Dave and Carla, then hops down and begins playing with some plastic trucks.*

Carla: We're really pretty flexible about decision-making, don't you think, Dave?

Dave: Uh, huh.

Carla: I make most of the household decisions. It's what I know best. I

## DATA COLLECTION: Visit 2—cont'd

| Interactions | Observations | Measurements |
|---|---|---|
| also make most of the decisions about Gabe because I'm with him the most. But Dave and I always talk it over first.<br>Dave: I make the decisions about the car, and we make joint decisions about how to spend our money and what to do when we go out.<br>Dave: How do I feel about family? You mean my mom and dad and brother and sister? The great thing about Mom and Dad is that they're giving us the money for my tuition, with no strings attached. It seems to me that after forking over that kind of dough they'd think they would have a right to tell us how to live our lives. But they don't. I always thought my parents were terrible dictators when I was in high school. I certainly have a different opinion of them now. I'm not sure how we'll ever repay them, even though I know they don't expect it.<br>I'll have to say that Carla is my best friend. Oh, I have buddies at work and at school, but I'm not real close to any of them. Gary and Sharon across the way are a fun couple, and we get together fairly often.<br>Carla: Of course you may come again. I'd especially like to discuss breastfeeding with you after I've had a chance to do some reading. But next time, let's make it in the evening when Gabe will already be in bed.<br>A week from today will be fine. | Gabe continues to go from toys to the couch, climbing on Dave and Carla and chattering constantly. Carla looks at Gabe and several times says, "shh" to Gabe and puts her finger over her mouth.<br><br>Dave puts his hand on Carla's shoulder. Carla smiles.<br><br>Dave nods his assent. | |

## ANALYSIS/SYNTHESIS OF DATA: Visit 2

### Analysis/Synthesis

I. The previous analysis of Carla and Gabe is still appropriate. To be consistent, the data will be analyzed according to Roy's model first, followed by the structural-functional approach to family life patterns. Only new pieces of data are addressed.
   A. Physiological Mode
      Dave gets adequate exercise at least some of the time and has been able to maintain a trim, muscular physique. He does not always get adequate rest, but does not appear tired. Carla is nutrition-conscious and Dave says that he enjoys her cooking. However, there is insufficient data to indicate adequate activity, rest, or nutrition. Data gaps exist in the area of elimination, fluids and electrolytes, oxygenation, and circulation, as well as regulation. Strengths are Dave's overall good health, determined from his health history and current health status.

B.  Self-Concept Mode

Dave's self-concept is a strength. He feels pretty good about himself, enjoys being a father and student, and takes care of his physical appearance.

C.  Role Function Mode

Data relating to Dave's role as a husband indicate that he considers his wife to be his best friend, is grateful for her support of his education, and wishes he could spend more time with the family. Dave's feelings about his roles as father and student are enjoyment. His positive attitudes toward his role show adaptation, which is a strength.

Data gaps: Dave's role as a worker, Carla's role as a wife

D.  Interdependence Mode

Dave, like the other members of the Smith family, openly gives and takes affection. He and Carla are adapting in the interdependence mode in that they can function and make decisions independently and yet confer with and support one another. Dave also appears to have appropriate interdependence with his extended family, accepting their help, yet "living his own life." These are strengths.

II. A.  Family Structure

1.  *Role:* Carla fears failure, as she experienced it with Gabe, at breastfeeding the new infant, yet expresses a desire to breastfeed. Data indicate that Carla has done little reading about breastfeeding and received misinformation or no information at all about breastfeeding from health professionals. There is a potential concern for repeated failure in Carla's role as a new nurturing mother.

2.  *Values:* Data gathered during the second visit show that Dave's values are the same as Carla's, which were identified as health, education, time together as a nuclear family, and extended family. The fact that Dave and Carla have no value conflicts is a strength.

3.  *Communication:* Dave is openly affectionate verbally and nonverbally with Gabe and Carla. Dave and Carla look at one another when speaking, they sit close to one another on the couch, they take turns speaking, and their communication appears to be open and honest with freedom to express feelings. According to Satir (1972), these are effective means of communication and a strength for the family.

4.  *Power:* Carla and Dave have separate areas of decision-making responsibility, but admit to flexibility, some joint decision-making, and some conferring before decisions are made. This can be considered a strength. More information is needed before a power hierarchy can be identified. The data gap of Gabe's power over his parents still exists.

B.  Family Functions

1.  *Affective:* A major strength of the Smith family is the open and free expression of verbal and nonverbal affection. A data gap still exists in the area of a response to members' needs.

2.  *Socialization:* Child-rearing practices were not discussed. However, data indicate that Dave takes an active role in Gabe's care. He readily helped Gabe use the toilet, gave him a snack, and seemed to enjoy playing with him. There is still no information on discipline and whether Carla and Dave agree on how Gabe should be raised.

There is no new data related to reproduction, family coping, economics, and provision of necessities.

The Smith family's strengths determined from this visit are:

1.  Dave's physiological adaptation
2.  Dave's positive self-concept
3.  Dave's adaptation toward his role as husband, father, and student
4.  Dave's appropriate interdependence with Carla and extended family
5.  No values conflict between Carla and Dave
6.  Open communication patterns
7.  Flexibility in decision-making
8.  Mutual expression of affection

**NURSING DIAGNOSES: Visit 2**

| Date | Diagnoses | Priority |
|---|---|---|
| 11/6/89 | 1.  Potential role conflict for Gabe related to inadequate preparation for new baby | 2 |
| 11/15/89 | 2.  Potential role failure for Carla related to lack of knowledge about breastfeeding | 1 |
| 11/15/89 | 3.  Incomplete data base | 3 |

## DATA COLLECTION: Visit 3

*Time*: Wednesday, November 22, 1989, 7:30 PM
*Place*: The Smith home. Dave answered the door. Gabe was playing on the floor, dressed in his pajamas. Carla was not on the first floor, and Dave called her down from upstairs. Carla greeted the nurse with tears in her eyes and stated that she found out at the clinic today that she will have to have a cesarean section. The visit lasted 45 minutes.
*Nursing goals*: To (1) fill in identified data gaps related to family life patterns, (2) evaluate previous nursing interventions, and (3) initiate at least one plan of intervention based on nursing diagnosis made during this visit.

| Interactions | Observations | Measurements |
|---|---|---|
| Carla: I do need to talk, but I'd rather talk about this thing after Gabe goes to bed.<br>Dave: I have some concerns, too. | Carla is fighting back tears, voice is quivering.<br><br>Gabe is playing with a puzzle with one hand while sucking his thumb on the other hand. He sits still, not moving about as during the last two visits. | |
| Carla: Yes, I've read one of the books on breastfeeding, and I've started a second.<br>The LaLèche League women were very nice and helpful, but some of them seem kind of fanatic. I'm not sure I'll go back to the meetings.<br>I am feeling more confident, but I'm still not sure about nipple preparation. I haven't really done anything about that. | Gabe begins to whine, but Dave picks him up and gives him a piggy-back ride upstairs after goodnight hugs and kisses to mommy. Gabe is giggling during the ride upstairs. | |
| I'd like to keep the books until after the baby's born, if you don't mind—especially now that I have to have a cesarean section. | Dave came downstairs, offered the nurse a drink of juice, got himself and Carla a drink of juice, then resumed his position next to Carla on the couch. Gabe came downstairs and Dave immediately took Gabe back upstairs to bed. | |
| I'm down to 1-week visits now, because my due date is so close. I went in for my regular visit this morning, and the doctor said "The baby's in frank breech position, and your pelvis is only borderline. You know, we had to use forceps to get Gabe out, and he weighed only 6½ pounds. This baby weighs much more than that. You're going to have to have a cesarean section." That's about all I remember. I was so shook up I couldn't even think of any questions to ask. But now I have a million. I'm so scared. | Carla takes a deep breath before beginning. | |

*Continued.*

## DATA COLLECTION: Visit 3—cont'd

| Interactions | Observations | Measurements |
| --- | --- | --- |
| I guess I'm mostly afraid of the pain. You hear so many gruesome stories. But I'm also afraid of not getting off to a good start with the new baby and not being able to take care of Gabe when I get home. I don't even know what frank breech position is. | Dave puts his arm around Carla's shoulder. She begins to cry again. | |
| (The nurse explained what breech position is and encouraged further exploration with the obstetrician.) | | |
| Dave: You mean talk to the doctor (in response to nurse asking what could be done to relieve the anxiety). I think he owes her a much better explanation of what's going to happen. I think I'll find some time and go to talk to him with you, Carla. Maybe he'll be more apt to give you the information you deserve. | | |
| Carla: I'm sorry! I was so shook up. | | |
| Dave: I'm not blaming you, honey. I just hate to see you so upset. And we're not dumb. We have a right to know. | | |
| Carla: Well, I need some time to think about what I'd like to ask him. I have an appointment next Wednesday. Do you think that would be soon enough? (in response to nurse asking when they would talk with the doctor). | | |
| Dave: Let's not take a chance of you going into labor. Let's call tomorrow and make an appointment for this week. Want to? | | |
| Carla: You're probably right. We'll call tomorrow. Maybe we should make a list of questions tonight. | Carla goes to the desk and gets a pad of paper and pen. | |
| Dave: Well, I want to know if I can still be in the delivery room and how long Carla will have to stay in the hospital. | | |
| Carla: As I said before, I'm afraid of the pain, so I want to know how much pain I'll have—both during the surgery and after—and what kind of scar I'll have. Will breast-feeding be harder? | | |
| It's good to know the different positions (in response to nurse showing her ways of positioning a baby for breastfeeding after a cesarean section). I hope the nurses in the hospital will help me. | | |

## DATA COLLECTION: Visit 3—cont'd

| Interactions | Observations | Measurements |
|---|---|---|
| Dave: Yes, I've read about the cesarean birth support group in the paper. | | |
| Carla: I guess we could call them. But I hope they're not as fanatic as LaLèche League. | | |
| I feel better now that we have a plan. | Carla smiled for the first time during this visit. | |
| Dave: All I want from the doctor and the hospital personnel and any other health person is the knowledge to make informed decisions and a healthy outcome for my wife and new baby. | | |
| Carla: I'll second that! | | |
| Dave: I'd have to say that I'm stricter with Gabe than Carla is. | | |
| Carla: But that's because you're with him less time. If you were with him as much as I am, he'd wear you down, too. | Carla raises her voice, sounds defensive. | |
| Dave: Oh, I agree with you, Carla, but you know how often we've talked about the importance of consistency. | | |
| Carla: I know you're right. It just doesn't always work out that way. | | |
| Dave: We do discuss how to deal with Gabe a lot. We'll probably do that even more when the new baby comes. | | |
| Carla: We agree on most things, too. We both think manners are important, and teaching Gabe responsibility. We're trying hard to get him to pick up his toys and take care of them. | | |
| Dave: We're not opposed to an occasional spanking, but it's not the only method of punishment we use, and we try hard not to do it when we're very angry. Right now, making him sit on a chair seems to work the best. | | |
| Carla: I'm always questioning if how we're raising Gabe is right. I fight the "guilts" a lot. | | |
| Dave: And I keep telling her that we're better parents than most. | | |
| Carla: Of course, we'll be glad and grateful to have you visit after the baby is born (in response to nurse's inquiry about a postpartum visit). | | |
| Dave: If you could visit in the hospital, that would be good too. | | |

## ANALYSIS/SYNTHESIS OF DATA: Visit 3

### Analysis/Synthesis

I. The previous analyses are still appropriate. No new information was obtained relating to Roy's adaptation model used to analyze the individuals. Only the categories from the structural-functional approach pertinent to new data are included at this analysis/synthesis.

II. A. Family Structures
Previous analyses remain relevant.

B. Family Functions

1. *Affective:* The open and free expression of verbal and nonverbal affection continues to be evident during this visit as a major strength of the Smith family. With regard to the previous data gap of a need-response, it was shown that Dave provided comfort, support, and help in developing a plan during Carla's time of need. Dave also admits to bolstering Carla's confidence when she has doubts about being a good parent. It is still not known if Carla provides the same for Dave during his times of need.

2. *Socialization:* Carla and Dave perceive themselves as agreeing on "most things" in relation to child-rearing practices. They use a variety of disciplining methods, and value manners and teach Gabe responsi-

bility. Dave and Carla feel that Dave is stricter with Gabe than Carla, but both understand the reason for this, and they try to be consistent. Overall, the child-rearing area of socialization in the Smith family is functional. This is a strength.

3. *Reproduction:* Carla's reproductive function has been altered because of the need for a cesarean section. Carla fears pain and the loss of control and is also stressed by her lack of knowledge. Dave is also stressed and is concerned about healthy outcome for his wife and baby. This is a concern.

4. *Coping:* A data gap still exists in the area of family coping. Dave appeared to use taking a definitive plan of action as a way of coping with stress, but a pattern could not be established on one incident, and coping was not discussed.

Data gaps previously identified that still exist are Carla's role as wife, Dave's role as worker, Gabe's separation anxiety, power hierarchy, sexual history, family planning, and provision of transportation.

The Smith family strengths determined from this visit are:

1. Functional affectional response by Dave for Carla
2. Functional child-rearing practices.

## NURSING DIAGNOSES: Visit 3

| Date | Diagnoses | Priority |
|------|-----------|----------|
| 11/6/89 | 1. Potential role conflict for Gabe related to inadequate preparation for new baby | 3 |
| 11/15/89 | 2. Potential role failure for Carla related to lack of knowledge about breastfeeding | 2 |
| 11/22/89 | 3. Stress related to need for cesarean section and lack of knowledge about cesarean delivery | 1 |
| 11/22/89 | 4. Incomplete data base | 4 |

## PLANS FOR IMPLEMENTATION

**Nursing diagnosis 1:** *Potential role conflict for Gabe related to inadequate preparation for new baby (11/6/89).*
**Goal:** *Gabe will be prepared for new baby to decrease potential role conflict by 11/15/89.*

| Objective | Nursing orders | Scientific rationale | Evaluation |
|-----------|----------------|----------------------|------------|
| 1. Client will list behaviors indicative of role conflict and possible strategies for dealing with conflict by 11/15/89. | 1a. Client will verbalize behavior expected of Gabe after baby is born by 11/6/89. | *Content:* Sibling rivalry. *Strategy:* Teaching and learning. 1a. New learning must be based on previous knowledge and experience (Pohl, 1981). | **Criteria statement:** Client will cite the following behaviors: Reversal of bowel and bladder control Attention-getting behaviors such as temper tantrums |

## PLANS FOR IMPLEMENTATION—cont'd

| Objective | Nursing orders | Scientific rationale | Evaluation |
|---|---|---|---|
| | 1b. Nurse will provide additional information to family about possible behaviors expected by Gabe after baby is born by 11/6/89. | 1b. Cognitive learning is the acquiring and development of concepts (Johnson, 1986). | Physical violence aimed at new baby (eg, hitting the baby, throwing things at the baby) Negative verbalization about the baby (eg, "Baby bad"). |
| | 1c. Client will verbalize possible strategies to use in dealing with above behaviors by 11/6/89. | 1c. Effective learning requires active participation (Pohl, 1981). | **Criteria statement:** Client will cite the following strategies: Put Gabe in new youth bed and take down crib |
| | 1d. Nurse will provide additional information about possible strategies to use in dealing with behaviors by 11/6/89. | 1d. Knowledge of what to expect increases the client's sense of control and powerfulness (Roberts, 1978). | Discuss with Gabe Carla's absence when the baby is born and who will stay with him Spend time each day with Gabe when baby is not around Include Gabe in care of baby (eg, getting a diaper, rubbing lotion on baby) Reinforce verbally to Gabe how good and special he is |
| | | | **Formative:** Nurse implemented plans 1b and 1d on 11/6/89. Client implemented plans 1a and 1c on 11/6/89. Carla mentioned all four behaviors and five strategies on 11/15/89. She had discussed them with Dave. Objective met. |
| 2. Client will take steps to prepare Gabe for coming of new baby by 11/15/89. | 2a. Client will decide which steps to take to prepare Gabe by 11/7/89. | 2a. An individual must be motivated in order to learn (Pohl, 1981). | **Formative:** Carla and Dave discussed and decided which preparatory steps to take with Gabe on 11/7/89. |
| | 2b. Client will obtain a youth bed, put Gabe in the youth bed at night, and take the crib down by 11/12/89. (Taking Gabe out of the crib and putting the new baby in the crib will be two separate events.) | 2b. Effective learning requires active participation (Pohl, 1981). Concept of centricism causes the child to think all events revolve around him (Hetherington and Parke, 1979). | Carla's mom did bring the youth bed down on 11/11/89, and the crib was taken down and Gabe put in the youth bed on 11/11/89. Gabe's apparent reaction to the bed was pride, but he had trouble staying in bed the first few nights. |

*Continued.*

## PLANS FOR IMPLEMENTATION—cont'd

| Objectives | Nursing orders | Scientific rationale | Evaluation |
|---|---|---|---|
| | 2c. Client will discuss Carla's absence with Gabe repeatedly, stressing not the time away but the assured return by 11/15/89. | 2c. Repetition strengthens learning (Pohl, 1981). | Carla and Dave discussed Carla's absence with Gabe many times since 11/6/89. Gabe says "Mommy go bye-bye, Gabe stay with Gram." |
| | 2d. Client will confirm that Carla's mom will stay with Gabe during Carla's hospitalization by 11/12/89. | 2d. Separation anxiety is high for the toddler (Matt, Fazekas, and James, 1985). | It was confirmed on 11/7/89 that Carla's mom would stay with Gabe at the time of birth. |
| | 2e. Client will leave Gabe with Carla's mom and then discuss with Gabe how that will be like when mommy goes to have the new baby by 11/12/89. | 2e. Separation anxiety is high for the toddler (Matt, Frazekas, and James, 1985). | Carla and Dave left Gabe with Carla's mom 11/13/89, and then discussed it with Gabe. |
| | | | **Summative:** Carla and Dave have taken steps to prepare Gabe. Actual effectivness of the steps will have to be evaluated after the baby is born. |

**Nursing diagnosis 2:** *Potential role failure for Carla related to lack of knowledge about breastfeeding (11/15/89).*
**Goal:** *Carla will use her increased knowledge about breastfeeding to decrease her potential for role failure by 11/30/89.*

| Objective | Nursing orders | Scientific rationale | Evaluation |
|---|---|---|---|
| 1. Client will discuss at least five new things learned about breastfeeding on 11/15/89. | 1a. Client will verbalize at least five points already known about breastfeeding by 11/15/89. | *Content:* Breast feeding. *Strategy:* Teaching and learning. 1a. New learning must be based on previous knowledge and experience (Pohl, 1981). | **Criteria statement:** Client will verbalize understanding five of the following: Supply and demand principle |
| | 1b. Nurse will provide several books about breastfeeding and the phone number of the LaLèche League leader by 11/16/89. | 1b. Cognitive learning is the acquisition and development of concepts (Johnson, 1985). | Importance of adequate fluid intake; importance of adequate rest Need for alternating breasts to begin feeding Importance of avoiding emotional upset Positions of mom and baby |
| | 1c. Client will select two breastfeeding books to read by 11/22/89. | | Engorgement Let-down reflex Breast/nipple care Amount of time to nurse |
| | 1d. Client will try to attend at least one meeting of LaLèche League by 11/22/89. | 1d. Effective learning requires active participation (Pohl, 1981). Learning may occur through imitation (Pohl, 1981). Provision of support group enhances learning. | Quality/content of breast milk Avoidance of drugs during lactation Importance of support person |

## PLANS FOR IMPLEMENTATION—cont'd

| Objective | Nursing orders | Scientific rationale | Evaluation |
|---|---|---|---|
| 2. Client will implement techniques to promote breastfeeding by 11/25/89. | 2a. Client will decide whether to breastfeed or bottle feed by 11/22/89.<br>2b. Nurse will support the client's decision on infant feeding by 11/22/89.<br><br>2c. Client, if she decides to breastfeed, will identify techniques to facilitate successful breastfeeding by 11/24/89.<br>2d. Client will begin prenatal nipple preparation (if breastfeeding) to reduce nipple soreness during nursing by 11/25/89. | 2a. The choice of infant feeding method is up to the mother (Jensen and Bobak, 1989).<br>2b. Support and encouragement may facilitate client's action on a decision. Therapeutic use of self (Stuart and Sundeen, 1987).<br>2c. Effective learning requires active participation (Pohl, 1981).<br><br>2d. Nipple preparation may reduce soreness when breastfeeding (Jensen and Bobak, 1989). | **Formative:**<br>Nurse implemented plan 1b.<br>On 11/22/89, Carla stated she had read all of *The Womanly Art of Breastfeeding* and had started *Nursing Your Baby* by Karen Pryor. She stated she enjoyed reading them, and sounded enthusiastic.<br>On 11/20/89, Carla attended a LaLèche League meeting. She was impressed with the knowledge and skill of the mothers, but was concerned about what she called "fanaticism."<br>Carla decided to try breastfeeding again, and stated that nipple rolling, a rough towel massage, and expression of colostrum prenatally may help with breastfeeding.<br>Carla sheepishly admitted that she had not done anything about nipple preparation. This was probably because she was not convinced of its value.<br><br>**Summative:**<br>Carla discussed five things she learned about breastfeeding on 11/22/89. She stated she felt more confident about trying it again, but was especially concerned about the effects of the cesarean section on her efforts to breastfeed. Carla has increased her knowledge, and the potential for role failure is reduced, although more support and evaluation should take place after the baby is born. |

**Nursing diagnosis 3:** *Stress related to need for cesarean section and lack of knowledge about impending cesarean delivery (11/22/89).*
**Goal:** *Carla and Dave will report decreased stress regarding the cesarean delivery by 11/30/85.*

| Objective | Nursing orders | Scientific rationale | Evaluation |
|---|---|---|---|
| 1. Clients will identify their specific stressors regarding cesarean delivery by 11/22/89. | 1a. Nurse will encourage Carla and Dave to express their feelings and concerns regarding cesarean delivery by 11/22/89. | *Content*: Stress/anxiety. *Strategy:* Therapeutic use of self (Stuart and Sundeen, 1987). | Nurse implemented 1a on 11/22/89. Carla and Dave stated their main concerns were the need for a cesarean delivery because of breech presentation; the effects of this delivery on the baby and on Carla; type of anesthesia; and duration of physical recovery for Carla. |
| | 1b. Clients will identify their major concerns regarding cesarean delivery by 11/22/89. | 1b. Areas of stress must be identified prior to handling them. | |
| 2. Clients will discuss at least five concerns about cesarean section during the next visit with the doctor by 11/28/89. | 2a. Client will make a list of questions and concerns about cesarean section by 11/22/89. | *Strategy:* Teaching and learning. 2a. Learning needs of the client must be determined (Pohl, 1981). | **Criteria statement:** Client will verbalize understanding of five of the following: Frank breech position Borderline pelvis Turn, cough, deep breathe Type of incision Type of anesthesia Length of hospital stay Pain medication available Consequences of cesarean birth to baby Consequences of cesarean birth to father Positions for breastfeeding after cesarean delivery |
| | 2b. Nurse will provide information about cesarean section by 11/22/89. | 2b. Cognitive learning is the aquisition and development of concepts (Johnson, 1979). Information reduces anxiety and fear. | |
| | 2c. Clients will visit the doctor and discuss questions and concerns by 11/29/89. | 2c. Information reduces anxiety and fear. | |
| | 2d. Clients will contact the cesarean birth support group in Bloomington before the birth of the baby, if possible. | 2d. Learning may occur through imitation (Pohl, 1981). Provision of a support group is one way of coping with stress. | **Formative:** Client implemented plans 1b and 2a on 11/22/89. Nurse implemented plans 1a and 2b on 11/22/89. Plans 2c and 2d not implemented because dates not yet occurring. Objective not met. **Summative:** Goal is not met. Evaluation will have to take place after the next visit to the doctor. |

## REFERENCES AND READINGS

Duvall EM: Marriage and family development, ed 5, Philadelphia, 1977, JB Lippincott Co.

Erikson E: Childhood and society, ed 2, New York, 1963, WW Norton & Co, Inc.

Friedman MM: Family nursing: theory and assessment, ed 2, New York, 1986, Appleton-Century-Crofts.

Hetherington EM and Parke RD: Child psychology: a contemporary viewpoint, 1979, McGraw-Hill Book Co.

Jensen MD and Bobak DM: Maternity care: the nurse and the family, ed 4, St Louis, 1989, The CV Mosby Co.

Johnson SH: High risk parenting: nursing assessment and strategies for the family at risk, ed 2, Philadelphia, 1986, JB Lippincott Co.

Matt SR, Fazekas NF, and James SR: Nursing care of children and families: a holistic approach, Menlo Park, Calif, 1985, Addison-Wesley Publishing Co, Inc.

Pohl ML: The teaching function of the nurse practitioner, ed 4, Dubuque, Iowa, 1981, Wm C Brown Co.

Roberts SL: Behavioral concepts and nursing throughout the life span, Englewood Cliffs, NJ, 1978, Prentice-Hall, Inc.

Roy Sr C: Introduction to nursing: an adaptation model, ed 2, Englewood Cliffs, NJ, 1984, Prentice-Hall, Inc.

Satir V: Peoplemaking, Palo Alto, Calif, 1972, Science and Behavior Books.

Stuart GW and Sundeen SJ: Principles and practice of psychiatric nursing, ed 3, St Louis, 1987, The CV Mosby Co.

# CHAPTER 17

# Nursing Process of the Community Client

KAREN A. SAUCIER

This chapter examines a hypothetical aggregate in the community of Rosetown, a small rural community with black and white mixed ethnic groups. The population has a low median income, high unemployment, and a high rate of teenage pregnancies. The aggregate is made up of pregnant teens enrolled in Rosetown High School.

The nursing care plan is presented using the Community-as-Client Assessment Framework as the organizing model (Stanhope and Lancaster, 1988).[31] This framework was selected to guide the assessment and analysis of this specific aggregate because of its emphasis on systems within a community and how each is related to the goal of health. The Community-as-Client Assessment Framework is useful in the examination of a community or aggregate located in a geopolitical community. Structure and process both are assessed with emphasis on structural components of an aggregate or community. Because the aggregate of pregnant teens resides in a geopolitical community, this nursing framework is an appropriate application. For a more complete explanation of the Community-as-Client Framework, see Chapter 6.

Most of the references for this hypothetical aggregate and community are fictitious but provide the reader with a sample format for documentation.

*Data collection.* Data have been collected using

the methods of observation, interaction, and measurement, and categorized into structure and interacting subsystems. The data were all collected prior to the analysis and implementation of plans.

*Data analysis.* During the analysis, models and principles are used. Data are compared with standards, and judgments are made as to strengths and concerns of a community's functioning. Health resources are analyzed by examining the direct services provided according to the three categories of services recommended in *Healthy People: The Surgeon General's Report on Health Promotion and Disease Prevention.* These categories are *preventive health services*—services that can be delivered to individuals by health providers; *health promotion services*—activities that individuals and communities can use to promote healthy lifestyles; and *health protection services*—measures that can be used by governmental and other agencies to protect people from harm.[34]

*Goal, objectives, strategies, and plans.* Knowledge regarding functioning of the community directs the appropriate change strategies to be used. The process of change according to Lewin is used, and involves three steps: unfreezing, moving to the new level, and refreezing at the new level.[30]

*Evaluation.* Evaluation data are not collected because this is a hypothetical situation. Questions that indicate appropriate data are provided, and criteria standards are established.

# DATA COLLECTION*

| Structure/Process | Interactions | Observations | Measurements |
|---|---|---|---|
| **A. Core structures** | | Adolescent pregnancy has been identified as a risk factor in this century as societal changes resulted in such trends as increased age at first marriage, increased need for advanced education, and increased life span resulting in changes in acceptable sexual experiences for teens.[3,4] Pregnant teens are not actively involved in school activities, such as clubs, sports, or recreational activities. Aggregate members are often observed in school with each other. | |
| *1. Self-concept* | "People in school looked down on me when I was pregnant, like I had done something shameful or something."[1] "I like being in a special class for pregnant girls 'cause they understand how I feel and the problems I am having."[1] | | |
| *2. History* | "When I became pregnant, I read all about the problems of having a baby when you're a teenager."[1] "The nurse at school told me about the things that have happened to pregnant girls in my school, like divorce and getting sick and dropping out of school and welfare."[1] | | |
| *3. Statistics* | | | |

Live births to women under 20 by race and ethnic group, in county of aggregate[36]

| | Total under 20 | Under 15 | 15-17 | 18-19 | % All births |
|---|---|---|---|---|---|
| All races | 292 | 7 | 135 | 150 | 20.1% |
| White | 59 | 1 | 15 | 45 | 17.4% |
| Black | 233 | 6 | 120 | 105 | 31.4% |

Age distribution of community[36]

| 18 and younger | 48.2% |
|---|---|
| 18-45 | 20.2% |
| 45-62 | 18.6% |
| 62 and older | 13.0% |

Total population of town and county of aggregate[18,36]

| Year | Rosetown | County | State |
|---|---|---|---|
| 1980 | 2,793 | 42,500 | 2,520,638 |
| 1989 | 2,791 | 45,034 | 2,598,000 |

*Continued.*

*See reference list for sources of data indicated by superscript numbers.

# DATA COLLECTION—cont'd

| Structure/Process | Interactions | Observations | Measurements |
|---|---|---|---|

**A. Core structures—cont'd**
3. *Statistics*—cont'd

Population of Rosetown High School[13]

| Year | Rosetown High |
|---|---|
| 1980 | 442 |
| 1989 | 450 |

Birth rate $= \dfrac{\text{No. live births per year} \times 1{,}000^{14,35,36}}{\text{average (midyear) population}}$

(See refs. 17, 35, 36.)

| Rosetown High | | County of aggregate | |
|---|---|---|---|
| No. | Rate | No. | Rate |
| 15 | 33.3 | 832 | 18.5 |

| State of aggregate | | U.S. | |
|---|---|---|---|
| No. | Rate | No. | Rate |
| 43,432 | 16.7 | 3,749,000 | 16.3 |

Mortality rates $= \dfrac{\text{No. deaths per year} \times 1{,}000^{35,36}}{\text{Average midyear population}}$

| Type of mortality | Rosetown | | State | | U.S. | |
|---|---|---|---|---|---|---|
| | No. | Rate | No. | Rate | No. | Rate |
| Neonatal deaths | | | | | | |
| White | 0 | 0.0 | 127 | 5.5 | | |
| Nonwhite | 12 | 21.1 | 241 | 11.8 | | |
| Totals | 12 | 16.9 | 308 | 8.5 | | |
| Infant deaths | | | | | | |
| White | 0 | 0.0 | 213 | 9.3 | | |
| Nonwhite | 14 | 24.6 | 383 | 18.7 | | |
| Totals | 14 | 19.7 | 596 | 13.7 | 39,500 | 10.5 |

Infant mortality rates by age of Mother, 1981, 1985, 1987 (state)[36]

| Age of mother | 1981 | 1985 | 1987 |
|---|---|---|---|
| 10-19 | 21.9 | 21.2 | 18.1 |
| 20-29 | 13.2 | 14.0 | 13.1 |
| All ages | 15.2 | 15.1 | 14.1 |

**Percentage of female-headed households, 1988[15,36]**

| Rosetown | County | State | U.S. |
|---|---|---|---|
| 61% | 47% | 34% | 25% |

**Sex distribution[13,18]**

| | Rosetown High | Rosetown |
|---|---|---|
| Males | 49.7% | 47.1% |
| Females | 50.3% | 52.9% |

**Income of families[18,36]**

| | Rosetown | State |
|---|---|---|
| Under $3,000 | 4.2% | 3.8% |
| 3,000-5,999 | 17.3% | 12.7% |
| 6,000-9,999 | 26.9% | 17.3% |
| 10,000-14,999 | 21.8% | 22.7% |
| 15,000-24,999 | 18.4% | 24.3% |
| 25,000 + | 11.4% | 19.4% |
| Median | $11,216.00 | $14,500.00 |
| U.S. median income = $25,300.00 | | |

**Education of persons 25 years and older[36]**

| | Rosetown | State |
|---|---|---|
| No schooling | 0.9% | 0.7% |
| H.S. graduate | 42.4% | 54.8% |
| Attended college | 16.4% | 19.4% |
| Median school yr completed | 10.6 | 12.2 |

**Unemployment rate, 1989[18,36]**

| Rosetown | State | U.S. |
|---|---|---|
| 12.4% | 10.2% | 8.1% |

**Leading causes of death in county of aggregate**

| Cause | White | Nonwhite | Total |
|---|---|---|---|
| Diseases of heart | 69 | 78 | 158 |
| Malignant neoplasms | 44 | 52 | 96 |
| Cerebrovascular disease | 14 | 40 | 54 |
| Accidents (all causes) | 9 | 16 | 25 |
| Atherosclerosis | 7 | 8 | 15 |

*Continued.*

# DATA COLLECTION—cont'd

| Structure/Process | | |
|---|---|---|
| Interactions | Observations | Measurements |

## A. Core structures—cont'd
### 3. *Statistics*—cont'd

**Interactions:**

"We have a real problem getting these girls in before the second trimester. They try to deny the pregnancy, pretend it doesn't exist. We don't have statistics on Rosetown, but a significant number of these girls' babies are small."[3]

**Observations:**

The pregnant teens are easily identifiable as the pregnancy advances.

### 4. *Culture*

"Pregnant girls are usually interested in childbirth and most are interested in baby care. They are aware that they are different than other girls their age."[3]

"I really want to finish high school even though I am pregnant. Some of the girls in my class have dropped out and gotten married and all they think about is being with a guy and having his baby. I want to be able to make sure my baby has what he needs so I need to get a job that pays money."[1]

**Measurements:**

High school completion rate by age at first birth for women age 20-26 (U.S.)[35]

| Age at first birth | Percentage of women who complete high school |
|---|---|
| 15 | 45% |
| 16 | 49% |
| 17 | 53% |
| 18 | 62% |
| 19 | 77% |
| 20 | 90% |

Birth outcome/prenatal care by age in the United States[35]

| | Under 15 | 15-19 | 20-24 |
|---|---|---|---|
| Percentage of babies born at low birthweight (5.5 lb or less) | 14.5 | 9.0 | 5.6 |
| Percentage of babies born at very low birth weight (3.5 lb or less) | 7.0 | 3.4 | 2.1 |
| Percentage of babies born to mothers who received early prenatal care | 33.0 | 53.0 | 71.1 |

Percentage of sexually active U.S. females who use contraception[35]

| Age | Percentage |
|---|---|
| 10-15 | 4% |
| 16-19 | 21% |
| 20-25 | 65% |

"I don't understand a lot of what is going on inside of me, but I know that my baby is going to be perfect and it will be all I want it to be (childbirth)."[1]

"The older people in our community are very religious, and most of their lives center around church meetings. The young are not as interested in church but still value religion. Whites value family, career, education, and good health. The black culture places much more emphasis on the rearing of children and recreation."[6]

"Rosetown is predominantly Southern Baptist. Values and customs vary among age and social groups."[6]

"We are seeing girls engage in sexual intercourse at a much younger age here in Rosetown. They talk about it more openly now, and they still believe that it (pregnancy) won't happen to me."[4]

5. *Social network/support*

"I am really scared about having a baby; I mean I can't believe all of this is happening. My mother is not really thrilled, but I know she is there for me anyway."[1]

"We have this special class at school for pregnant girls and they help us with doctor appointments and food stamps and things like that."[1]

"I don't know where I will put the baby if I come back to school. My mother works and I don't know anybody who can keep it."[1]

"We all kind of stick together like we all understand what this is all about cause we have the same problems."[1]

"We really don't have much help for these girls in Rosetown. The health department has the prenatal clinic and baby clinic and WIC, and we have a welfare office. I meet in a support group for girls out of school. There is really no

There are five Southern Baptist churches and one Episcopal church in Rosetown.

**Percentage of adolescents aged 15-19 who have had sexual intercourse (US)[35]**

|        | 1970 | 1975 | 1985 |
|--------|------|------|------|
| White  | 23.2 | 33.6 | 42.3 |
| Black  | 52.4 | 64.8 | 71.4 |
| Total  | 27.6 | 46   | 53.4 |

Continued.

# DATA COLLECTION—cont'd

| Structure/Process | Interactions | Observations | Measurements |
|---|---|---|---|

**A. Core structures—cont'd**

5. *Social network/support—cont'd*

baby care and very little follow-up if the girls drop out of school."[4]

"My boyfriend isn't too good about this whole thing. When I'm scared or need something I call my teacher or my mother, not him. He don't know what to say or do."[1]

**B. Interacting subsystems**

1. *Physical environment*

**Appearance:**

Rural farming community bordered by Strong River on western boundary and surrounded by farmland, artificial boundaries on east, north, and south. State routes 61 and 8 divide the area. Area is combination of residential and farmland.

Many houses in need of repair; houses very close together, particularly in black segregated areas. One neighborhood observed with larger lots and houses in good condition, lawns well maintained with shrubbery and flower gardens. New housing projects provide low-cost housing for lower income families. Animals roaming free in streets. Farm houses older than housing in town; many houses do not have adequate plumbing or pro-

"Some of our houses are in real bad shape. We have a federal grant which will help us remodel for some of these folks."[6]

"We are real proud of our housing projects in town. They help out our poor a great deal."[6]

"We have the richest soil in the world here in the Rosetown area. We can grow anything."[2]

"The unemployment situation is very serious in our town. Folks just stand around with nothing to do."[2]

Rosetown—4.52 square miles with an estimated population of 2,793.[5]
Topography—flat terrain at an average of 150 inches above sea level.[5]
Nearest neighboring towns—25 miles to the east and 20 miles to the north.[5]
822 housing units in Rosetown; 316 tenants occupied.[8]
Value of houses in Rosetown—from $8,500 to $150,000; average—$21,400 ($90,000 median for the US).[9]

| | |
|---|---|
| Average temperature | 64.2° F |
| Maximum temperature | 85.5° F |
| Minimum temperature | 48.3° F |
| Average rainfall | 26.2" |
| Average relative humidity | 57.7% |

tection from weather. Roofs in bad condition. Yards littered with old cars and farm equipment. Streets in degrees of repair. Speed limit is 35 mph in rural areas, 15 mph in town. No center line markings on streets other than highway. Children seen riding bikes on streets. People observed "hanging around" bars and stores all during day and night. High school built in 1921 and in need of repair. Inadequate lighting, no air conditioning, gas heat, crowded classrooms. Students seen laughing and talking quietly outside building. Class change quiet and orderly. Parenting class for pregnant teens held in spacious home economics classroom with fetal models, growth charts, and pelvic models present. Audiovisual equipment observed and used. Students in class actively participating in activities with obvious interest. No neighborhood watch. Business district located in center of town.

"We desperately need more room in our high school, and our buildings need repair."[13]
"We have a very friendly school with well-behaved students. We don't have the problems that a lot of the city high schools do, with drugs and guns."[14]

"We can walk to our doctor's appointments from school, which helps a lot. The welfare office is only 10 minutes from school, too."[1]

"I have been trying to get a neighborhood watch up for 2 years without success; no one seems concerned or interested."[10]

Continued.

## DATA COLLECTION—cont'd

| Structure/Process | | |
|---|---|---|
| **Interactions** | **Observations** | **Measurements** |

**B. Interacting subsystems**—cont'd

*1. Physical environment*—cont'd

"We have a real friendly, quiet little town."[11]

"We fry everything around here, and we tend to use salt pork in all of our vegetables. We really eat a lot of salty foods."[12]

"My favorite foods are hamburgers and pizza and my doctor won't let me eat them while I'm pregnant 'cause of my blood pressure. I can't wait until I can have my mother's french fries again."[1]

*2. Health and welfare services*

The city has applied for a federally funded physician and clinic.[6]

"Most of our patients in Rosetown do not pay fees because of their income."[3]

"The girls from the high school use the prenatal and well child health dept. services and are encouraged to do so by their teachers. They rarely miss appointments. The problem as I see it is that they don't come to family planning. They just don't seem to want to prevent pregnancy. We just aren't getting to them."[3]

**Sounds:**

No heavy industry present in town; loud cars without mufflers evident.

**Tastes:**

Southern style cooking preferences: fried chicken, fried vegetables, steak, and tamales. Fast food hamburgers and pizza establishments frequented by teens. People very friendly in local restaurants, eager to share recipes and ingredients.

**Smells:**

Pleasant smell of flowers. Noxious odors noted in rural areas from aerial spraying of pesticides on crops. No pollution index available. Gas fumes noted around highways. Health department and physician's office within walking distance of school. Welfare office—3 blocks away. No hospitals in Rosetown. A 135-bed regional hospital is 21 miles away in neighboring city. Physician's office within five blocks of high school.

No emergency center services in Rosetown.

Medical/health services, including dental and eye clinics, are provided free by the Levee Clinic, which is federally funded. There are 2 physicians, 1 nurse, 2 dentists and a part-time optometrist. There are 2 pharmacists in 2 different drug stores. Ambulance service is available within a 25-mile radius of Rosetown, 24 hours a day housed in the fire department and staffed with 4 EMTs.

The health dept. offers comprehensive services 5 days a week:
- Immunizations
- Midwife and MD services 2 days a week at prenatal clinic (Tue and Thurs)
- TB screening at schools once a year and 3 times a week at clinic
- Well child clinic, 2 days a week (nurse practitioner, pediatrician)

Large number of persons in waiting room of health department and welfare office.

There is 1 school nurse, but her services are limited to the elementary and junior high schools. Home health care services available, on referral from physician.[8]

All health and social services are available on a sliding scale with most residents classified as "A", which means they are below poverty level and do not pay fees.[16]

Mental health services are available free in the county seat 21 miles away. Includes all counseling: drug abuse, teens, children, and psychiatric referral.[8]

No counseling available in Rosetown except through local ministers.[16]

No parenting classes for community at large.[3]

"Sometimes I think that Rosetown is in the middle of nowhere. I have problems with my blood pressure and sugar diabetes so I have to go to the medical center 100 miles away once a month. I have to miss school for a day, and my mother or aunt has to miss work to take me. I wish we had these special doctors closer."[1]

No crisis intervention, except in neighboring town's mental health center and hospital emergency room.[16]

No telephone hot line services within 100 miles.[16]

Meals on Wheels by the Commission on Aging for the town's elderly residents.[16]

*Continued.*

# DATA COLLECTION—cont'd

| Structure/Process | Interactions | Observations | Measurements |
|---|---|---|---|
| | **B. Interacting subsystems**—cont'd<br>2. *Health and welfare services*—cont'd | Occupational safety services are provided in various industries. There is no occupational health service in Rosetown. For developmentally disabled children and adults: services available on referral from State Mental Health and through local school system.[8] | |
| | | For ages 5 years to 21 years: developmental classes, physical and speech therapist services, psychological services.[8] | |
| | Audiologist and speech pathologist 20 miles away. Available through referral from health dept. and school system.[3] | No health profession training available within 50-mile radius; nearest nursing school (A.D. and B.S.N.)—62 miles; nearest medical school in state medical center—150 miles away. | |
| | Services for mentally handicapped in school and through mental health center in town 21 miles away.[14] | Rosetown Connection bus with full load. By calling federally funded bus line (Rosetown Connection) 1 day in advance, any resident may be picked up at home and transported free of charge to any health or social service location. | |
| | "We could really use one more bus. The people in Rosetown depend on us since most all services are in Cleveton."[17]<br>No utilization statistics readily available.<br>One private day care center accepts children over the age of 9 months.[16]<br>No low cost child care services are available for children under the age of 4. Headstart available at 4 years free to all residents.[16]<br>Health promotion activities:<br>• Physical education classes in junior and senior high schools<br>• Stress management taught in home economics | | |

- Smoking and drug education offered twice per year at high school
- Recreational activities primarily organized by individuals
- Nutrition classes offered in home economics and through home demonstration office[13]

Welfare services:
Welfare department has a branch office located in Rosetown, which is open 5 days a week and dispenses food stamps and welfare payments.[16] "I worry that too many of our residents, particularly our young girls, get dependent on the welfare system. I like to see this as temporary assistance only until girls can get education and get a job. The office really needs to encourage education for pregnant girls more than they do."[6]

High degree of usage, as indicated by full waiting room in welfare office each day.

3. Economics
"We need more jobs for our young men and women. They have to move away to get off welfare."[2]

Farming is the leading occupation, and industry is second. Leading crops are soybeans, rice, cotton, and catfish.[5]

County unemployment rate (1988): 11.6%[18]; state unemployment rate: 10.2% (1988).[36]
Unemployment rate 18 and under: 72% (1988).[18]
Unemployment rate for aggregate: 100% (1989).
No pregnant high school girls are employed.[4]
Median family income: $11,216.00[18]; state median family income: $14,500.00.[36]
50.2% of families are below poverty level (1988).[18]

Shopping facilities:
4 grocery stores, 4 appliance/hardware supply stores, 3 gas stations, 2 banks with combined assets of $32,828,000.00, 2 drug stores, 3 attorneys, 1 CPA, and 1 insurance agent.[6]
Three major industries are located in Rosetown: Apco Metal Products employing 260 persons: 175 females and 85 males; Riverco, a marine construction company employing 139 persons: 135 males and 4 females; Searight, a grain processing company employing 100 persons: 85 males and 15 females.[6]

4. Safety and transportation
"Sometimes I feel unsafe in the crowded halls of school, like I could fall or something and hurt my baby."[1]
The crime rate is low in Rosetown with no murders or homicides recorded in the past 6 years.[19] "We have a quiet, safe little town. No one really bothers anyone else here. Our biggest crime problem is with petty theft and breaking and entering."[19]

Transportation is primarily through private car or on foot.
Bus service is available free to surrounding towns for needed services.

Police protection: 5 full-time and 2 part-time police officers; 3 police cars with 2-way radio contact with county police department.[19]
Fire protection: 35 man volunteer fire dept. two 500 gpm (gallons per minute) pumper trucks, 1 utility truck available in town; ambulance housed in fire department building.[20]
Flouridated water via 3 wells. Water is treated at waste water treatment plant. Plant has 1,663,200 gpd (gallons per day) and peak capacity of 420,000 gpd. Plans are to overhaul complete system to update equipment.[21]

Continued.

# DATA COLLECTION—cont'd

| Structure/Process | Interactions | Observations | Measurements |
|---|---|---|---|
| **B. Interacting subsystems**—cont'd | | | |
| *4. Safety and transportation*—cont'd | An airport and a Greyhound bus station are 25 miles away; train services 30 miles away.[17] Handicapped services not readily available except through welfare services in town 21 miles away. Rosetown Connection is accessible for wheelchairs.[17] | | |
| | "Our treatment plant is quite adequate since we are using it at 50% capacity."[21] | Compact treatment plant with a 0.4 million gpd capacity.[21] | |
| | Entire community has access to sewage disposal.[22] | | |
| | Garbage disposal is done with city trash collection. Sanitary landfill five miles outside city limits.[21] | | |
| | Mosquitos are continuous vectors: problem is due to the rice fields. Spraying to control mosquitos is done in city limits weekly during peak season of summer.[21] | | |
| *5. Politics and government* | Weekly town meetings open for the first hour.[6] Mayor and 4 council members form the Rosetown city government structure. Current issues: attract a clinic from federal government and decrease unemployment.[6] | No political activism observed. | Informal leaders: 2 ministers and a local café owner. |
| | "We are pretty much conservative Southern Baptists here in Rosetown."[2] | | |
| | "If you want to get anything started or finished talk to Reverend Taylor, everybody respects and listens to him."[23] | | |
| | "We listen to our teacher when she directs us; she knows better what we need than any of us. She's looking out for us."[1] | Aggregate leadership not formally identified. Teacher of class for pregnant teens holds formal leadership position. | |
| *6. Communication* | "Sometimes the only people I can talk to are the girls in my parenting class—they understand what I'm going through better than anybody."[1] "If you want to know something about our town, hang out at Hank's Barber Shop—you'll soon find out."[2] | Aggregate members communicate through parenting class experiences and through common experiences at clinic. | |

Barber shop is center of information dissemination for residents of Rosetown.[24]
Bulletin boards in local supermarkets and businesses advertise parenting class at high school for girls who have dropped out of school.[4]
Rosetown News published weekly, carries pictures and announcements of local events.[24]
About ¾ of the community residents receive the local newspaper.[24]

*Informal communication:*
Billboard advertisements frequently are of liquor and restaurants.
The newspaper contained no stories about available contraception services or risks of teen pregnancy.
National media observed focusing on teen pregnancy.
No members of aggregate visible at community meetings.

*Formal communication:*
School paper produced monthly.
Two radio stations accessible to community.
Three television stations accessible to residents.
75% of residents have telephones.[5]
90% of residents have televisions.[5]

The average number of years of education in the US for an adolescent who has a child prior to age 20 is 10.8.[28] This information was unavailable from Rosetown.
One public library in Rosetown, open 9-12 am Mon–Fri.[25]
There are 2 elementary schools, 2 junior high schools, and 1 high school.

Public recreational facilities:
- 3 ball fields
- 1 swimming pool
- 4 tennis courts
- 2 local parks

There is 1 private country club available to members only with the following facilities: 1 golf course, 1 tennis court, and 1 swimming pool.[27]

7. *Education*

One class per day at Rosetown High offered to pregnant girls and to girls with infants up to 1 year of age. A night parenting class has been available for girls who have dropped out of school for 6 months. The teacher reported that at least 3 students from the night class have started back to school. Number of students varies from 6-9 per class.[4]

Special services available for physically and mentally handicapped students. Bus services provided free to students living within the district.[13]

"I like having classes with all of the students but I also like having a special class for pregnant girls. I look forward to hearing from the other girls about how they're getting along."[1]

8. *Recreation*

"I usually don't feel much like getting out in shorts anymore and going out for gym. I would rather walk after school."[1]

"I get enough exercise out in the fields—I just want to rest when I'm off."[26]

Rosetown has no physical fitness center.
No organized recreational program in Rosetown. Physical education is available as an option to all high school students. Recreational facilities are widely observed to be used at a high rate.
All pregnant teens at Rosetown High are or have been enrolled in physical education classes.

## ANALYSIS/SYNTHESIS OF DATA

### Core Structure

The aggregate of pregnant teens of Rosetown High School participates in very few community activities and appears to be marginal to the community structure. The *self-concept* of these pregnant teens varies from feeling special to feeling ashamed. *Historically*, adolescent pregnancy has been demonstrated by national and state statistics to be a risk factor in terms of low birth weight infants, infant mortality, unemployment, poverty, and low educational achievement. Nationally, the number of teens who engage in sexual intercourse has steadily increased to an estimated 53%. *Culturally*, Rosetown is an ethnically mixed community with a large percentage of the population under the age of 45. The total population has remained essentially unchanged at 2,791 persons. The population of the high school has remained consistent. The infant mortality for the county of the aggregate is high, the percentage of teens who gives birth is high, and the state infant mortality rate of the aggregate is high.

Rosetown teens seek prenatal care later than adults and are much less likely to use any type of birth control before or after the first pregnancy, according to the local public health nurse. The birth rate for the aggregate based on number of *known* pregnancies is more than twice that of state and U.S. rates and significantly higher than the county rate. The median number of years of school completed by the aggregate is 10.6 compared with 12.2 for the state.

*Statistics* show that the greatest number of residents is in the 18–45 age group. Almost half (48.2%) of the population is under the age of 18 years; the sex ratio is about equal. The aggregate has a birth rate twice that of the national and county birth rate average. The percentage of female-headed households in Rosetown is over twice the U.S. average, and the median income is $11,216, well below the state average of $14,500 and the national average of $23,300. The unemployment rate is 12.4%, higher than the state average of 10.2% and the national average of 8.1%. The aggregate of pregnant teens has a 100% unemployment rate of those in high school.

Teen pregnancy exposes the young female to economic, social, and biological risks based on research and statistics from national and state sources. Consequently, teenage pregnancy is considered a stressor that has the potential for causing disequilibrium in the system. Pregnant teens are much less likely to complete high school, more likely to deliver a low birth weight infant, and less likely to seek prenatal care during the first trimester.[28] Pregnancy affects the teenager's future and, according to Neuman's system model, would cause a significant degree of reaction.[29] *Degree of reaction* is the amount of disequilibrium or disruption that results from stressors affecting an aggregate's lines of defense.[29]

*Social support* is provided to pregnant teens through special classes, prenatal clinic, family, and WIC. However, no child care is available for teens who want to complete high school after giving birth.

These statistics reveal that Rosetown is *economically* and socially depressed and that the aggregate is at specific risk. The age distribution and birth rates for the area provide documentation of the need for specific health care facilities and services for females of childbearing age.

The leading causes of death in Rosetown are in the same rank and order as that for the nation, as indicated in the Surgeon General's Report on Health Prevention.[34]

### Interacting Subsystems

Rosetown is a rural community interspersed with farmland, housing developments, and business. The *physical environment* is adequate and in a temperate climate. Community residents have an adequate supply of clean water for drinking, bathing, and recreational needs. The area is adequately supplied with telephone service and energy sources. The pollutants were identified as pesticides and gasoline odors. The positive environmental aspects of pure water and clean air is congruent with Nightingale's environmental standards.

There is adequate police and fire protection. *Safety* is a major community strength.

The rural isolation of Rosetown affects the members of the community and members of the aggregate, specifically regarding health care services for specific needs. The primary mode of *transportation* is the private car, with the Rosetown Connection free bus service available for transport to social and health services in nearby cities.

The community of Rosetown is *governed* by a mayor and elected aldermen. Council meetings are poorly attended and *political* interest appears low. Decision-making power is concentrated in the leadership of the community, formal and informal, with little involvement of the community residents. The aggregate of pregnant teens has very little power within the school and the community. Their needs are represented through a spokesperson, a teacher in the high school.

*Communication* exists through both formal and

informal channels. The aggregate members communicate with each other in a class specifically designed for their special needs. A variety of modes are used to transmit information to the community residents. Citizens and aggregate members appear to be informed about social and health services available to them. Community meetings are not well attended; no aggregate involvement was observed. A school newspaper and community newspaper are published for school and community residents, respectively.

*Educational* services are delivered through a total of two elementary schools, two junior high schools, and one high school. Special services are available for mentally and physically handicapped students. Free bus service is provided to all students living in the school district.

*Recreational* facilities are limited, primarily restricted to public parks. Protective services are provided by Fire and Police Departments. Services appear to be adequate to cover Rosetown's needs. Housing varies in quality with much of the population living in substandard living conditions. The average value of a house in Rosetown is $21,400 compared with $90,000 for the U.S.

*Health and welfare services* for pregnant teens are described under preventive health services, health promotion, and health protection.

*Preventive health services.* Childbearing during the teenage years is a high risk experience for both the mother and the child; it also presents social risks for the community. A major concern that urgently needs addressing is underutilization of contraceptive counseling and services available free 5 days a week at the health department. These services serve as *lines of resistance*, which, according to Neuman's model, are internal mechanisms that act to defend against stressors. They represent a community strength. Special needs of the adolescent mother, as a result of biological risks and child care services needed, are not available in the local community.

Comprehensive prenatal care services are available in Rosetown through the health department and private clinics. Clinics are within walking distance of the high school. Infant care is available after the age of 9 months through a private day care center. Child care for low income persons is not available until the child reaches 4 years of age. Well child care is available through the health depart-

ment. Special health care services are available in neighboring towns with transportation provided free. The residents and members of the aggregate were aware of the availability of services.

*Health promotion services.* Health promotion activities for the aggregate are primarily offered at the high school, including nutrition classes, physical education classes, and stress management. Health promotion activities are sporadic in Rosetown. The high school offers special programs twice a year on tobacco and drug use. Sports are organized by residents with no planned recreational program. Facilities for recreation are limited to public parks and to the country club (members only). Benefits of these recreational activities are low costs, open participation, promotion of community cohesiveness, and family involvement. Constraints are the time and energy required for the organization and execution of the activities.

Residents of the community who are involved in farming engage in physical exertion activities. Other occupations do not require physical activity, and the aggregate members do not reflect an interest in the benefits of exercise. No community effort has been made to educate the public regarding these types of health promotion activities.

*Health protection.* Environmental protection services are provided by the health department, including sanitation and environmental inspection. Vector control is a significant problem in Rosetown, and mosquitoes are prevalent. Accident safety and education are offered in all grades of the schools. Occupational safety services are provided for workers in the local industries.

## NURSING DIAGNOSIS

Two nursing diagnoses have been identified and arranged in order of priority. Plans have been formulated for only the first diagnosis.
1. Potential for increased incidence of teen pregnancy related to increased sexual activity and nonuse of contraceptive services
2. Potential for increased school dropout of teen mothers related to inaccessibility of child care services for children under the age of 4 years

## PLANS FOR IMPLEMENTATION

**Nursing diagnosis:** *Potential for increased incidence of teen pregnancy related to increased sexual activity and non-use of contraceptive services (3/12/90).*

**Goal:** *The Rosetown High School population will have a decreased pregnancy rate by June 1992.*

| Objectives | Nursing orders | Scientific rationale | Evaluation |
|---|---|---|---|
| 1. Community will have access to information regarding the risks of teen pregnancy by October 1990. | 1a. Interview health care providers regarding perception and incidence of problem. | *Content*: Teen pregnancy. *Strategy*: Change process and principles of community health nursing practice.<br><br>**Unfreezing**<br><br>1a. Implies that for change to take place, community has to become dissatisfied with status quo.[30]<br>    Local health care providers often serve as community gatekeepers; community residents tend to respond to those with informal power.[33]<br>    Empirical rational mode of change implies that humans are rational and will make informed decisions after information is presented.[32] | **Outcome criteria:**<br><br>1. Media will communicate informative news stories concerning the incidence, risks, and prevention of teen pregnancy.<br>2. Community residents will acknowledge and respond by discussion with each other about above information.<br>3. Specific community organizations and groups will request programs to inform the aggregate of teen pregnancy risks.<br><br>**Formative:**<br><br>Who was contacted and what was their response? |
| | 1b. Contact local newspapers regarding incidence of teen pregnancy in community. Offer to write series of articles regarding<br>    Incidence and risks of teen pregnancy to teen and community<br>    Interviews with local leaders, physicians, teachers, clergy, school board members, and public health officials regarding the problem | 1b. Essential elements for reducing teen pregnancy include education of public to understand economic, biological, and social risks.[28] | Was newspaper contacted? Were articles printed? |
| | 1c. Solicit several people to write to newspapers commenting on the problem and suggesting measures to decrease incidence of teen pregnancy. | 1c. Quoting community residents and leaders promotes concern necessary for social action.[31] | Were letters to newspapers written and printed? |

| Objectives | Nursing orders | Scientific rationale | Evaluation |
|---|---|---|---|
| | 1d. Encourage aggregate and community residents to call local talk radio station and comment on articles. | 1d. Keep isssue before public to raise consciousness of community residents.[31] | Were radio stations contacted? What was the response? Did health professionals participate in community talk shows? |
| 2. Community will take action to inform the aggregate population of the risks of teen pregnancy by April 1991. | 2a. Encourage school board to form a task force to plan sex education, including contraceptive counseling, to be offered in junior and high school courses: Task force to be composed of parents, teachers, clergy, physician, nurse, and other health professionals and aggregate members Task force to look at specific content and the options of program: Elective or required With parental permission During school or after school hours. 2b. Support total community involvement and acceptance by supporting task force effort in local media. 2c. Contact health department, local health care providers, and service organizations regarding available services, cost, and community acceptance of this type of service. 2d. Suggest to school board the formation of a citizen's task force to look further into the concern. | **Moving to the new level** 2a. Community involvement will influence whether change will be accepted.[30] Formal and informal community leaders as well as aggregate members need to be involved in decision-making.[33] It is important to encourage collaboration between and among groups.[33] 2d. Decisions regarding content and course planning by community facilitates community acceptance.[33] | **Outcome criteria:** 1. School board will have teen pregnancy as an agenda item at monthly meeting. 2. A task force will be formed with active participation by members. 3. The program will include information on incidence, risks, and prevention. 4. A contraceptive counseling course will be implemented in the junior and senior high schools. 5. A citizen's task force will be formed with active participation by the members. **Formative:** Was a task force formed? When? Who was on the task force? Was there interest evident by task force members? What content will be taught? Where and when will course be taught? Who will teach it? Who will be required to attend? Was health department contacted? Was information shared with members of aggregate? What was the response? Was a citizen's task force formed? Why or why not? Was there interest evident by task force members? |
| 3. Community will provide contraceptive education in junior and high schools by August 1991. | 3a. Act as resource for implementing contraceptive education, including class involvement and evaluation. | **Refreeze at new level** 3a. Provided change has been brought about through community forces, it should continue.[30] | **Outcome criteria:** 1. There will be an increase in contraceptive services by the health department. |

*Continued.*

## PLANS FOR IMPLEMENTATION—cont'd

| Objectives | Nursing orders | Scientific rationale | Evaluation |
|---|---|---|---|
| | 3b. Encourage school staff to share information about progress of contraceptive education with parents and community residents through the following: PTA meetings, Media, Written and oral correspondence | 3b. Essential elements of controlling teen pregnancy are sex education, contraceptive counseling, and decision-making.[28] Rosetown has demonstrated active participation in community decisions; acceptability of services is more likely when community is involved in decision-making.[31] | 2. Everyone in the community will have access to such services, regardless of ability to pay. 3. Confidentiality will be ensured. **Formative:** Was program implemented as planned? If not, why not? What modifications were made in the original program? Who was contacted? By whom? When? What facilities available? What was cost? Community acceptance? Did meeting evaluation criteria lead to goal achievement? |
| | 3c. Monitor contraceptive services of health department utilization by aggregate members and sexually active teens. | 3c. Essential to successful program planning is determining what community residents perceive that they need and the motivation to achieve these needs.[31] | **Summative:** Were evaluation criteria met? |

## REFERENCES*

1 Aggregate members: Interviews.
2 Community residents: Interviews.
3 Rosetown Health Department nurse: Interview.
4 High school faculty member (teaches class for pregnant teens): interview.
5 Chamber of Commerce: This is Rosetown (pamphlet).
6 Mayor of Rosetown: Interview.
7 National Weather Service: National Weather Service Bulletin.
8 Rosetown Bureau of Social Service: Resource Directory.
9 President of Board of Realtors: Interview.
10 PTA president: Interview.
11 Rotary Club President: Interview.
12 County home economist: Interview.
13 Rosetown High School principal: Interview.
14 Rosetown High School guidance counselor: Interview.
15 United States Bureau of the Census, 1988.
16 Social worker, Rosetown Welfare Department: Interview.
17 Rosetown transportation manager: Interview.
18 Rosetown annual report.
19 Rosetown Police Chief: Interview.
20 Rosetown Fire Chief: Interview.
21 Health Department environmental engineer: Interview.
22 Rosetown City Manager: Interview.

*References 1-27 are fictitious.

23 Rosetown Town Council member: Interview.
24 Newspaper editor, *Rosetown Review:* Interview
25 Rosetown Public Library Director: Interview.
26 Community resident, farmer: interview.
27 Rosetown Recreational Services Director: Interview.
28 Alan Guttmacher Institute: Teenage pregnancy: the problem that hasn't gone away, New York, 1981.
29 Neuman B: The Neuman systems model, 1982, Norfolk, Conn, Appleton-Century-Crofts.
30 Lewin K: Field theory in social science, New York, 1951, Harper & Brothers.
31 Stanhope M and Lancaster J: Community health nursing, 1988, ed 2, The CV Mosby Co.
32 Bennis WG et al: The planning of change, ed 3, New York, 1976, Holt, Rinehart, & Winston.
33 Klein DC: Community dynamics and mental health, New York, 1968, John Wiley & Sons, Inc.
34 US Department of Health, Education, and Welfare: Healthy people: the Surgeon General's report on health promotion and disease prevention, Washington, DC, 1979, US Government Printing Office.
35 US Department of Health and Human Services: National Center for Health Statistics, Monthly Vital Statistics Report, 1988.
36 Research Development Center: Handbook of selected data (state and US), 1988.

**accountability** Ability to explain rationale for actions taken that is consistent with the responsibility for which the nurse contracted.

**advocate** One who acts in the interest of the health care consumer.

**assessment** Ongoing process of data collection and analysis/synthesis of data that results in conclusions about the client's health concerns and strengths.

**autonomy** The freedom to develop and control oneself.

**behavioral objective** Statement describing a specific expected observable behavior of the client that is relatively short-term.

**biomedical domain** Collaborative, interdependent nursing actions related to the client's pathological condition or medical treatment.

**caring** Concerned with or interested in another.

**catalyst** Person who promotes actions and reactions and enables them to proceed under optimum conditions.

**client** Individual, family, group, or community.

**collaboration** Joint effort for the purpose of creating change toward a mutually desired goal.

**colleague** Peer functioning in a group in which each member openly shares knowledge and has equal opportunity to exercise power and authority.

**communication techniques (facilitative)** Methods used to promote open dialogue between people.

**clarifying** Asking the client what was meant by a particular statement or question.

**consensual validation** Asking the client the meaning of a particular word that was used in the conversation.

**focus** Restrict discussion to obtain specific information.

**open-ended statements and questions** Statements and questions that cannot be answered with a "yes" or "no" answer.

**reflect feelings or content** Share with the client your (interviewer's) thoughts or feelings of the content spoken.

**related questions** Questions that are relevant to previous statements for the purpose of obtaining more information about the topic.

**restate, repeat main idea** Restate what the client said verbatim or pull together the main idea of what the

client said and state it. This is used to promote elaboration on the topic or validation of what was said.

**sharing perceptions** Telling the client what your (interviewer's) impressions are of a given statement or situation.

**summarize** Share with the client succinct impressions or conclusions drawn from data.

**verbalize the implied** State what the client implied to validate the interviewer's impressions.

**community** Specific population living within a defined perimeter; or group that has common values, interests, or needs.

**community process** How the components of a community system function.

**community structure** Arrangement of animate or inanimate properties or parts of a community at a given moment.

**comprehensive** Reflecting the totality or wholeness of the client's life experiences.

**concept** Complex mental formulation of objects, events, or ideas that can be symbolized by a word.

**conceptual model** Matrix of concepts, theories, or ideas that are interrelated but in which the precise interrelationships among the concepts are not clearly defined.

**concurrent evaluation** Ongoing examination of activities as they occur.

**consultation** Invited communication with an expert who serves in an advisory capacity for the purpose of information exchange or analysis.

**continuum** Continuous whole whose fundamental common character is discernible amid a series of variations.

**coordination** Regulation and combination of effort for harmonious performance.

**criteria statement** Statement reflecting the expected qualities, attributes, or characteristics that measure a client's performance.

**data** Units of information obtained through the use of the senses and the designated methods of observation, interaction, and measurement.

**dependent** Relying on or requiring the support of others for the authority to perform activities.

**depleted health** Alteration in the dynamic pattern of

functioning whereby there is an inability to interact with internal and external forces as the result of a temporary or permanent loss of necessary resources.

**developmental needs** Any requirement arising from the natural process of situational concerns of growth and differentiation.

**diagnosis** Clear, concise, definitive statement of the client's health status and concerns that can be affected by nursing intervention.

**empirical knowledge** Knowledge obtained through the conscious use of the senses and grounded in scientific investigation.

**evaluation** Systematic, continuous process of comparing the client's response or observable behavior with the established goals and objectives.

**family** Dynamic system of two or more individuals who consider themselves a family and share a history, common goals, obligations, instrumental and affectional bonds and ties, and a high degree of intimacy.

**family process** Functions and group interactions by which the family operates; salient features that differentiate it from another collection of individuals.

**family structure** Names, ages, health states, and occupations of family members.

**formative evaluation** Ongoing process for determining the completion of the objectives and nursing orders.

**goal** Broad or abstract statement of client performance that is relatively long-term.

**health** Dynamic pattern of functioning whereby there is continued interaction with the internal and external forces that results in the optimal use of necessary resources that serve to minimize vulnerabilities.

**health care system** Organized distribution of services and personnel to meet the health needs of others.

**health care team** Organized group of health care workers who have common goals, cooperative relationships, and coordinated activities related to the health care needs of the client or group of clients.

**health concern** Actual or potential health problem, disability, deficit, or limitation.

**health maintenance** Act of protecting and preserving patterns of maximum potential for health.

**health promotion** Advancement of patterns of functioning that foster and encourage optimal health.

**health restoration** Advancement of patterns of functioning from depleted or impaired health to health maintenance.

**health status** State of health.

**holistic** View that an integrated whole has a reality independent of and greater than the sum of its parts.

**impaired health** Alteration in the dynamic pattern of functioning whereby there is a diminished ability to interact with internal and external forces as the result of a reduction in necessary resources.

**implementation** Nurse and client executing the plans.

**independent** Assuming autonomous authority to perform activities.

**inference** Judgment made from data obtained compared with health norms, concepts, principles, or standards.

**interdependent** Mutually collaborative effort in performing health care activities with other health care professionals and the client.

**interpretation (personal)** Individually biased perception of a given event that may be judgmental.

**interviews** Transitory relationships or exchanges of information that are goal directed.

  **directive-interrogative** Discussion between client and nurse for the purpose of obtaining information.

  **open-ended** Discussion between client and nurse for the purposes of obtaining information and building rapport.

  **rapport-building** Discussion between client and nurse for the purpose of establishing a relationship.

**intuition** Awareness of meanings, relationships, and possibilities by way of insight without conscious knowledge.

**leader** Person with foresight who is able to influence others in a positive direction, who is accountable for his or her own beliefs, who is willing and able to take risks, and who accepts power and uses it judiciously.

**leadership** Complex relationship between individuals whereby interpersonal influence is exercised through the process of communication toward the achievement of specific goals.

**maximum potential for health** Client's ability to achieve or develop the highest pattern of functioning possible within his or her health perimeter.

**measurable** Able to be determined in terms of extent, dimension, rate, rhythm, quantity, or size; used for a given behavior, performance, or characteristic.

**methods for data collection** Means by which the nurse obtains data from the client.

  **interaction** Mutual or reciprocal exchange of verbal information.

  **measurement** Use of all the senses as well as instruments to allow quantitative value of observations.

  **observation** Use of all the senses to obtain information about a client.

**multifocal** View that clients are composed of multiple foci, such as biophysical, spiritual, psychological, developmental, and sociocultural.

**nonjudgmental** Free from personal interpretation and bias.

**norm** Generally accepted range of behavior, performance, or characteristics.

**nursing domain** Independent nursing actions related to health promotion, health maintenance, health restoration, and referral.

**nursing orders/nursing prescription** Actions chosen by the nurse and client to achieve the goals and objectives.

**nursing process** Deliberate intellectual activity whereby the practice of nursing is approached in an orderly, systematic manner. Components consist of assessment, diagnosis, planning, implementation, and evaluation.

**objective** See behavioral objective.

**objective domains** Categories on which to base objectives.

**affective domain** Reflects interests, attitudes, values, or feelings.

**cognitive domain** Reflects knowledge or intellectual abilities and skills.

**psychomotor domain** Reflects ability to perform a manipulative or motor skill.

**optimal health** See maximum potential for health.

**outcome or performance evaluation** Examination of the result of nursing actions according to the client's change in behavior and health status compared with objectives and goals.

**pattern** Composite sample of traits or behaviors that is characterized by rhythm, rate, intensity, duration, and amount.

**perception** Individual's idea of an event or situation that is based on the use of all senses and past experience.

**performance** Any behavior or outcome of a client that can be directly or indirectly assessed.

**personal knowledge** Knowledge gained through introspection, intuition, and the intentional development of self-awareness.

**philosophy** Statement of a person's beliefs, values, and assumptions about a given phenomenon (eg, nursing).

**planning** Determining how to assist the client in resolving concerns related to the restoration, maintenance, or promotion of health.

**principles** Guiding rules or laws that have been supported over time through research.

**process** Interaction of the components of a given system.

**process evaluation** Examining the actions and interactions of the nurse.

**reliable** Stable, dependable, accurate, consistent, and relatively predictable.

**research** Systematic inquiry to discover facts or test theories to obtain valid answers to questions raised or solutions for concerns identified.

**resource** External or internal source of strength or assistance.

**responsibility** Obligation to fulfill the terms of implied or explicit contractual agreement in accord with professional and legal nursing standards.

**retrospective evaluation** Examining the nurse's actions for effectiveness after the client is discharged from care.

**role** Dyad that is an actual or expected behavior pattern determined by socialization, including the interaction and interpretation of given norms, status, or position.

**spiritual** Internal essence or quality that gives meaning to a client's existence.

**standard** Acceptable, expected level of performance that is established by authority, custom, or general consent.

**strategy (nursing)** Overall method or approach that serves as a guide for individual nursing orders.

**structure** Arrangement of animate or inanimate properties or parts of a given system at a given moment.

**structure evaluation** Examining the physical facilities, types and availability of equipment, and organizational components.

**summative evaluation** Description of whether and to what degree goals have been met.

**synthesis** Integration of theories and concepts into varied patterns.

**systematic** Organized and planned method of completing a given project.

**theoretical framework** Collection of concepts whose interrelationship describes or explains phenomena that have not been proven.

**theory** Internally consistent body of relational statements and concepts that describes, explains, controls, or predicts phenomena.

**unique** Way clients differ from each other by virtue of heredity, environment, particular experiences, perception of such experiences, and the manner in which they react to such experiences.

**valid** Quality of data or data collection method to accurately reflect what was intended to be reflected.

**validation** Process of determining accuracy of data.

**verifiable** Capable of having authenticity of data confirmed through a variety of sources.

**vulnerability** State of being at risk or susceptible.

# Guidelines for the Nursing Process

A. Assessment
   1. A systematic format is used for data collection.
   2. The data are comprehensive and multifocal.
   3. A variety of sources is used for data collection.
   4. Appropriate methods are used for data collection.
   5. The data are verifiable.
   6. The data reflect updating of information.
   7. The data are recorded and communicated appropriately.
B. Diagnosis
   1. Analysis and synthesis of data
      a. Data are categorized.
      b. Data gaps and incongruencies are identified.
      c. Cues are clustered into patterns.
      d. Appropriate theories, models, concepts, norms, and standards are applied and compared with patterns.
      e. Health concerns and strengths are identified.
      f. Etiological relationships are proposed.
   2. Diagnostic statements
      a. The nursing diagnosis is a statement of an actual or potential health concern.
      b. The nursing diagnosis is written as a descriptive and etiological statement.
      c. The nursing diagnosis is concise and clear.
      d. The nursing diagnosis is client-centered, specific, and accurate.
      e. The nursing diagnosis provides direction for nursing interventions.
      f. The nursing diagnosis is the basis for independent and collaborative nursing actions/interventions.
      g. The list of nursing diagnosis statements reflects the client's current health status.

   h. The list of nursing diagnostic statements is validated.
C. Plans
   1. Priorities
      a. Actual or imminent life-threatening concerns are considered before actual or potential health-threatening concerns.
      b. Temporal, human, and material resources are examined deliberately.
      c. The client is involved in determining the priority of concerns.
      d. Scientific and practice principles provide rationale for decisions.
   2. Goals
      a. Goals are client-focused and reflect mutuality with the client.
      b. Goals are appropriate to their respective diagnosis.
      c. Goals are realistic, reflecting the capabilities and limitations of the client.
      d. Goals include broad or abstract indicators of performance.
      e. Scientific and practice principles guide the establishment of goals.
   3. Objectives
      a. Objectives are client-focused and reflect mutuality with the client.
      b. Objectives are appropriate to their respective goal.
      c. Objectives are realistic, reflecting the capabilities and limitations of the client.
      d. Objectives include specific indicators of performance.
      e. Objectives are numbered in appropriate sequence to achieve the goal.
      f. Scientific and practice principles guide the development of objectives.
   4. Strategies
      a. Major strategies for implementation are identified.

b. Strategies are appropriate to their respective goal and objectives.

c. Strategies are based on scientific rationale.

5. Nursing orders

a. Nursing orders are appropriate to their respective goal, objective, and strategy.

b. Scientific and practice principles provide rationale for orders.

c. Nursing orders incorporate the autonomy and individuality of the client.

d. Nursing orders indicate specific intended behaviors, giving direction to the nurse, client, and others.

e. Nursing orders reflect consideration of human, temporal, and material resources.

f. Nursing orders are numbered in sequence to achieve the objective.

g. Nursing orders are dated and include the signature of the responsible nurse.

h. Nursing orders are kept current and are revised as indicated.

i. Nursing orders include plans for termination of nursing services.

D. Implementation

1. The actions performed are consistent with the plan and occur after validation of the plan.

2. Interpersonal, intellectual, and technical skills are performed competently and efficiently in an appropriate environment.

3. The client's physical and psychological safety are protected.

4. Documentation of actions and client responses is evident in the health care record and care plan.

E. Evaluation

1. The nurse continuously monitors, appraises, and reassesses the client's response to nursing actions.

2. The client's response to nursing implementation is compared with the client's objectives to determine the extent to which the objectives have been achieved (formative evaluation).

3. The client's progress toward goal attainment is determined (summative evaluation).

4. The nursing care plan is revised to reflect changes in the client's condition or when the goals or objectives have not been adequately met.

# Index

Elimination—cont'd
   hospitalized client and, 238, 241, 244, 251-252
   individual in community and, 258, 262
Emerging family; *see* Family
Emotional
   expression, 300
   patterns, data collection and, 81
Employment, data collection and, 90
Endocrine function
   analysis/synthesis and, 144, 146
   data collection and, 69
   individual in community and, 259, 263
Energy
   data collection and, 90
   in systems theory, 24
Energy fields, 41
England's sanitary reform acts, 111
Environment
   analysis/synthesis and, 153-155
   data collection and, 83, 105
   in Johnson's behavioral system model, 25
   in King's theory, 29
   in Leininger's transcultural nursing, 31
   in Neuman's health-care systems model, 33
   in Parse's man-living-health model, 37
   in Peplau's interpersonal model, 39
   in Roy's adaptation model, 42, 44
Environmental Protection Agency, 151
Environmental stressors, 31
Equilibrium of a system, 24
Erikson's developmental stages model, 4, 22, 315
Ethnocaring, 31, 33
Ethnonursing, 33
Etiology, statement of and nursing interventions, 167-169
Evaluation, 220-231
   of assessment, 224
   characteristics of, 224-226
   community client and, 229-230, 348-350
   concurrent, 221-224
   criteria and standards, 221
   of diagnoses, 225
   family client and, 228-229, 296-303, 326-330
   formative, 225-226
   forms of, 221-224
   guidelines for, 226-227
   historical perspective, 221
   of implementation, 225
   individual client
      example of, 227-228
      hospitalized, 245-253
      non-hospitalized, 265-274
   in nursing process, 8
   outcome, 223-224
   of planning, 225
   process, 222-223
   retrospective, 221-224
   structure, 222
   summative, 226
   of teaching and learning process, 193

Excretion; *see* Elimination
Exercise
   data collection and, 76
   analysis/synthesis and, 144
Explanatory theory, 14
Exploitation, in Peplau's model, 39

**F**

Family; *see also* Family client
   actualizing, 46
   boundary, 103-104
   change, 88
   composition, 103
   coping, 298
      analysis/synthesis and, 149
      data collection and, 82, 102
   crystallizing, 46
   culture, 105
   definitions of, 86
   development, 50, 106
   emerging, 46
   extended, 105
   external structure, in Calgary's family model, 50
   health history, data collection and, 78-79
   interacting, 46-47
   internal structure, in Calgary's family model, 49-50
   nursing models for use in diagnosis, 172
   principles of nursing practice and, 202
   structure of, in Friedman's model, 94, 96
   subsystems, data collection and, 103
Family client; *see also* Family
   assessment of, 86-110
   nursing process of, 276-331
Family functions, 50
   affective, 316, 322, 326
   coping, 316, 326
   economic, 316-317
   reproduction, 316, 326
   socialization, 316, 322, 326
Family models, 44-51
   developmental, 88-94
   eclectic, 97, 102-109
   for data collection, 87-88
   interactional, 89, 94
   structural-functional, 94-109
Family structure
   communication, 316, 322
   power, 316, 322
   role, 315-316, 322
   values, 316, 322
Feedback
   among components of nursing process, 9
   data collection and, 117
   in systems, 115-116
   in systems theory, 24

System—cont'd
    process, 114-117
    structure, 114, 116
System linkage, analysis/synthesis and, 153, 154
Systems
    interpersonal, 30
    personal, 29
    social, 30
Systems approach, analysis/synthesis of family data, 147
Systems theory, 10, 23

**T**

Tanner, C.A.
    clinical problem solving, 132
    decision making in diagnosis, 134
Target system, data collection and, 116
Tasks, developmental for family, 88-89
Taxonomy of nursing diagnoses, 163
Teaching and learning; *see* Strategy
Theile, J.E., 138
Theoretical model, 12-13
    King's theory of goal attainment, 29-31
    Parse's man-living-health model, 36-39
Theory
    definition, 12, 13-14
    description of, 12-17
    functional components of, 14-15
    King's, of goal attainment, 29-31
    in nursing, history of development, 10-12
    Parse's man-living-health, 36-39
    predictive, 14
    Rogers' science of unitary human beings, 40-41
Theory-based nursing practice, 1-52
    overview of, 20-52
    relevance of, 3-19
Therapeutic use of self; *see* Strategy

Throughput
    data collection and, 117
    in systems, 115
Time, data collection and, 90
Transcultural nursing, 31, 33
Transportation, community assessment and, 125-126
Triangulation, 113
Trust versus mistrust
Turkoski, B.B., 162

**U**

Unitary human beings, 41

**V**

Value systems, 48
Values, data collection and, 84
Vital signs, normal ranges of, 139

**W**

Walsh, M.B., 5
Watson, J., 11, 195-196
Wellness-illness continuum, 33-34
Wilcox, B., 127
Windshield survey, 114, 152

**Z**

Zderad, L., 11